T0221615

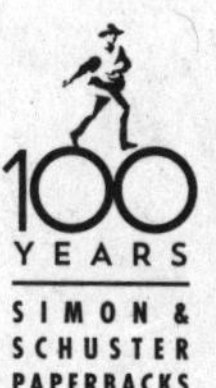
100
YEARS
SIMON &
SCHUSTER
PAPERBACKS

ALSO BY DAVID B. AGUS, MD

The Lucky Years

A Short Guide to a Long Life

The End of Illness

The Book of Animal Secrets

Nature's Lessons for a Long and Happy Life

DAVID B. AGUS, MD

Simon & Schuster Paperbacks

New York London Toronto Sydney New Delhi

An Imprint of Simon & Schuster, LLC
1230 Avenue of the Americas
New York, NY 10020

This publication contains the opinions and ideas of its author. It is intended to provide helpful and informative material on the subjects addressed in the publication.

It is sold with the understanding that the author and publisher are not engaged in rendering medical, health, or any other kind of personal professional services in the book. The reader should consult his or her medical, health or other competent professional before adopting any of the suggestions in this book or drawing inferences from it.

The author and publisher specifically disclaim all responsibility for any liability, loss or risk, personal or otherwise, which is incurred as a consequence, directly or indirectly, of the use and application of any of the contents of this book.

First Simon & Schuster trade paperback edition December 2024

Simon & Schuster: Celebrating 100 Years of Publishing in 2024

Interior design by Ruth Lee-Mui

Manufactured in the United States of America

1 3 5 7 9 10 8 6 4 2

Library of Congress Cataloging-in-Publication Data is available on file.

ISBN 978-1-6680-4357-8
ISBN 978-1-9821-0304-0 (pbk)
ISBN 978-1-9821-0307-1 (ebook)

To my dear Georgie,

You are a better person than I,
even though you are a dog.
Without your companionship, kisses, and desire to play,
this book would have been completed many months sooner.
But time with you was—and always is—worth it!

Thank you for the oxytocin boosts . . .

Contents

Introduction

Look deep into nature, and then you will understand everything better.

—ALBERT EINSTEIN

What if, for the rest of your life, your body could be ten to fifteen years younger than your birth certificate says? What if you could safely edit your genes to avoid getting the Alzheimer's or heart disease that notoriously runs in your family? What if I could assure you that you'd never develop cancer or some rare, abominable illness with no meaningful treatment? What if you could know exactly which diet and exercise regimen to follow to stay lean and fit? What if you could avoid ever feeling depressed, achy, foggy, and "old"?

What if.

What if.

What if.

This book was born out of frustration. I read scientific and medical journals daily to stay ahead of all the latest developments and innovations. But I'm always somewhat dismayed as I follow the progress of medicine. We're having breakthroughs, no doubt about it. I'm seeing diseases that were once deadly now being managed for long periods of time. And yet when I learn about another species that has adapted in the same environment we have but has done so much better—an elephant that will avoid cancer in spite of its size, a giraffe that will never experience cardiovascular problems regardless of high blood pressure, a queen ant that can outlive its genetically similar comrades by a factor of eighty—I start to wonder what we can learn from those adaptations and how we can leverage them in our own lives to live longer, healthier, and happier. How can we hack our system?

You're about to find out.

The Cancer Doctor Who Opened His Eyes

I'm a cancer doctor. That's usually the first thing I say to people when asked what I do. I've found the work has really come to influence my personality—I'm always seeking, searching, questioning, and regularly being deflated by my lack of success. I'm up against a wily disease. For the past thirty years, cancer has been public enemy number one for me, and yet it is an adversary that I must confess I've learned so much from. Cancer in all its forms surprises me every day and teaches me new things about its habits and behavior. I watch cancer evolve before my eyes—the same process that happens in every living being but accelerated. Every treatment causes a reaction, a change in the cancer, many times leading to resistance to the therapy. This is the one artful disease that gets stronger and more aggressive with every potential remedy and counterattack. It doesn't weaken over time; it is infuriatingly resilient. Watching cancer truly is like spying on Mother Nature's evolution in high speed.

I once had a patient with newly diagnosed cancer that had spread throughout his lung, liver, and brain. When I sequenced and analyzed the DNA of his tumor, I discovered that a gene called ALK was amplified; it was in an active state that appeared to be the driving force of the growth of this cancer. Yet when I prescribed an oral pill that blocked ALK, essentially turning off the growth signal of the ALK gene, the tumor disappeared, and scans of his body showed no cancer at all. It was so quick that nobody at his workplace knew he'd even had cancer, and all of his symptoms had resolved.

Ten months later, the cancer reappeared. The cancer cell had adapted to grow in the presence of the drug that turned off its signaling molecule. Either the ALK molecule of the tumor changed so the drug wouldn't bind to it, or a new pathway arose to enable the cancer to continue to grow without being stimulated by ALK. That the cancer's beguiling nature found a way to survive made me wonder how humans could learn from this so that we might become this resilient. We try to change our bodies through medications and lifestyle modifications, and although their benefit is real, it is generally limited. We need more change at a much more rapid pace than science is generating to lessen the tolls of the myriad diseases we face. I also started wondering whether there are clues in nature to more efficient approaches.

This is a book about what we can learn from other creatures—those we love and those we detest and those we don't think about much—to inform our own health, longevity, and even ways of thinking and relating to others. Human evolution has happened over millions of years, and while we've been studying that, one of the things we've missed is that every other creature on Earth has also been evolving, figuring out how to handle threatening stressors, procreate, and thrive. Many have had vastly more time to perfect themselves and adapt to their and our environment. Many never get cancer, grow obese, suffer from anxiety and depression, contract infections, show symptoms of cardiovascular disease, experience glitches in their neurology like dementia or Parkinson's disease, become diabetic, fall ill with autoimmune disorders, or even develop outward signs of aging like thin gray hair, wrinkles, and arthritic joints. Some life-forms can hear without ears, see without eyes, remain fertile until death, regenerate lost limbs, revert to a younger stage in the life cycle, communicate with one another without speaking or even using what we'd consider language, and think without a brain.

Most of us don't often ponder evolution, but it is very much worth considering. Evolution can help us understand ourselves better and learn how to live better too. It can provide a framework for navigating what often appears to be a difficult, chaotic world; offer guidelines for making good decisions and accepting harsh realities; and explain both wellness and disease. This book will open you to a new perspective.

I was not planning to be a cancer doctor. I began my career as a laboratory researcher. I was a student immunologist studying mostly T-cell biology, which is a key part of our immune system and where much of the scientific understanding of immunology started in the last century. My father was a kidney doctor who also conducted research, and watching his love for science surely had an impact on me as a teenager. The first time I met other kids who liked science as much as I did was when I participated in a summer program between my high school sophomore and junior years away from home in Gainesville at the University of Florida. It was extraordinary to be with other kids who had the same passion for science as I did, and it had an important influence on me. So did reading books like Michael Crichton's *Andromeda Strain*.

The following school year, I had the opportunity to continue the research I had begun the summer before with scientists at the University of Pennsylvania who studied kidney disease in rats. I'd go to the lab after school, weigh the rats, and inject them with a drug. Watching the experiments work was intoxicating.

In 1984, when I was nineteen, I made my first public scientific presentation at the annual meeting of the American Federation for Clinical Research. It reflected the culmination of my work at Penn the previous three years in Eric Neilson's laboratory. My presentation that day at the Omni Shoreham Hotel was at the last session of the four-day meeting. By the time I ambled nervously up to the podium to give my rehearsed and memorized talk, most of the participants had already left. But it didn't matter to me. I gave a ten-minute talk with my 35 mm slides, answered a few questions, and then went to the bathroom and closed the door in a stall to let the moment sink in: I had presented research to doctors and scientists—and they listened to me! The following year, my first scientific paper was published. I had found my life's work.

Laboratories are exciting places, but I realized that I didn't want to be isolated from patient care. Most researchers don't get to see patients or witness a disease they are studying, such as cancer, unfold in living, breathing humans. I had a deep desire to do both: be in the lab and see patients.

My focus on cancer grew out of my desire to have a direct impact on people—to be on the front lines treating patients, talking to them, learning from them, and following their long-term prognoses. Whenever I appear in the media to deliver the latest news in health, I'm acutely aware of the disconnect between the esoteric world of medicine and people's regular, everyday lives. Whether I'm describing an advance in treating or understanding cancer or other life-threatening illnesses, I am keenly aware that every patient with the disease who is watching is asking themselves: "Why aren't I benefiting from this advance he's describing? Why am I still suffering?" What we learn from the news about health can be meaningless if we can't benefit from it. Learning the secrets to living a good, long life should not be hoarded by a few who have resources—hence my motivation to keep doing what I'm doing by connecting the two worlds. And nature, it turns out, is the ultimate connector, our common denominator. Nature is everyone's master, mother, and the holder of life's best-kept solutions, solutions rigged by evolution.

• • •

I begin with the story of the legendary British naturalist and explorer Alfred Russel Wallace, who found a different way of looking at the world around him. And since we'll be spending so much time over the next twelve chapters learning about all the incredible ways in which the creatures of this planet have evolved—just as he realized they did—we should pay our respects to him.

An Idea Takes Root

In January 1858 while he was ill, most likely from malaria, Wallace was thinking about Thomas Robert Malthus's ideas on population dynamics. Malthus, a British philosopher and scholar, wrote extensively on what would become known as the Malthusian catastrophe: the end of the world was coming because the planet would not be able to keep up with its ever-expanding growth in population. Famine and war would eventually result, keeping the numbers in check. Perhaps slightly delusional from his fever or imaginative because of it, Wallace was struck by an idea as he pondered the concept of natural selection: that forces are at work on every living creature in nature.

As a biologist and naturalist who traveled to remote places in the world to observe animals in their natural habitats, Wallace was used to being consumed by thoughts about how animals change over time to survive. But this day in January 1858 was a pivotal moment for him. Like good scientists then and now, he drew parallels between Malthus's ideas and his own, asking himself if environmental pressures and a limit to available resources could provoke alterations in a species. And could such pressures render changes to its biology and ability to breed, which would allow certain living things to survive while simultaneously knocking off the weaker or, better described, less fit ones? He began to take notes that bore striking similarities to what we call the theory of evolution today, with its classic survival of the fittest model.*[1]

At the time of this sudden spark of mind, Wallace was renting a house on a volcanic Indonesian island deep in the South Pacific where he was conducting fieldwork to study the local fauna and collecting beetles and bird bones. Wallace was an expert naturalist as well as a geographer and pioneered combining the two disciplines.

These questions were no doubt swirling in Darwin's head too, though he had yet to publish on the subject. The two men knew each other, but they were not close friends. Wallace was fourteen years younger than Darwin and more adventuresome in his travels, though chronically broke. Darwin enjoyed a higher social status than Wallace, which may have played a part in his ascendance to fame. But while the two naturalists were not equal peers in a socioeconomic sense, they were equals in their scientific inquiry and curiosities. Both were thinking alike, albeit unconventionally, and to some extent, each was reaching similar conclusions on his own. Or maybe their independent conclusions came from the intellectual volley of letters they exchanged, which stimulated each other's ideas. Science is, after all, about collaboration. We may never know how much their correspondence influenced each of their thinking processes and who was truly first to figure out the whole theory, but we all know that Darwin eventually enjoyed the most credit. As another notable English

*Charles Darwin was not the first to consider the possibility of evolution. He was not even the one to coin the phrase "survival of the fittest," which was introduced by Herbert Spencer, another English biologist and philosopher who came up with the wording after reading *On the Origin of Species*. The idea of transformation from one species to another had been around long before Darwin and had even been suggested by his own paternal grandfather, the physician, philosopher, and poet Erasmus Darwin, who wrote a two-volume medical work, *Zoonomia; or, The Laws of Organic Life*, in 1794 that includes early ideas about the theory. According to Erasmus, God was a "first cause," setting the universe in motion. But after that, creation had been left to run and improve itself.

explorer, Sir Francis Galton, quipped in their era, "In science credit goes to the man who convinces the world, not the man to whom the idea first occurs," a quote that remains largely true today.

The mystique of this controversial bit of history revolves around a now famous essay that came out of Wallace's journaling and that he sent to Darwin the month after he developed the idea when he was ill. He did not use the term *natural selection*, but he did draft some details as to how an evolutionary divergence of species from similar ones could happen under environmental pressures. Wallace trusted Darwin's opinion and likely hoped that Darwin's clout would be helpful in disseminating his ideas. Wallace wanted Darwin to pass the essay on to Darwin's close friend Charles Lyell, a well-known Scottish geologist who could help facilitate publication. It took several weeks, until June 18, 1858, for the essay to reach Darwin.

Darwin did indeed send the manuscript to Lyell and included a note saying, "He could not have made a better short abstract!" It was presented to the Linnean Society of London on the first of July, but the reaction to the reading was nothing extraordinary. In fact, the president of the society said later that the year had not been marked by any striking discoveries. The following year Darwin would go on to publish *On the Origin of Species*, which would change everything.

Darwin and Wallace were actually friends. Wallace met him when he returned from a trip to the South Pacific in 1862. Wallace, in fact, became one of Darwin's staunchest defenders later in life. Whether Darwin stole any of Wallace's ideas from that essay has been a fierce topic of debate among historians, though most agree that Darwin deserves his place in history. I do wonder how Wallace could remain so humble and deferential if he contributed so much to a paradigm shift in scientific thought. He struggled mightily to support himself and his family and frequently sold specimens he'd collected on his expeditions and, worse, edited some of Lyell's and Darwin's works to get by. Darwin did stand up for Wallace and even lobbied to help get Wallace a government pension for his career science work. Did this lobbying stem from guilt? If given the chance, I'd ask Darwin if Wallace's essay held the missing key he needed to unlock the entire theory of evolution and introduce it on the world stage.

The Power of Evolution

Evolution is one of the most powerful forces on the earth. We humans have been under the same laws of natural selection that have governed life for the past four billion years. Most of us have wondered about our last moments on Earth, silently questioning where, when, and how they will take place. It's probably human nature to do so, unlike the trees, birds, and bees around us that do not have that cognitive capacity and live, for the most part, in the moment. Yet the curious thing is that we are relatively new on this planet. The vast majority of creatures predate us by tens of millions, and even hundreds of millions, of years. We need to use our intelligence not just to imagine the future but also to learn from these other "more experienced" species that are smart in their own special ways and have been gaming Earth for eons.

Do these "old" earthlings hold the secrets to living long and robustly? The answers astounded me as I began to dig in. In a world where there are seemingly more naysayers and doomsday events than positive, optimistic news, I'm thrilled to tell you that possibilities for a better, healthier tomorrow in fact do exist if we learn where to look to find the clues that can inform us how to change what we are doing today to benefit us tomorrow. What would happen if we tried to think like an octopus, communicate like an ant, love like a vole, hold on to our memories like a pigeon, parent like a chimpanzee, dodge cancer like an elephant, live in the moment like a dog, and—excuse the pun—drink like a fish? The idea of learning from nature isn't necessarily new, as many scientists from Darwin on down have delved into this domain before, including Barbara Natterson-Horowitz and Kathryn Bowers, who talked about studying animals to find solutions to our mental and physical health issues in their 2012 book, *Zoobiquity*, but I hope I can shed some important new insights. I am not going to give you cure-alls in this book, but rather novel ways of thinking and, I hope, a fresh and revitalizing understanding of health and longevity.

Human studies are sorely limited by the nature of their experiments. It's very difficult to conduct meaningful studies on humans (and their laboratory surrogates such as mice) that give us clues as to what we should be doing to live longer and better. Clinical trials that test drugs or the impact of certain lifestyle habits can take an excruciatingly long time to come to fruition and yet still be inconclusive. By the time we have the answer, many of us will not be here and the technological revolution may have made the results obsolete.

Studying lifestyle habits is extremely challenging and in some cases impossible. We can't, for one example, deprive a large group of people of access to exercise for years to then show its benefits through the group allowed to break a sweat regularly. And even the experiments we can conduct are fraught with challenges due to confounding factors in testing lifestyle habits. This is why we need to look toward other things in nature for answers. Nature already provides a lot of ready-made randomized trials. We just have to go looking. If an elephant can defy cancer despite its size, if an octopus can instantly become invisible, if a species of jellyfish can rebirth itself and be immortal, and if a bird can fly home over thousands of miles without any map or GPS device, then who are we to say we humans are the smartest living things on this planet?

In this book, you'll meet people who think radically differently than I do, and probably you too. As a cancer doctor, I tend to observe science through a lens that often involves cellular and molecular biology. I'm not pitching a tent to watch chimpanzees in Tanzania or digging through ant colonies to find the long-lived queen, for example. So I went out and spoke to (and sometimes Zoomed with) the amazing scientists around the world who do these kinds of experiments, and what I uncovered was astonishing. It has changed how I approach problems, how I see the world, and how I choose to live, from how I parent and mentor to how I get rid of ants in my kitchen or bees in my backyard. I have a love for the classic scientific laboratory with its coal-black countertops and Erlenmeyer flasks, but now I see the entire world as a gigantic laboratory in which to discover and extrapolate lessons that can be applied to human health.

I have made a career out of stimulating the convergence of a number of disciplines—biology, physics, math, engineering, technology, and the clinical sciences—to better understand both wellness and cancer in one place: the Ellison Institute for Transformative Medicine, which I helped create. Our mission is to bring collaborators from both conventional health and wellness fields, as well as from a broad range of other fields of specialties, to study cancer and potential ways to prevent, detect, and treat the disease. Why wellness and cancer? One of my favorite quotes is by Captain B. H. Liddell Hart, a British soldier and military historian who wrote in 1967, "If you wish for peace, understand war." The war is fighting cancer, and from this, my team and I have learned much about wellness, a dichotomy that provides a new perspective to studying each. Hanging on the wall at the entrance to the institute are three large fossils of plants and fish, one as large as eight feet by five feet that is over fifty million years old. I want everyone working in the building to take notice of this and be reminded to have a respect for and learn from nature, which speaks to us every day. We just have to listen.

I can't yet cure my patients of cancer, Alzheimer's, or heart disease, but the frustration motivates me to keep seeking. The first time I lost a patient, I was a resident at Johns Hopkins working in the clinic where people usually didn't have health insurance. A tall, beefy man in his midthirties with congestive heart failure frequently came in. We'll call him Joe. His heart was too large, and its pumping of blood was not keeping apace. Fluid routinely collected in his body, and despite our insisting that he stick to a strict diet and his medications, Joe continued to come into the clinic or wound up in the ER

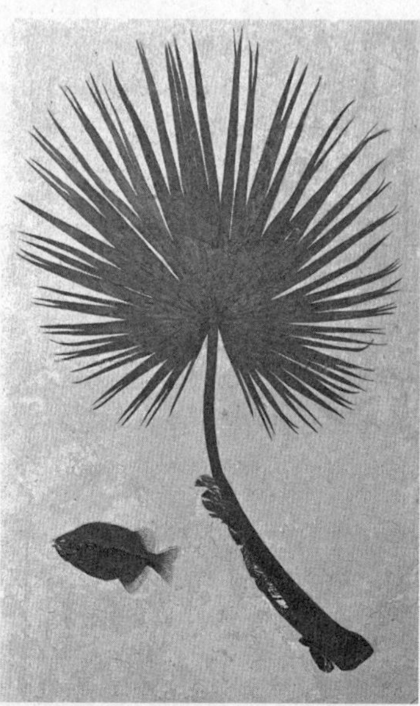

Palm fossil featured at the institute from Lawrence J. Ellison's collection. Fifty million years ago, this palm was on the edge of a warm freshwater lake in Green River, Wyoming. Fossils of plant material are rare, especially a palm as large as this one. The top of the frond is fifty-five inches in diameter.

after eating a meal high in salt or forgetting to take his medications. He was one of our "frequent flyers," as we fondly called patients who were admitted too regularly. All of the interns and residents knew him, and most learned to manage congestive heart failure from him as he instructed the new doctors in what to do to help him.

The last time I admitted him, in the middle of the night, I recall getting a page from the Hopkins ER, which usually meant, when I was on call, that there was a patient for me to admit. I called the ER and was told it was Joe. I rushed to him and noticed that he looked worse than usual. I stabilized him as best I could and started his usual cocktail of medications to treat his heart failure. My shift was over late the next morning, so I went home to catch some sleep and returned the following day. As was the norm, my colleagues and I gathered together to go on rounds with the doctor who had been on call the previous night and hear the events of the night so the new shift could take over everyone's care. We went room by room. When we passed the room Joe had been in, I realized that Joe was gone. He had died the night before after suffering a heart arrhythmia. Nothing worked to resuscitate him.

I retreated after rounds alone to my call room, where I would get occasional stretches of sleep while still on call, and I cried. The sense of loss was immense. I felt that we had failed him. Joe's death in fact marked the beginning of a long trail of losses that motivates me every day to work toward solutions and better treatments to save lives. Knowing what I know now, my hunch is that lessons from the giraffe might one day help us keep someone like Joe suffering from heart disease alive.

Each of the next twelve chapters is structured as a deep dive into one animal or a complementary set of animals that offers a handful of extraordinary secrets to life, most of them adaptable for our purposes, but others explored for entertainment value (and fodder for conversation at your next dinner party). Each chapter is replete with stories and subject matter that may at first seem a little disjointed, but which come together around a dominant theme to make for a surprising lesson or two. Just as it may seem counterintuitive to study cancer to understand wellness or war to know peace, excitingly eclectic ideas gather around a center of gravity that can speak volumes. In the years of research for this book, I came across some facts new to me. Some of these morsels could be tucked into the narrative, while others too far afield have been organized into short footnotes and longer endnotes with the addition of important citations.

I hope that you come away from this book with both a profound appreciation for the nonhuman world around us and some practical strategies to benefit your life. These are listed in Creature Cheat Sheets at the end of every chapter. They aren't the final answer to preventing or treating disease and they won't make you immortal, but you can use them now to help you live longer and better (and hopefully die fast without a prolonged illness). In addition, this book might change not only how you think and live each day, but also how you lead, parent, work, teach, discipline, make decisions, show affection, love, play, collaborate, create, relate with others (strangers included), deal with challenges, cope with stress, forgive the past, be in the present, plan the future, and even prepare to die. And through the lessons, we may all gain a richer understanding of one another and ourselves.

Evolution used to get rid of people in their fifth, sixth, and seventh decades, but now we live longer through a combination of medicine and lifestyle. We can, as it were, cheat death by mimicking or copying some of the techniques other species have used to survive. And we continue to evolve. At the close of *On the Origin of Species*, Darwin wrote, "There is grandeur in this view of life, with its several powers, having been originally breathed into a few forms or into one; and that, whilst this planet has gone cycling on according to the fixed

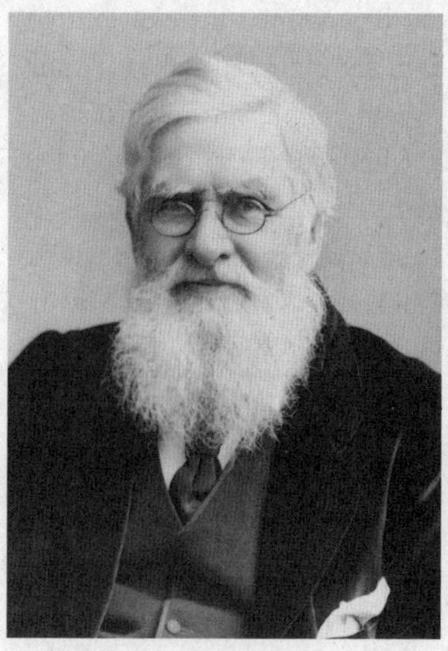

Alfred Russel Wallace (1823–1913)

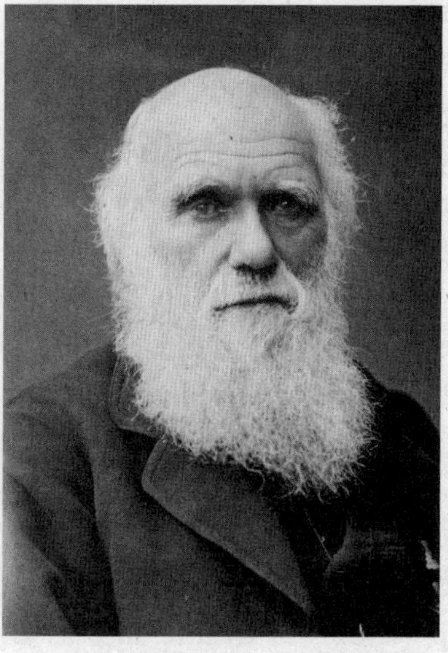

Charles Darwin (1809–1882)

law of gravity, from so simple a beginning endless forms most beautiful and most wonderful have been, and are being, evolved."

Darwin may have won the popularity contest in scientific circles, forever eclipsing Wallace in history as the lead authority on evolutionary theory, but today the pair are memorialized in London's Westminster Abbey side by side. And it was Wallace who would win the longevity race: he lived to the age of ninety, making it to the twentieth century. He even looked like Darwin in his old age, long white beard and all. By the end of his life, he was known as "the Grand Old Man of Science." Perhaps some of the secrets he picked up during his extensive global travels and work in nature came to good use. What did the bats and eucalyptus trees of Southeast Asia whisper to Wallace? We'll never know. But let's bend an ear and see what they have to tell us.

I am excited for you to read *The Book of Animal Secrets* and hopefully gain a new understanding of the creatures we share this earth with, as well as some insights into yourselves.

The Book of Animal Secrets

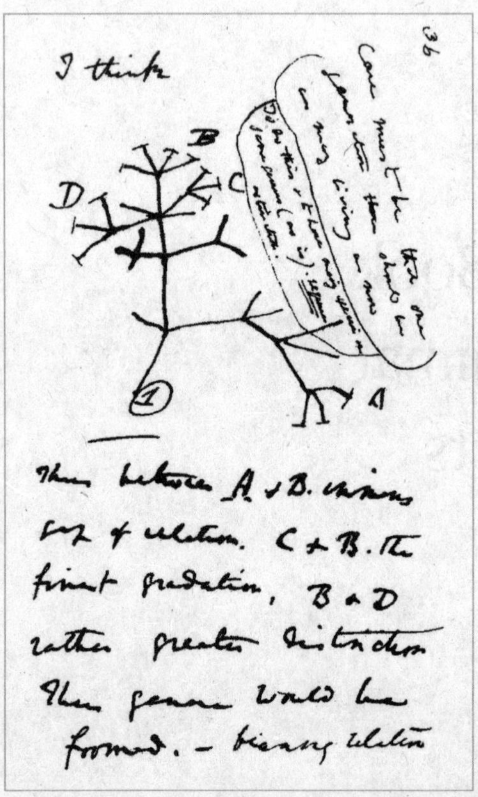

This is a copy of Charles Darwin's 1837 sketch twenty-two years before the publication of *On the Origin of Species*. He wrote, "I think . . . case must be that one generation then should be as many living as now. To do this and to have as many species in same genus (as is) requires extinction. Thus, between A + B the immense gap of relation. C + B the finest gradation. B + D rather greater distinction. Thus genera would be formed." This now iconic, rudimentary draft of the "tree of life" went missing for twenty-two years with another one of Darwin's early notebooks. Both books, small and leather-bound, were mysteriously and anonymously returned to their home at Cambridge University Library in 2022. They were found in a bright-pink gift bag on the library's floor with a typed message:

"Librarian
Happy Easter
X."

1

Living in a Zoo Cage

What Wild Animals Can Teach Us about Living Stronger, Wiser, and Longer

The city is not a concrete jungle, it is a human zoo.

—**DESMOND MORRIS**, *zoologist and sociobiologist*

You awaken abruptly at three o'clock in the morning. You try not to look at the bedside clock, hoping to roll back into sleep. But you can't help yourself, and your obligations that will begin in a few hours fill your thoughts in the dark. You tell yourself that now is the time to sleep and that you will take care of everything once it's light out, but nothing you think about calms you down. You can feel yourself warming up, your body priming for action: conversations you need to have, emails you must write, and notes you should make march in your head. The minutes go by.

An hour later, your anxiety reaches new heights as your thoughts turn to why you haven't scheduled that long-overdue appointment to have a checkup with your doctor. Maybe she could give you something to help you sleep through the night. Wait, you don't even have a doctor because it's been so many years since she retired. You haven't felt particularly energetic lately. This insomnia must be a sign of something worse. Maybe there's something horribly bad brewing, like dementia or cancer. Panic sets in. Your brain continues to ruminate and obsess. You don't know when you eventually fall asleep, but you do, and then soon enough, the sun is streaming through a window and it's time to get up.

Most of us have experienced some version of this scenario. It's a similar dilemma that Stanford neurologist Robert M. Sapolsky describes perfectly in his seminal book, *Why Zebras Don't Get Ulcers.*[1] And why don't they? Because they and other animals don't suffer the kind of chronic stress we place on our bodies. And to that I add that they don't think like us either. When I greet Georgie, my dog, in the morning, I know she hasn't been tossing and turning all night long over an argument she had with another pooch on the previous day's walk or over worries that cancer might be in the cards. (Golden retrievers have a notorious history of the disease.[2]) She has the luxury of living a relatively stress-free life. You and I, however, have a lot to contend with. And while we like to think we're a wild species—free from constraints—we are living captive in our own zoo of sorts.

We've built sophisticated societies, but they are confined by structure, laws, social norms, geographic borders, and physical impediments to roaming freely like we used to. Not many of us spend much time outdoors. Indeed, Americans spend a remarkable 87 percent of their day inside and another 6 percent in their cars.[3] In 1900, there were about seven people living in rural environments for every one urban dweller. Today, more than one out of every two people—roughly half the global population—live in an urban center. By 2050, 70 percent of us will live in cities.[4] We are, as it were, an indoor species, like a domesticated pet.

We no longer have to forage for food or fend off predators. Food is available 24/7 in our kitchen cabinets and refrigerators (or around the corner down the street). And we are increasingly tethered to our electronic devices, which can deliver virtually anything we want at the touch of a button or swipe of a finger. No other animal on the planet comes close to having such technology, not even our closest relatives. Picture a chimpanzee scrolling through a smartphone while munching on a gooey cheeseburger.* Over the past century, technology has radically shifted how we experience life and extended our life expectancy by about thirty years. It has made our lives easier and afforded us opportunities to live better in advanced age. But technologies do have their downsides, including making us more likely to suffer from an array of preventable diseases.

Most of the diseases that kill us today are not seen in the wild. Dementia, heart disease, high blood pressure (hypertension), type 2 diabetes, obesity, autoimmune disorders, and osteoporosis are extremely rare outside our species, if they exist at all. Together, these ailments have become known as "diseases of civilization." They are diseases of our human zoo, and they're on the rise. Yet they are largely preventable, especially given what we know about how to use modern technology and medicine to avert them entirely, years or even decades before a single symptom shows up. The three biggest culprits leading to diseases of civilization are chronic toxic stress; our penchant to sit all day long despite our body's design for constant movement; and unhealthy eating habits that go against millions of years of evolution. To fully appreciate these ideas, let's go on safari.

Fear and Lounging in the Wild

We all learn about survival of the fittest in middle or high school as if it were a theoretical concept. But there's nothing like seeing it in action. A few years ago, I went on safari to Africa, a trip that put survival

*When the San Diego Zoo renovated its orangutan exhibit, the zookeepers had to keep the animals occupied in a hospital where they didn't have the same entertainment as in their normal environment. The primates were thrown popcorn parties and given iPads to watch nature videos, which they loved. They were especially drawn to images of horses and dogs and apparently did a number on the security system—breaking all the cameras.

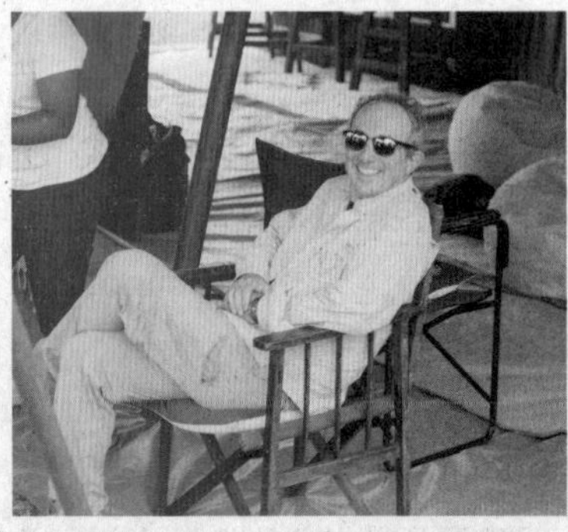

Me on safari in July 2014 with my family (not pictured).

of the fittest into context, especially as it relates to our own human zoo cages.

Equipped with binoculars and cameras and dressed in safari clothes, we spent our days on "hunts"—going out early from a base camp to observe wildlife. Fear was the prevailing theme I could sense all around me among the animals like a familiar aura. Every animal is in a survival game. Some were afraid of being eaten by a predator, some of being attacked by a stronger animal in their own group, and others were on alert to protect their young.

Fear, one of the dominant emotions that powers life, drives everything in nature. It's an emotion that is meant to protect us as it enables us to avoid harm. There are many benefits to fear when it's used positively and is short-lived. The biological reaction that stimulates our nervous system during temporary fear-inducing experiences, including that adrenaline rush, can help us think more clearly, be more motivated and psychologically resilient, and achieve new heights. It may also boost the immune system. Studies dating back nearly two decades show that psychologically stressful events, assuming they're temporary, can lead to an increase in white blood cells in circulation.[5] White blood cells are key sentries in the immune system to protect against infections and respond to injury or illness.

On the other side of fear can be a better mood, reduced baseline anxiety, and even a relaxation response on par with mindfulness meditation. This may be why many people love putting themselves into a frightening moment they can control, such as watching horror movies or taking a thrill ride at a theme park—what's called a "safe scare," without real danger. You can't enjoy being scared unless you know you're in a safe environment. In 2019, when scientists at the University of Pittsburgh put fear to the test with participants in a haunted house, most admitted to feeling a "significantly higher mood" after the experience.[6] Sociologist Margee Kerr, the study's lead author, who explores the nature of fear, hypothesizes that remarkably scary activity may shut down parts the brain, which may actually lead to an overall improved feeling. Obviously the brain is not "turning off," but it's reacting to a fearful event in ways that induce a type of euphoria. And this calculated pause could be the biological mechanism for the beneficial effects of fear. There's also something to be said for the triumph of overcoming a scary moment: we prove to ourselves we can survive, not let our emotions win, and respond appropriately for self-protection.[7] (In chapter 11, we'll see how the balance between pleasure and pain also comes into play.) Fear can help us manage pain or change our experience of pain when it turns chronic so it's less disruptive to our quality of life. It also can help us bond with others. Have you ever walked out of a haunted house with a smile on your face and high-fived a total stranger who just went through it too? That's partly due to the chemical oxytocin flooding your body, another phenomenon we'll explore in this book. This is the same molecule that gets pumped out during sex and childbirth; it's how we connect with others and forge powerful friendships (and delight in being freaked out).

The animals I saw in Africa seem to have adapted to the fears they face, enabling them to live an optimized life. They don't look as if they are in high-alert mode all the time; even animals that are prey for others can spend much of their day lolling about. Unfortunately, the kind of fear we humans experience today is nothing like that of species in the savannas. Lions fear death every day in their own way, but for the most part, they do not ponder their own mortality the way we do or lament yesterday's letdowns and worry incessantly about tomorrow's to-do list. I watched a lot of lions lounging in the savanna that weren't thinking about money, marriage, or work-life balance. Nor were they living in a constant state of guardedness like many people do, which affects every system in the body. Long-term fear (another way of saying chronic stress) has adverse effects, such as prolonged increased blood pressure and the flood of stress hormones, overly tensed muscles, defensive behavior, and ulcers that zebras don't get.

The World Health Organization has deemed chronic stress the "Health Epidemic of the 21st Century"[8] and for good reason: it's one of the leading proximal causes of death, bringing about heart disease and strokes, anxiety, depression, addiction, obesity, and serious memory loss that can tumble into dementia. Wild animals show us to live in the moment, and as we'll see in the next chapter, some domesticated animals tell us even more about the value in this way of living to ease anxiety and manage and reduce our stress levels.

Now let's meet your inner fish.

Our Inner Fish

University of Chicago evolutionary biologist Neil Shubin coined the term "Your Inner Fish" in his 2008 book (with the same title) about the amazing history of the evolution of structure of the human body. So the next time you've had one too many cocktails and lose your coordination, you'll have to blame your inner fish. Prosanta Chakrabarty is an ichthyologist (*ichthys* is Greek for "fish") and professor at Louisiana State University who has discovered over a dozen new species of fish, including previously undocumented species of anglerfishes and cavefishes. Anglerfishes are among the crankiest-looking deep-sea dwellers, like something out of a sci-fi movie; cavefishes, as their name suggests, live in caves and other underground habitats, and many are blind. One of Chakrabarty's findings, the Louisiana pancake batfish, was named a "Top 10 New Species" in 2011 by the International Institute for Species Exploration at Arizona State University.[9]

This rather unsightly pancake batfish is flat like a pancake and spiky, has huge bulging eyes, and can jump around on its fins. Like the dark-dwelling anglers and cavefishes, it lives in some of the most inhospitable habitats on the planet, where it's lonely and lightless. Chakrabarty probably would never describe any fish as being "ugly" or "heinous," but you can't help but wonder why these creatures turned out the way they did.

Chakrabarty fell in love with fish in his youth. Growing up in Queens, he volunteered at the New York Aquarium on Coney Island and eventually earned a PhD at the University of Michigan. He's been in Baton Rouge, Louisiana, for the past decade. When I interviewed him, he was driving south toward the Gulf of Mexico with one of his twin daughters to search for salamanders.

The first surprising thing Chakrabarty shared with me is that he sees fish as having "perfect bodies." Their vertebral column allows them to move swiftly through water without feeling the consequences of gravity. We humans have to defy gravity all day long

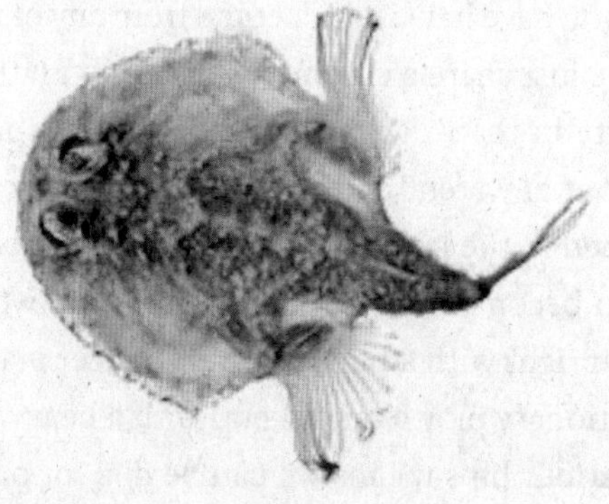

to stay upright—hence our tendencies to bad backs, knee pain, and osteoarthritis.

Chakrabarty is the one who first suggested to me that we're all "living in captivity" now. And he would know: he instructs one of the largest evolutionary biology classes in the country, where he dispels lots of misinformation about our past. He set me straight too. When I think about evolution, I picture the classic image of a four-legged, apelike furry animal turning into a two-legged naked caveman. But to understand our origins, it's important to look back further still. "Knowing you're a fish and not a monkey is actually really important to understanding where we came from," Chakrabarty said in his TED Talk, before reminding the audience that humans are not the goal of evolution.[10] We're not perfectly evolved creatures at the end of a long line of more primitive forms changing under the forces of natural selection.

He added, "About three billion years ago, life-forms made up of more than one cell (called multicellular eukaryotes)—fungi, plants, and animals—evolved. The first animals to develop a backbone were fishes. So technically all vertebrates are fishes, so technically you are and I are fish. So don't say I didn't warn you." One fish lineage moved onto land and gave rise to, among other things, mammals and reptiles. Some reptiles became birds, some mammals became primates, and some primates became monkeys with tails, while others became the great apes. From the great apes evolved a variety of human species. So there you have it: we didn't come from any of the monkeys we know today; we just share a common ancestor with them.

Chakrabarty in that TED Talk urged us "to think of [ourselves] as a little fish out of water," and poorly constructed ones at that. Our gills transformed to the larynx and middle ear. Our aquatic vertebral column had to become stronger to support our two-legged stance. But standing upright with a big head and flat feet may not have been the best evolutionary ploy. Standing up with a heavy head and a center of gravity at our hips means we can be due for orthopedic issues later in life. The key for us is to focus on our alignment, standing up straight, and especially building our core muscles that support our head and skeletal system.[11]

If you still can't see yourself as a fish, go back to the idea of losing your balance after drinking too much. Apart from causing aches and pains, our upright bipedalism makes it extra difficult to maintain our balance, especially when it's under the influence of alcohol. When you indulge, the alcohol that ends up in the bloodstream finds its way into the fluid of the inner ear, as blood naturally flows to the inner ear—and that flow increases when you imbibe. The fluid that's normally in the ear (and it's not that much) to help with your balance is denser than the alcohol, so once the alcohol is added to it, the fluid becomes less dense. And this is what triggers problems as tiny hair cells, neurons inside the gel-like fluid, become stimulated and your brain gets the wrong message: it thinks you're moving when you're not. The eyes depend on the vestibular system to stabilize them against any head movements. Your brain's ability to detect motion is an aquatic trait, a vestigial leftover from evolution. You experience the spins, and the brain sends a message to your eye muscles, which then twitch in one direction—typically the right. (This is called positional alcohol nystagmus, PAN, and it's one of the signs police are looking for when they pull over drivers they think might be drunk.) The abnormal changes in the inner ear's fluid also stir a cascade of effects that ultimately cause the nausea and vertigo that intoxicated individuals feel. Our bodies weren't designed for too much alcohol, and there is a danger to continued use—as the expression goes, drinking like a fish. When someone has repeated, long-term exposure to alcohol, damage accumulates in their central auditory cortex, the part of the brain in the temporal lobe that processes auditory information. When the central auditory complex is damaged, the processing of sound can be delayed, which would mean you might have trouble distinguishing someone talking in a noisy environment or even understanding if someone is speaking very quickly.[12]

In addition, the eyes of those who are experiencing a painful hangover may twitch, a result of that alcohol diffusing back into the bloodstream from the tubes in their ears. Your liver will have already taken care of the blood-alcohol levels in your bloodstream from the night before, but the next day, the spins can happen again. And this time, when your eyes twitch, they might do so *in the opposite direction*, as the alcohol is removed from the ear more quickly than from the body, so its concentration is actually lower in the ear canal.[13]

While we don't consider ourselves aquatic species today, we can't forget the fact we all begin bathed completely in water, surrounded by the amniotic fluid of our mother in the womb. And then we take our time gaining our bearings on land, learning to crawl, then walk, and eventually run. Our vertebral column supports our movement just as it does for fish with "perfect bodies," but these days, we don't respect our body's design the way we should. Being able to walk on two feet rather than four offers us many energy-efficient advantages: it improves our ability to cool off, survey our surroundings, carry tools and tots, and travel longer distances, for example. But these advantages can be outstripped by our proclivities toward too much sitting, slouching, slumping, and general sedentariness. We are designed to move.

Prolonged sitting and poor posture are twin enemies to our skeletal health, but it's more than about maintaining spinal alignment to prevent neck, shoulder, and back pain, not to mention injury as well. Standing up straight helps with breathing, swallowing our food, overall blood circulation, and preventing maladies such as skeletal pain (joint stiffness—predominantly neck, shoulders, and back).[14] An amazing study out of the University of Auckland in New Zealand demonstrated that when people with depression were either randomized to sit like they usually do or told to have better posture, the ones who sat up straight had more energy, less anxiety, and a better outlook. Posture can have a pretty significant impact on health, including mental health.[15]

Posture is easy to work on: establish and maintain a sturdy core (no extreme six-pack required); be mindful how you hold yourself when you're walking, sitting, and standing (straight and tall, shoulders back and relaxed, stomach in); wear comfortable, low-heeled shoes; and use posture-friendly devices when possible (e.g., ergonomic chairs and standing desks). It also helps to own a mattress that supports your body's sound sleep to prepare for another gravity-defying day.

One of the biggest cues we can take from bony fish in particular is this: they are constant swimmers. It's how they breathe. You won't find fish resting for too long, because swimming allows them to keep a constant flow of water moving past their gills, which is helpful for maintaining a proper oxygen level in their bodies. Most fish keep moving even while they sleep. Although we don't rely on movement to breathe, it's something to think about—and we do rely on movement to pump our lymphatic system, the body's drainage pipes that have everything to do with the strength of our immune system. Some call it the body's sewerage system that complements the circulatory system. The lymphatic system's main role is to manage the body's fluids by ushering excess fluid and proteins leaked from blood vessels back into the bloodstream via the lymph nodes. But its actions also serve to produce white blood cells called lymphocytes (and their antibodies) to fight infections. This is why the lymphatic system is considered a star player in the body's adaptive immune response. It also happens to serve an important role in the gut and intestinal function, where it aids in the absorption of fats and fat-soluble vitamins.

Lack of sufficient movement has plenty of repercussions. But what if those repercussions were more immediate than, say, losing mobility, reducing immunity, and gaining weight over time? If we could remember that preferring to be sitting makes it difficult to breathe, we'd certainly have more incentive to move—and move more often. We should keep in mind that we're not so very different from our ancestors the fish.

Outstripping Natural Selection

Most of us may be living in a zoo cage today, but that's not necessarily a bad thing. We're no longer kept up at night by the lion strolling by our tent, like the one I saw on safari. We don't have to worry too much about how we will procure our next meal and drink of water. But modern living can be stressful for other reasons. Although it can be quite comfortable, sometimes it is too comfortable.

Daniel E. Lieberman is a paleoanthropologist at Harvard University, where he chairs the Department of Human Evolutionary Biology. He too devotes his time to understanding our evolution and is particularly fascinated by how we developed the bodies we possess today. Lieberman is alarmed by the pace of our "evolution" in recent decades, as cultural change has outstripped natural selection. In his 2013 book, *The Story of the Human Body*, Lieberman makes the case for the prevalence of chronic disease in our current society being the result of a mismatch between our evolutionary roots and modern lifestyles. He writes, "We still don't know how to counter once-adaptive primal instincts to eat donuts and take the elevator."[16] Food was limited through most of our evolution, so expending calories without purpose wasn't an advantage. At the same time, our "anatomical and physiological systems" were optimized to function based on our regular movement. All of this changes when we are in the zoo cage of today's society, as we are not adapted for long periods of inactivity. Nor are we adapted to be constantly exposed to a cornucopia of sustenance. Our inner fish can only swallow so much.

In 2019, one of the medical industry's finest journals, the *Lancet*, published a study showing that one in five deaths globally can be attributed to a poor diet.[17] That's more deaths than from tobacco usage or high blood pressure. And it's not due to a lack of education or resources. The study took into consideration age, gender, country of residence, and socioeconomic status to show that people are affected by poor dietary habits *despite* these factors. That's eleven million deaths a year globally due to consuming a diet high in salt and low in whole grains and fruits. It's ironic because we have the ability to grow or produce any food we want and acquire foods from around the world no matter the season. Survival of the fittest today isn't about getting enough calories through hunting and gathering to survive; it's about choosing to consume the right foods from the bounty.

Another study that came out in 2019 put the spotlight on ultraprocessed foods, something else we did not evolve to eat.[18] In a fantastic, well-designed "zoo-like" experiment, twenty adults were brought to the National Institutes of Health (NIH) Clinical Center for four weeks. They were each given two weeks of food that was unprocessed and two weeks of a diet dominated by ultraprocessed food. The ultraprocessed food is described as "formulations mostly of cheap industrial sources of dietary energy and nutrients plus additives," including high-fructose corn syrup, preservatives, sweeteners, artificial coloring, refined carbohydrates, chemical flavoring and texturing agents, salt, and refined oils and trans fats. Think of packaged

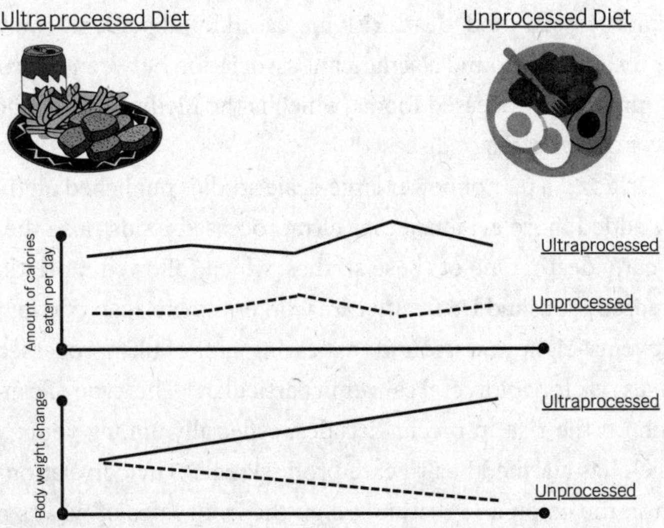

Unprocessed foods beat ultraprocessed foods for weight loss over a fourteen-day period.[19]

baked goods and snacks, soft drinks, sugary cereals, instant noodles, dehydrated vegetable soups, processed cheese products, microwaveable dinners, and reconstituted meat and fish products (e.g., sausages, fish fingers, hot dogs). The participants were given the same amount of food daily during each two-week segment and allowed to eat as much as they wanted. While on the two-week ultraprocessed period of the study, participants ate five hundred excess calories a day and gained almost two pounds, while the same people lost two pounds on the unprocessed diet.

This was a small study, but others have confirmed similar findings. On the heels of this NIH study came two large studies from France and Spain that both demonstrated a direct correlation between the amount of ultraprocessed foods consumed and heart disease and death.[20] These European studies covered tens of thousands of people, and the Spanish study showed that eating more ultraprocessed foods (more than four servings daily) was associated with a whopping 62 percent increased risk of death compared with eating less (fewer than two servings daily). For each additional daily serving of ultraprocessed food, death risk increased by 18 percent. Conversely, the researchers found a significant association between unprocessed or minimally processed foods (which is the Mediterranean diet) and lower overall risks of disease.[21]

In 2022, a pair of newer large-scale studies published on the same day added more evidence that ultraprocessed foods raise the risk of an early death. One of these studies, which followed more than two hundred thousand US health care workers over a span of twenty-four to twenty-eight years, found that eating a lot of ultraprocessed foods spikes risk for colorectal cancer in particular.[22] This type of cancer has been on the rise in recent decades, especially among young adults, which has alarmed health care professionals. The correlation makes sense: the colon and rectum are on the front lines of what's moving through your digestive system. And ultraprocessed foods more easily contribute to obesity, another risk factor in all this mortality.

These results may not seem surprising, but we hadn't had scientific data like this previously. And although these studies are observational and don't establish causality, they point out how much lifestyle factors into our health. Ultraprocessed foods are recent. They came on the evolutionary scene in the last microsecond and are nothing close to what nature intended for us to consume. I can only imagine what our ancient ancestors would think if they came across us gobbling up a midday meal with sugary ketchup and a milkshake. We'd probably look as ridiculous as that imaginary chimpanzee devouring a drippy burger while scrolling on a touch screen—and you know we'd also be eating over our smartphones.

The reason that ultraprocessed foods are so problematic is not that we cannot digest them, but that they are exceedingly palatable (tasty), so we have trouble with portion control. They also contain ingredients that are unhealthy in large quantities, such as sugar, salt, and saturated fats. These foods can tinker with our satiety signals, and some of them can mess with our hormonal system to the extent they change how we store fat, burn calories, and maintain humming metabolisms. They also lack the fiber and nutrients our bodies need to thrive, like essential fatty acids, healthful plant compounds that exert anti-inflammatory and anticarcinogenic effects, and protein. So when we eat ultraprocessed foods, they replace what our bodies truly need. Most people consume fewer than two cups of whole fruits and vegetables a day, far below the four to six cups we should be getting. The more fruits and vegetables you consume, the less likely you'll replace them with nutrient-poor, health-depleting options.

The University of North Carolina at Chapel Hill's Gillings School of Global Public Health attempted to study the percentage of Americans who are metabolically healthy, which they define as having optimal levels of five factors without the aid of taking pills: blood sugar, triglycerides (blood fats), high-density lipoprotein cholesterol (HDL, the "good cholesterol"), blood pressure, and waist circumference. Their study queried National Health and Nutrition Examination

Survey (NHANES) data from 8,721 people in the United States between 2009 and 2016 to determine how many adults are at low versus high risk for chronic disease. The result is that only 12.2 percent of us, or one in eight Americans, are achieving optimal metabolic health.[23] The news got gloomier when another calculation was made by a group at Tufts University's Gerald J. and Dorothy R. Friedman School of Nutrition Science and Policy.[24] They used some of the same representative NHANES data, but this time from about fifty-five thousand US adults from 1999 through 2018. The number published in 2022 suggested we're going in the wrong direction, with only 6.8 percent of us living with optimal cardiometabolic health (that's fewer than one in fifteen adults).

If we were to make the same calculation on animals in the wild, my bet is the percentage would be closer to 100. Part of this has to be related to the fact that we keep tinkering with the food we evolved to eat. Whether it was from Gregor Mendel's experiments on peas in the 1860s, which accelerated breeding for produce with certain traits, or the introduction of foreign genes to produce GMO foods, or the move to low cost and convenience with ultraprocessed foods, we've significantly changed the food we evolved to eat. We'd be better off if we ate food in the way it was meant to be eaten—including eating whole fruits and vegetables rather than in juiced or processed forms.

I've long been an adversary of juicing. You may think that fresh, pressed juices are nutrient bombs, but pulverized produce has been stripped of its fibrous surroundings that help us feel full and contribute to digestive health by aiding in the movement of food through the system. And we change the whole chemistry of a produce's flesh—and the nutrition that goes with it—when we subject it to the disruptive power of a blender and exposure to light and air, which may lead it to become oxidized, thereby losing its nutritional punch. Put simply, juice from a blender is not whole food; it's processed. What's more, many juices contain added sugars that further disrupt and adulterate the whole nutritional equation. The result is an insult to anyone's metabolic health.

When the factors of metabolic health I just described are unfavorable, meaning you've got high blood pressure, elevated blood sugar, excess body fat around the waist, elevated triglycerides in the blood, and abnormal cholesterol levels, it's called metabolic syndrome (also called MetS or syndrome X). It is a constellation of risk factors that increases the risk of heart disease, stroke, diabetes, sleep apnea, liver and kidney disease, cancer, and Alzheimer's disease. And it even immensely hikes the chances of dying from an infection because the downstream effects dampen immunity. If you have unhealthy numbers for at least three of these factors of metabolic health, then you are considered to have metabolic syndrome. It's thought that metabolic syndrome may be the most common and serious condition people have never heard of, and yet it's the greatest public health threat in the twenty-first century. It's the ultimate disease of civilization not seen in the wild.

Lieberman, in his book, gives a simple summary for increasing the chances of living a long life without disease: "Men and women aged forty-five to seventy-nine who are physically active, eat plenty of fruits and vegetables, do not smoke, and consume alcohol moderately have on average one-fourth the risk of death during a given year than people with unhealthy habits."[25] Those tenets, all of which are achievable even in our cage, can help us counter the negative effects of living in a zoo. We have to behave like animals in the wild that still consume what they evolved to eat and lead vigorous lives. And we must understand where our maladaptive behaviors are coming from. We can take risks in our careers but we can't with our behavior. I would add to Lieberman's list, though, because he's missing a critical habit that we sorely need to work on: a habit that your dog is likely much better at keeping than you are.

Creature Cheat Sheet

Wild animals may not have the benefits of modern technology, but neither do they suffer from diseases of civilization. All creatures must jump into alert mode when threatened. But we humans have a tendency to let stress get the best of us and keep us rigged for battle when there's nothing really to fight other than insomnia, cravings for junk food, and a weakness for the couch. We would do well to manage healthy levels of transient stress (including indulging in the occasional "safe scare"), respect our physiology to maintain good posture, move frequently as if our breath relied on it, and eat as close to nature as possible.

Remember your inner fish: don't drink like one, but do glide through the world upright with a strong core that supports your center of gravity, promotes ideal posture, and helps prevent atrophy of bones and muscles. And watch out for signs of metabolic syndrome, all of which are modifiable and treatable. These basic tenets will help us to adapt to our modern environment and enjoy living in our collective, cozy zoo.

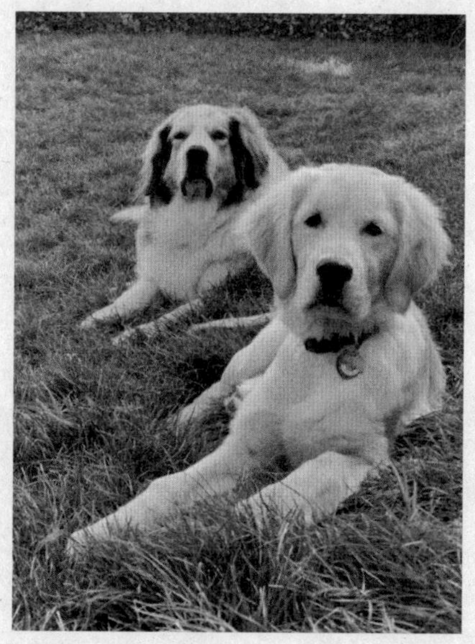

Georgie and the late great Sadie (far back).

2

Oh My Dog!

More Than Man's Best Friend

> *To his dog, every man is Napoleon; hence the constant popularity of dogs.*
>
> —ALDOUS HUXLEY

Seventy-eight million households in America have four-legged, fleecy family members. My family is one of them, and my endearment with these marvelous furballs goes way back. My wife, Amy, and I had been married barely a year when we decided we were ready for our first child—a canine one. Amy and I had been set up on a blind date by my aunt Edna, whose husband was the first cousin of Amy's father. I was a student at the National Institutes of Health and going to give a presentation at Yale University, where Amy was in grad school. Neither of us wanted to be set up on a date, so rather than going out for dinner, we met up for a cup of tea at the Atticus Bookstore Cafe in New Haven. The rest was history.

The inspiration to get a dog first occurred as we were walking in Madison Square Park in New York City and came across a young woman walking an adorable Bernese mountain dog. We then contacted a breeder upstate. Berneses are large and beautiful, originating from Bern, Switzerland, with teddy-bearish features and a distinctive tricolored coat in bold patterns of tan, black, and white. Two small rust-colored patches sit over their eyes (resembling comma-shaped eyebrows), popping out against ink-black facial hair. The spots are meant to mislead prey or perpetrators as part of their guard uniform. Because the spots can look like eyes, Berneses can be deceptive as to the direction of their gaze. Even when they are sleeping, their eyes almost seem to be open. Originally used to guard farms and drive cattle, they are mellow workhorses and affectionate, loyal, and protective. The breeder we called happened to have a puppy ready for a home, and we arranged the trip for our first wedding anniversary.

We were instantly smitten with Arthur, who sat on our laps the entire car ride back to our home in Brooklyn. As he grew, gregarious Arthur earned a reputation around town and became known as the mayor of Brooklyn Heights—he knew everyone, and everyone knew him. Always the worker, he loved to help us out when he could. When we went to the market, he carried the shopping bag proudly in his mouth back to our apartment, and even once managed a cardboard pizza box! Two years later, our daughter, Sydney, was born; she spent many hours drinking her bottle lying on Arthur's soft, furry belly.

Arthur moved with us when we ventured West, but he lived only six years, dying of gastric torsion. Bernese mountain dogs are prone to this condition in which the stomach twists on itself and fills with gas, which cuts off blood supply to the stomach. Our next Bernese mountain dog, Yogi, suffered from a short life too, succumbing to cancer.

We had learned the lesson. Though still smitten by the loyalty and love of Berners, we hoped this time to avoid the heartbreak of losing another dog too soon. Our next dog, Sadie, was half Bernese mountain dog and half Great Pyrenees. Sadie got up with me early every morning and sat with me as I wrote or worked. She was the sweetest dog, although not a small dog, coming in at 125 pounds, and I really don't think she realized she was that big, hence the recurrent knocking things over with a bushy sweep of her tail. Shortly before her death in 2021, we welcomed Georgie into our home.

It's astonishing that there are so many varieties of dogs (at least 150 breeds) that all belong to the same species (*Canis familiaris*) and come from the same ancestor, the gray wolf (*Canis lupus*). This is the outcome of intense, purposeful interbreeding in just the past roughly 150 years.* No other species on the planet comes with such extensive genetic variability. Dogs are the product of one of the largest genetic experiments ever conducted by humans, which makes them uniquely fascinating to study. And they are increasingly being studied (in dog-friendly settings) to inform human health. Because dogs age much like we do but far more rapidly, research scientists have come to respect dogs as superior models of human aging.

Michael Kent is a respected veterinarian at the University of California, Davis, where he studies cancer in dogs. Like many other scientists, he appreciates canines as models of human disease. If he can figure out why dogs generally develop cancer so much sooner than humans do, relatively speaking across the life span (and barring the anomalies of childhood cancers, which are rare and unusual), maybe that can help inform ways for us to avoid cancer altogether. He is also a strong believer in the dog-longevity link: people who have dogs enjoy a higher quality of life and live longer and happier lives.

We often think of dogs as companions rather than conduits for

*Despite his brilliance, Darwin was incorrect about dogs: he thought their remarkable diversity was from interbreeding with several types of wild dogs. The modern DNA findings prove otherwise. All current breeds of dogs are descendants of wolves. This domestication may have happened twice in the history of dogs, producing groups of dogs from two unique but common ancestors. Darwin in fact owed a lot of his observations in nature as a serious scientist in his adulthood to his early love for dogs in his youth. The role of dogs in Darwin's work isn't discussed often, but he was significantly affected by his experience with canines. What we forget about in the twenty-first century is that dogs were much more than companions in Darwin's Victorian England. They were essential to daily country life, herding livestock, guiding hunters to their prey, and controlling vermin.

making sense of the natural world, but they can be surprising sources of wisdom. If Darwin had never taken to dogs, it's possible he never would have pursued natural sciences. His interactions with dogs helped shape his scientific approach in his formative years. He observed his dogs' behavior, studying their role in nature, their breeding, and the relationships among all of these things.

David Allan Feller probably knows more about Darwin's dogs than anyone else in the world today. After a career as a lawyer, he went on to study the history of biology and animals in science, writing a master's thesis in 2005 titled "Heir of the Dog: Canine Influences on Charles Darwin's Theories of Natural Selection." In this thesis, he describes how "surprisingly little attention has been given to the influence of dogs in Darwin's work" and that Darwin owed much of his scientific outlook to his canine observations.[1] He then pursued a PhD at Darwin's old stomping grounds at Cambridge University in the Department of History and Philosophy of Science. According to Feller, who himself has three dogs, the foundations of natural selection, evidenced in Darwin's journals and notebooks, rest on canine analogies. In fact, Darwin's 1842 essay, which laid out the principles of *On the Origin of Species*, uses the model of the greyhound as an example of adaptation and selection. Greyhounds are well adapted to running down rabbits, but breeding greyhounds through careful selection is not the only factor in their behavior. Darwin also imagined the dogs as natural, predatory, and feral—selected for by nature too. Before long, Darwin's keen observations moved to other animals as well.

The question becomes: Can the dogs we keep today help us to better understand the world and make more perceptive observations—and not just about others but also about ourselves? My guess is yes. We've evolved to need dogs in our lives. But what about their needing us? There's a common yet surprising misconception I've encountered: Perhaps dogs are not *our* companions; rather, we are *their* companions. They evolved *because of us* but not necessarily *for* us. In other words, the old theory that some hunter-gatherer found a litter of cute puppy wolves and took them in until they eventually evolved into obedient dogs in subsequent generations is probably bunk. What probably happened is *they* approached *us* (and domesticated us to some degree).

And yet we have made them our best friends, growing ever more accustomed to having them in our lives as important companions who help us live longer. As a group of Finnish researchers summed up nicely in 2021, "The domestication of dogs has increased the success of both species to the point that dogs are now the most numerous carnivore on the planet."[2] And they contribute mightily to our livelihoods through a variety of ways, one of which is simply the "feel-good" vibes they give us to help us forge onward.* But before we get to the benefits of dog ownership, let's first get to know where our furry friends came from.

Survival of the Friendliest

The timeline for the domestication of dogs is still up for debate. Some say the domestication of dogs happened 40,000 years ago. DNA analysis published in 1997 in *Science* suggests the domestication began more than 130,000 years ago. That's a large discrepancy. We don't even know for sure if dogs were domesticated more than once or where it happened (Europe? Asia?). But here's something we

*Dogs were the first species to forge a bond with humans. They went from wild wolves to willful pets. One of the first pet dogs whose name is known was Abutiu (also transcribed as Abuwtiyuw), who belonged to an Egyptian pharaoh in the early third millennium BC. But signs of dog-human dyads date back to Paleolithic times. In search for clues to human evolution, archaeologists have unearthed burial sites where early humans, including young children, have been found with their four-legged companions. As the *Wall Street Journal* pointed out in 2020, "Humans kept animals as companions long before we domesticated livestock like sheep, goats, and cattle some ten to twelve thousand years ago. By contrast, horses were only tamed in Eurasia only around six thousand years ago. Though they weren't considered household pets, they inspired passionate feelings in their owners."

do know: such a timeline for the transformation of wolves to dogs has monumental implications because it means that wolves began to adapt to human society centuries before we settled down and began planting seeds and herding animals, which happened only some 10,000 to 12,000 years ago. The discrepancy is important as it calls into question the explanation passed on for many generations that humans domesticated dogs to work as their protectors or helpful comrades.

The lore of the solitary hunter befriending an injured wolf is just that—folklore. What's more likely to have happened is that wolves domesticated themselves among hunter-gatherer people. They may have gotten humans to take them in out of the cold and feed them. Put another way, the dogs warmed up to us rather than the opposite. It's unlikely that humans tamed wild wolves into pets for our own good, as wolves are not easily tamed or approachable. (Despite the fairy tale of "Little Red Riding Hood," there is no such thing as the Big Bad Wolf; wolves are shy and fearful of people.) And according to Brian Hare, founder of Duke University's Canine Cognition Center and coauthor of *The Genius of Dogs*, the physical changes that appeared in dogs over time, such as floppy ears, curly or short tails, and patterned fur coats follow a process that reflects self-domestication.[3] These physical changes are driven by friendliness because the friendliest animals gain an advantage. Call it survival of the friendliest. This selection can happen relatively quickly in only a few generations. The most remarkable evidence for self-domestication comes from a now famous experiment from Russia where captive foxes were bred to be comfortable getting close to humans over the course of just forty-five years.[4] The researchers also found that the foxes got skilled at picking up on human social cues (e.g., pointing), which is something seen in dogs but not wolves or even other primates like chimpanzees. And they even began to look increasingly adorable—like dogs.

Evolutionary biologists also have an idea about the genetic forces at work in self-domestication. In 2017, researchers at Princeton

University and UCLA suggested that we share genetic variations with dogs that drive our hypersocial behavior.[5] Studies show that social dogs have a disruption to a region in their DNA that remains intact in wolves, which are more aloof. And, intriguingly, there's a genetic variation in the same stretch of DNA in humans, a condition called Williams-Beuren syndrome, a rare genetic disorder characterized by being overly friendly and trusting, along with troubling physical abnormalities including heart and musculoskeletal defects, pointing to there being genetic underpinnings to social behavior.

We also have new evidence that those "puppy-dog eyes" we've come to love evolved in dogs to gain our attention. In 2019, a paper published in the *Proceedings of the National Academy of Sciences* noted that dogs' faces are structured for complex expression in a way that wolves' faces are not, owing to a special pair of muscles framing their eyes.[6] These muscles are responsible for that "I'm so cute, adopt me" look that dogs give by raising their inner eyebrows. It's the first biological evidence scientists have found that domesticated dogs might have evolved a unique ability to communicate better with humans. Our desire to breed certain traits into dogs has also influenced their behavioral evolution. The traits humans have chosen most in their selective breeding of dogs? Childlike characteristics such as floppy ears and snub noses, which has contributed mightily to making dogs look different from fierce-looking wolves.

Over millennia, our relationship with dogs has grown so close that even our brains are attuned to one another. Studies have shown a stunning phenomenon: dogs can positively tap into the human brain's maternal bonding system. When we look adoringly into our dog's eyes, each of our brains secretes oxytocin, a hormone linked to bonding between a mother and child, as well as trust. As we'll see in chapter 12, other mammalian relationships feature oxytocin and bonding too, but the human-dog example of this intimate two-way relationship is the only case seen so far between two different species. This ultimately means that by studying dogs, we may also learn much about human cognition and mental well-being. We share more biology with our canine comrades than with other creatures we use in studies, like rodents and flies.*

In addition, the concept of survival of the friendliest applies to us humans as well. Brian Hare's work with his wife, Vanessa Woods, a research scientist also at Duke's Center for Cognitive Neuroscience, has argued that self-domestication occurred in us too. Late in our evolution, their theory goes, we underwent a process of extreme selection for friendliness that helped us outcompete other species of humans. As they discussed in a *Scientific American* article (and in their 2020 book, *Survival of the Friendliest*), "This friendliness evolved through self-domestication. Domestication is a process that involves intense selection for friendliness. When an animal is domesticated, in addition to becoming much friendlier, it undergoes many changes that appear completely unrelated to one another. This domestication syndrome shows up in the shape of the face, the size of the teeth and the pigmentation of different body parts or hair; it includes changes to hormones, reproductive cycles and the nervous system. Although we think of domestication as something that we do to animals, it can also occur through natural selection, a process known as self-domestication."[7]

The provocative theory has met its critics, but it's still worth considering how being prosocial, cooperative, and friendly—as opposed to aggressive and despotic—aids us, and not just in our evolutionary survival but also in our daily lives. So think about that the next time you're tempted to be abrasive or adversarial to other people, even when they vex and annoy you. In chapters 7 and 11 we'll see

*Interestingly, our own DNA does not always reveal parts of prehistory that we can see with dog genomes. Pontus Skoglund, a population geneticist at the Francis Crick Institute in London, who co-led a study published in 2020 on canine evolution, noted in an interview in *Nature,* "Dogs are a separate tracer dye for human history." He added, "Sometimes human DNA might not show parts of prehistory that we can see with dog genomes."

how helping others—altruism—can have lifesaving benefits. Future research will have to answer the question: Can friendliness also breed success in health and in life? We know that friendships are crucial to well-being and even for staving off cognitive decline, so I'm betting the answer is yes.

I don't think our four-legged friends would be at all surprised.

Canine Medicine to the Rescue

When he was growing up, Michael Kent never saw himself as a veterinarian. In the early 1990s, he had aspired to be a photojournalist and was the first in his family to go to college. His dad was a plumber in Rockland County, New York, and his mother worked all kinds of odd jobs. But he had science in his background: his grandfather had been a tech writer for the engineering company Northrop Grumman (formerly called Grumman Aerospace) and had written one of the manuals for astronauts going to the moon. Kent briefly trained his efforts at engineering in his first year at Boston University then soon switched his major to political science, but that wasn't for him either. Neither were any of the jobs he took after college while finding his way in Los Angeles, until a dog entered his life that he adored. He then took a job at the zoo, signed up for his first biology class through UCLA's adult education program, and volunteered at a large veterinary hospital in downtown. From there, he entered the University of California, Davis in Northern California, where he earned his veterinary medicine degree and now works as a professor of surgical and radiological sciences.

Kent focuses on what he perceives as the best model for human health and aging: dogs. Unlike rodents and other animals used in laboratory settings, dogs have complex physiology and share disease processes with us, meaning that certain ailments manifest and progress in them as they do in us. This makes dogs better models for study and testing novel therapies for both effectiveness and toxicity.

Not only do dogs get cancer, but they can also develop diabetes, epilepsy, Alzheimer's disease (known as canine cognitive dysfunction), and Crohn's. Moreover, pets are often exposed to the same disease-causing environmental factors as humans. We share more viruses with dogs than with any other animals, and a dog's immune system is incredibly the same as ours. For a long time, we moved medicine from humans to dogs, treating them based on us. Now we're going in reverse. In 2017, STAT News noted that now "veterinarians are working closely with medical and other doctors around the world to further clinical research in a host of intractable diseases using a broad range of animals. . . . Many veterinary schools refer to their work in comparative medicine as 'One Health.'"[8]

The US Food and Drug Administration has sought to decrease the number of dog clinical trials to reduce unscrupulous experiments that ignore animal welfare, but I think a lot of good comes from studying dogs using safe and humane methods.* Many of these studies are not cruel to animals. Animal patients often have fervently devoted owners who want to do anything to save their pets. Kent takes the informed consent process seriously so pet owners understand the risks.

Many of the recent advances in immunotherapy that are helping human patients with cancer began their testing in spontaneous models of dog cancer. ("Spontaneous models" refers to cancer that arises naturally, without being artificially induced in a lab.) Certain tumors in humans and dogs are indistinguishable under the microscope. Kent has successfully partnered with radiation oncologists who work

*Over summer 2022, thousands of beagles were rescued from a breeding facility in Virginia that were destined to be sold to research groups. But the facility had violated many animal welfare laws, including those against deficient veterinary care, insufficient food, unsanitary conditions, and euthanasia without anesthesia. I applaud such a move and hope new regulations emerge to end the unethical treatment of dogs in research and testing settings and promote their positive participation in safe scientific settings where they thrive.

with humans to test new therapies that harness the immune system to combat metastatic lung cancer and bone cancer in dogs—cancers that behave in a similar way in humans. Many of these dogs are living years longer because of these treatments. These canine findings can lead to breakthroughs in human medicine much quicker than traditional trials, which can take an excruciatingly long time and leave desperate patients with no solutions. Dogs have a much shorter life span than humans, so it doesn't take as long to glean insights from interventions and noteworthy experiments.

To grasp how this works, let's take the example of bone cancer (osteosarcoma), which has a bleak prognosis in both dogs and humans with few advances in recent decades. Osteosarcoma is an aggressive cancer of the skeleton that typically spreads (metastasizes) to other parts of the body beyond the main site. Untreated, 90 percent of dogs with osteosarcoma develop metastases within one year, and 85 to 90 percent of humans do so within two years.[9] Once that happens, survival is dismal; fewer than 20 percent of human patients survive five years, and fewer than 5 percent of dogs survive two years with the disease.

Because dogs and humans share extensive similarities in the genetic features of the disease and in the complex ways our immune systems interact in the presence of cancer, we may be able to treat the disease using the same therapies. One therapy already undergoing clinical study in dogs homes in on novel methods to manipulate specialized immune cells called natural killer (NK) and T cells. These cells interact with cancer cells and other immune cells in complex ways, leading to changes in pathways that can work both for and against the tumor.[10] Natural killer cells in particular are known for their ability to target cancerous cells, effectively preventing them from proliferating. These clinical studies in dogs have already shown the use of leveraging the power of NK cells to treat osteosarcoma, making them valuable precursors to clinical trials in humans. If we can successfully treat osteosarcoma in dogs using these new immunotherapies, we could possibly do the same in humans. The field of immunotherapy is one of the most exciting for advanced cancers.

I met Elinor Karlsson by Zoom in our respective offices. Elinor studies dogs at the Broad Institute of MIT and Harvard, where she is director of the Vertebrate Genomics Group. (She is also a professor in bioinformatics and integrative biology at the University of Massachusetts Medical School.) Born in Sweden and raised in Rhode Island, she calls herself a "genomicist"—someone trying to understand the genome. She has been hooked on genetics since learning about Gregor Mendel and his garden peas in high school. Although she studies the DNA of hundreds of species to understand how the genome works and why things sometimes go wrong, dogs have played a central role in her work. One project in particular that has gained attention is her Darwin's Ark initiative (https://darwinsark.org), which recruits people's pets to become part of a collaborative research venture seeking answers to common health and behavioral issues. If you have a dog, purebred or mutt, you can sign up as a citizen scientist with her lab and answer a survey of roughly one hundred questions about your pet's personality and behavior (and you can rest assured she does not own or sell these data). If you want to participate in this amazing project, you can order a kit and send in a mouth swab from your pooch. Her lab uses the swab to isolate and then sequence the DNA and will send back to you the genetic and ancestry information about your pet—just like the personal genomics available today for all of us from sites such as 23andMe.com and Ancestry.com. That information is also added to their enormous data bank, shared freely (with privacy protection) throughout the scientific world.

From the more than twenty-two thousand dogs registered in the program, more than 2.5 million answers have been collected. So far, the DNA sequence of a boxer named Tasha has been completed, with more work underway to understand variations in the dog genome among different breeds and how those variations relate to the human genome. By understanding the patterns of variation in the individual breeds and how those relate to, say, golden retrievers' notoriously high risk of cancer, researchers can gain insight into complex diseases that are difficult to map in human populations, which aren't as genetically homogeneous as our furry friend.[11]

A Primer on Genomes: Your Life-Giving Software

Genome, another word for our DNA, refers to the entire set of instructions every cell in a body has for every function that bodies perform, as well as all of the information to pass life on to the next generation. Every cell has the entire instruction manual; in the case of humans, the manual is 3 billion letters long. It's an important concept in health circles, especially now that we're hearing so much about CRISPR, the technology recently developed to edit DNA. Each species has its own distinctive genome—the shark genome, the rose genome, the streptococcus genome, and so on. But individuals within a species also each have a unique genome that's ever so slightly different from the standard genome for the species. In other words, the "human genome," or, by the same token, the "dog genome," represents a general shared foundational framework of DNA for each species in which there are variations that confer higher or lower risk for certain traits or diseases.

It helps to think of DNA as a list of parts or ingredients rather than a complete manual that explains how those parts work together. Consider someone you know who has a chronic or degenerative disease such as cancer or a form of dementia. That person used to be somebody who didn't have cancer or dementia, and he or she still has the same DNA. The difference between having and not having cancer or dementia does not solely reside in the genome. Most of that person's cells are not turning into cancer or fueling dementia. Both illnesses are dynamic processes that are indeed happening, but they are happening far from the confines of a static piece of DNA. There could be a genetic vulnerability to these maladies, but the diseases are not themselves inherited. The person merely inherits a predisposition. Whether the individual develops a disease is due to other factors that come into play, chiefly from that person's environment.

Among the groundbreaking findings uncovered by the Human Genome Project, which completed mapping our genome in 2003, was that approximately 99.9 percent of DNA sequences are similar across the human population. Single nucleotide polymorphisms (SNPs, typically pronounced "snips") represent variations in DNA sequences and occur every one hundred to three hundred bases along the three-billion-base genome. A base is one of the rungs of DNA's well-known double helix structure. The human genome is made up of approximately three billion base pairs, composed of four chemical bases or nucleotides known most commonly by the letters A (adenine), G (guanine), C (cytosine), and T (thymine). These nucleotides are key structural elements that make up the genes that individually or in combination determine everything from your eye color to your predisposition for, say, Parkinson's disease. SNPs are alterations in the set of genetic instructions that are thought to provide the genetic markers for our response to diseases, environmental factors, and drugs. For example, an A instead of a G on a particular gene may indicate a trait for male-pattern baldness or attached earlobes. Other variations in nucleotide sequences may provide a marker for cystic fibrosis, breast cancer, sickle cell anemia, or psoriasis, for example.

What is interesting about Elinor Karlsson is that while I pictured someone who wrangled six or seven different dogs down the street after work—the pugs and Chihuahuas getting all tangled up with the Labs and golden retrievers in their long strappy leashes—she has never had a dog and never considered herself a "dog person." But her admiration for them is visible in her cherubic, youthful face and upbeat personality that any dog would gravitate toward, with a sunny disposition and innate curiosity.

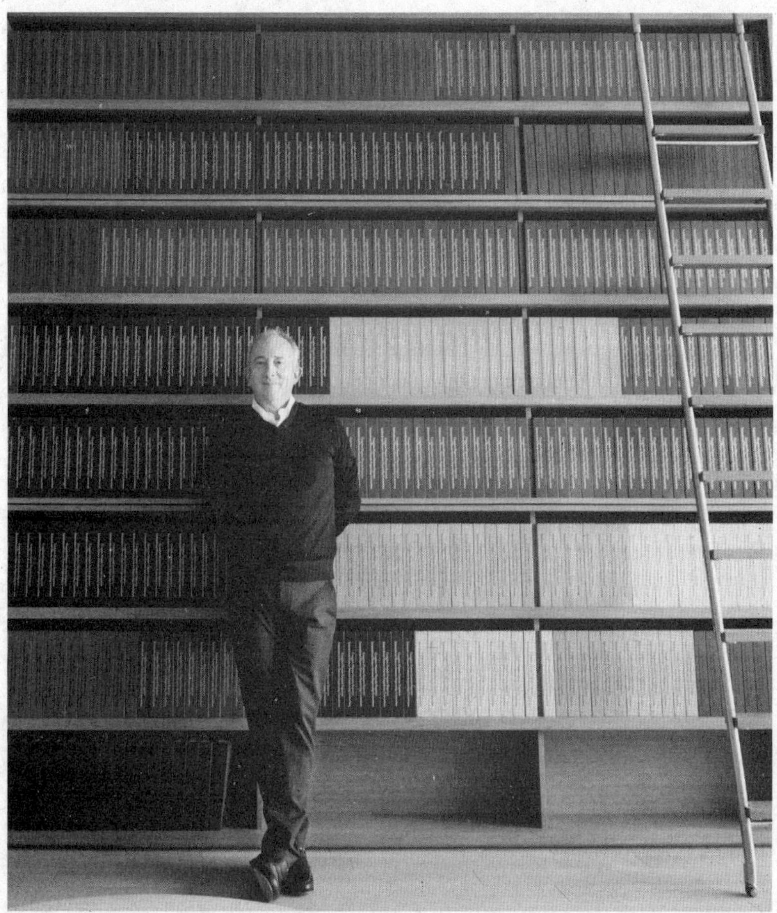

At the institute, we have a large bookcase whose shelves are filled with colorful tomes organized in such a way that, as a whole, they symbolically reflect the twenty-three pairs of human chromosomes that hold a library of information for your life. Each cell in our body has the entire contents of this bookcase in its nucleus.

In the early days of her work in genomics more than a decade ago, obtaining enough samples was a challenge. It was when she met people with dogs that she saw an opportunity to gather a treasure trove of data. Karlsson is studying more than cancer in her dog project. She wants to know how the dog genome has changed as dogs evolved from predatory wolves to beloved companions. And she is quick to point out that "domestication" is a poorly defined process. The notion of domestication carries with it a semblance of being well behaved, civilized, or even intelligent, but that's a vague and specious definition. Wolves are actually smarter than dogs; they can solve puzzles, whereas dogs will give up on solving a problem, appealing to their master with a "help me out" look. Dogs also lack a nuclear family, while wolves travel in packs in which parents stay together and raise their pups, with wolf fathers invested in rearing their offspring. Even without humans around, male dogs are not involved in their pups' upbringing. That is not to imply that dogs are relatively stupid or neglectful; they are simply different from wolves in their behavior. Wolves are independent and would never look to a human for affection or guidance. Dogs view *us* as their family.

What's so valuable in studying the dog genome is that it has gone through many changes in a relatively short period of time. Not only did dogs evolve away from their ancestral *Canis lupus* gray wolf tens of thousands of years ago, but they have also been under the potent influence of purposeful breeding to arrive at different types of dogs to perform various tasks—herding, hunting, fetching, guarding, and playing. Humans have been breeding dogs for intended outcomes for about four thousand years, but only in the past two centuries have we taken the selective breeding mill to the extreme, rendering dogs with very specific physical features and attributes. We've tampered with the laws of nature and even bred dogs for pure vanity. This has involved a lot of mating dogs with their family members, which fosters the spread of genetic disorders and heightened risk for certain health issues such as early-onset cancer, hip dysplasia in big dogs, and persistent dislocation of the kneecap in miniature dogs. This is not natural selection under Mother Nature's watch. But it sets the stage for some captivating genomic investigative science, where we can learn what genes and alterations of genes actually do. One area in particular that Karlsson is scrutinizing is sorely desperate for answers: psychiatric issues.[12]

We don't think of dogs as having psychiatric issues, but some dogs chase their tail or chew it to no end—or act sad and even depressed. They can show signs of obsessive-compulsive disorders (OCD), anxiety, and even posttraumatic stress disorder. By comparing portions of the genomes of ninety Doberman pinschers suffering from OCD with the genomes of sixty non-OCD-behaving Dobermans, Karlsson and her colleagues have documented several key differences.

Studies described in 2014 in *Scientist* noted that by "scanning the genomes of bull terriers, Shetland sheepdogs, and German shepherds, the researchers narrowed the field down to four genes with high rates of mutations in dogs that tend to exhibit OCD behaviors." What makes this research so staggering is that it has been hard to find genes associated with psychiatric diseases in humans, despite many studies being done, yet we know that psychiatric illnesses tend to be heritable.[13] Now the question becomes: Can we leverage our current knowledge of genetics to pinpoint what brain pathways go wrong in these diseases? And can we design therapies that target those pathways in safe, healthy ways? The piece in *Scientist* continued, "Indeed, finding an effective treatment for OCD is a great medical need, as current therapies, which typically involve antidepressant medications, only help about 50 percent of patients, both human and canine. Karlsson and her colleagues proposed that if the genes identified in OCD dogs can be linked to pathways involved in human OCD, the dogs may serve as a good model for the disorder."[14] Traditional psychiatry hesitates at the thought of looking toward other animals to understand the human psyche, but results like these are telling us something. We should investigate further.

Psychiatric issues are common in the world today. Estimates are that approximately a quarter of the globe has these issues that can have major impacts on learning, behavior, social relations, and personal well-being. The largest genetic map of psychiatric disorders so far was published in 2019 and covered about 230,000 patients and half a million controls worldwide.[15] The study describes over one hundred gene associations with eight common psychiatric issues: obsessive-compulsive disorder, ADHD, anorexia nervosa, schizophrenia, bipolar disorder, depression, autism, and Tourette's syndrome. The genes are not diagnostic of the disorder, just associated—and in the future, it may be helpful to predict who will respond to what drugs and at what dose, but these are still early days with technologies like this.[16]

Interestingly, many health problems that we encounter can be reflected in our dogs. If your dog is anxious, chances are you are too. If your dog is overweight and out of shape, you may want to look in the mirror. And if your dog has allergies, do you? As family physician Daphne Miller discovered by talking to a number of veterinarians, and described in a *Washington Post* article, one's pet's health can often match one's own; furthermore, "anxiety, allergies, gastrointestinal infections, even insomnia are all disorders that can exist in pet-owner dyads."[17] (One big reason to have a dog in the first place: they show us who we are.)

The Benefits of Parenting a Dog

Scientists are just beginning to study pet-human pairs, but the research has highlighted interesting initial findings. In the Netherlands, for example, studies have shown that overweight dogs are more likely to have owners who are also overweight. The authors of the study suggest the amount of time taking walks together is the best predictor of the duo being overweight. This is not too surprising because the same phenomenon occurs with children and their parents: a child with obese parents has an 80 percent chance of obesity; a child with one obese parent has a 50 percent chance of being obese.[18]

While it may seem odd to link allergy diagnoses between a dog and her human parent, a 2018 study from Finland found that people and their dogs who live in an urban environment and are disconnected from nature and other animals have a higher risk for allergies than those who live on a farm or in a household with many animals and children or who regularly stroll through a forest.[19] Allergies in dogs are often diagnosed as canine atopic dermatitis, which is similar to human eczema, and is one of the most common reasons dogs go to the vet.

Dogs also serve us well in many ways, from helping us to keep better schedules (they must be fed and walked on cue) to protecting our families and sensing danger. They can detect an earthquake minutes away by hearing seismic activity underground that precedes the actual quake, and they can smell environmental changes in the air that signal a major storm or tsunami coming. Their keen senses make them excellent helpers in tracking down criminals, finding illegal drugs and explosives, and locating people trapped or dead. They can be trained to sniff out cancer and COVID-19, dangerously low blood sugar, and even pregnancy in humans. They may even help children develop stronger immune systems. The exposure to pet dander and what's in their fur, including bacteria, dust, and soil, may fortify a developing immune system and lower the risk of allergies or autoimmune disease later in life.

More recently, we've learned that dogs can smell when we're stressed out—they detect changes in our breath and sweat indicative of psychological turmoil.[20] Dogs also can help alleviate the stressors of adolescence, a time often riddled with self-doubt, peer judgment, unwanted adult expectations, and emotional turmoil.[21] A pet pooch provides comfort, cuddles, and unconditional love. And because dogs know only how to live in the present, they can help us all focus on the now, sometimes hard to do. Even the bond we feel when we play with our dogs and enjoy those almost inevitable licks is like therapy on the brain and nervous system: it calms and connects. Touch therapy with dogs is now being used in some health care settings to help patients get through tough treatments. The dogs provide their love and affection with physical touches (and kisses) that soothe as well as distract from otherwise stressful situations. Although it can be more challenging to receive such cuddly endearment from other animals, some people can benefit from having any kind of pet nearby to bolster emotional support and lower anxiety, be it a rabbit, cat, bird, turtle, or minipig. But dogs will probably always win the contest for being the best all-around "therapists."

People who own dogs live longer: dogs reduce loneliness and the risk of cardiovascular disease—two big killers the older we get. A 2019 study in *Scientific Reports* suggests that dog owners may be more active and in better health in general.[22] I do think there is something to be said for the responsibilities of taking care of a dog. Fido won't let you sit on the couch all day eating madeleines. What's more, the 2019 study revealed that dog owners have a lower reactivity to stress and faster recovery of blood pressure following stressful events.[23] I'd take an educated guess that dogs help keep their owner's blood pressure down overall. I feel my whole body relax when I enter my home and am greeted by Georgie's exuberant hugs, kisses, and very vocal remarks. One habit, however, we would do well to avoid is to sleep like a dog.

Don't Sleep like a Dog

You may have heard the phrase "sleep like a dog" to refer to getting a good night's sleep, but that's not an accurate description of how dogs rest. Georgie can definitely keep me up if something startles her in the night. She springs into protective action—hence the proverb "let sleeping dogs lie" that dates as far back as biblical times and derives from the observation that dogs can be unpredictable when disturbed from sleep.

Most people stay awake for the whole day and have extended sleep at night, spending up to a quarter of their sleep in rapid eye movement (REM)—the stage of sleep in which we dream and areas of the brain that are essential in learning and making or retaining memories are stimulated. Our eyes dart about during this stage because of the brain activity going on; research suggests that the rapid eye movements allow us to change scenes while we dream. Our pulse, blood pressure, and breathing also speed up during this phase.

Dogs are only in REM for about 10 percent of their sleep time because of inconsistent sleep schedules. According to the American Kennel Club, "Dogs tend to spend as much as half of their days asleep, 30 percent awake but relaxing, and just 20 percent being active." But unlike humans, who have the best sleep outcome when on a regular schedule, dogs can sleep anytime and anywhere. They can fall asleep out of boredom, wake easily, and become immediately attentive to the situation at hand. This ability means they end up needing more total sleep to make up for lost REM. The average dog sleeps for about twelve to fourteen hours per twenty-four-hour cycle. And puppies, who expend a lot of energy exploring and learning, may need as much as eighteen to twenty hours. Older dogs, and certain breeds among them, also tend to need more rest.[24]

Sleep is equally as important for dogs as it is for humans; in addition to cataloging our memories, it allows us to fine-tune our immune systems, regulate our hormones, and spur cellular renewal. Our bodies can power up during sleep for these biological "housecleaning" chores because while our bodies are physically at rest, there's more energy to devote to critical tasks. It's when our brain is triggered to fire up its own secret immune system, the glymphatic system, to break down cellular waste products and flush them out (accumulation of the waste products may be linked to a higher risk of developing brain disease). Sleep also provides the main reset button for our circadian rhythm, the body's internal clock that lords over our sleep-wake cycle and roughly correlates with the solar day. The term comes from the Latin for "about" (circa) and "day" (dies). A healthy rhythm directs normal hormonal and other enzymatic secretion patterns, from those associated with hunger and fullness cues to those that relate to stress and cellular renewal, as well as fluctuations in body temperature, blood pressure, and even brain chemicals. Your body is not the same now as it was earlier today or last night, and it won't be the same in an hour or tomorrow. After a restless night of sleep, your circadian rhythm will play into not only your tiredness and feeling "off" in general but also your cravings for carbs (notably sugar) the next day.

In studies on canine sleep, dogs experience short bursts of electrical activity, called sleep spindles, during non-REM sleep like we do.[25] Similar to us, retaining learned information is tied to the frequency of these sleep spindles in dogs. Studies in humans similarly link quality sleep to how well we remember things that have happened and new information. Sleep spindles are how we, and our dogs, commit learned information to long-term memory and prepare to learn new things; when spindles happen during sleep, the brain is focusing on one thing, which makes information retention easier. Unfortunately, we don't have the luxury of intermittently sleeping throughout the day like dogs do. We have to get all of our sleep in one long slumber. So if you want to "sleep like a dog," make sure you're banking at least seven to nine hours a night. That idiom, in fact, is meant to refer to getting lots of sleep (not necessarily sound sleep). And to have maximal spindly sleep, keep your bedroom as quiet and dark as possible to reduce the risk of light- or noise-induced interruptions. You're going for quality foremost, not necessarily quantity. You're better off sleeping like a log for eight hours than like a dog for nine.

What is interesting is that we literally sleep like a dog our first night traveling, whether it is in the same time zone or not, in Aunt Edna's house or a hotel. Our brains recognize the sleep location as foreign: the bed feels different, and there are different visual cues, noises, and light. We don't sleep that deeply, and we feel it the next day, no matter how long we've slept. It's a protective mechanism. Our brains are saying, "Hey, this bed isn't usual, so let's not get that deep sleep in case something happens and we have to flee." There are ways to get around this. I use my smartphone as my night clock for several weeks before I travel. That way, when I look at the clock at night, the sight is familiar to my brain. I also travel with a travel pillow (the same shape and density as mine at home), again to make my brain feel comfortable in the new location with the feel and smell of the pillowcase. These small details make a big difference in my sleep: I sleep less like a dog and more like myself when I'm on the road. I am one of those geeks who measure their sleep cycles with various devices, and this little hack has made a difference to me. Like the wisdom offered by our fun-loving, nonjudgmental four-legged companions, it may not be millions of years old but it's nonetheless wonderfully practical.

Creature Cheat Sheet

Dogs are more than our best friends. They are models for human medicine, sometimes mirrors to ourselves, and masterful mentors of well-being. Perhaps no other species can tell us to live in the moment, jump for joy when happy, engage in playtime daily, stay curious and seek new experiences, be observant and on guard for dangerous situations, act affectionately and friendly even toward strangers, and drink lots of water.

That leash is a two-way street: health can travel both ways, and we can learn from dogs in carefully designed research settings too. We can also learn to hack our sleep when traveling and sleep less like a dog to get the restful sleep we need. Although pre-dog wolves likely cozied up to us eons ago as they scavenged around garbage dumps on the edge of human settlements, we've since coevolved long enough to know we need each other. And despite the demands that dog ownership places on us—from picking up poop and finding dog sitters once in a while to tending to their daily ritualistic feedings, walks, and naps—the benefits of dog ownership are infinite and infinitely welcome. So get your own pooch, plan to adopt one someday soon, or join a dog-walking friend or neighbor on an evening stroll. Then enjoy the all-around companionship and the joy it will bring.

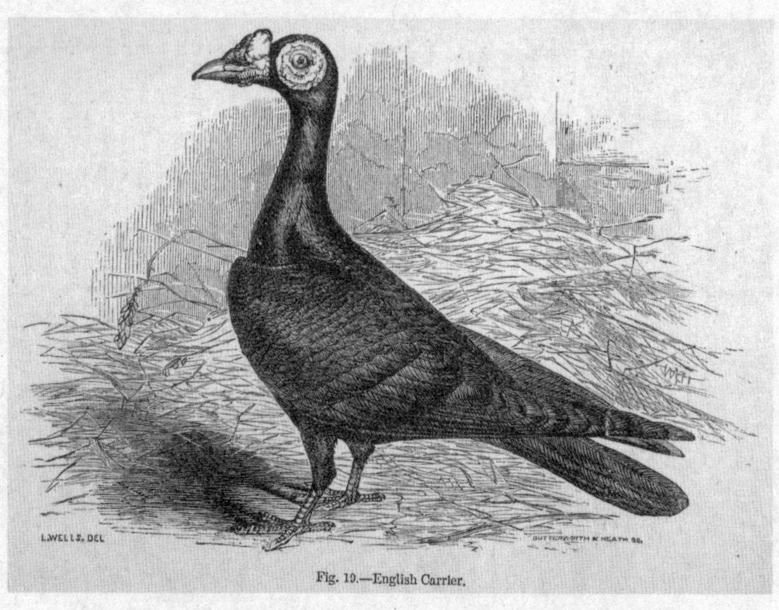

Fig. 19.—English Carrier.

Charles Darwin's illustration of the English carrier pigeon, 1890.

3

Take the Long Way Home

The Power of Pattern Recognition and the Perils of Overthinking

One must have a good memory to be able to keep the promises one makes.

—FRIEDRICH WILHELM NIETZSCHE

Perhaps nothing is more powerful in our day-to-day living—and ability to stay healthy—than our habits. Studies show that nearly half (upward of 47 percent) of the actions we perform each day are not decisions; they are routines.[1] Although we like to think we have agency over ourselves and live exciting, ever-changing lives, we keep similar habits day in and day out, from the time we get up to the people we interact with; the foods we gravitate toward (and not); the words, phrases, and intonations we use; the routes we take when we drive; the way we carry ourselves (your gait is as unique to you as your fingerprints); the behaviors we exhibit at work; and the sequence of events that unfold when we end the day and prepare for sleep. Our lives are not as spontaneous and dramatic as we'd probably like them to be; they are repetitive. But in that repeating echo lies a sense of security and comfort.

Probably you have reached a destination from the driver's seat of a car and not recalled the actual ride or even thinking about how to drive—when to turn your head to check the side-view mirror before banking a right turn, where to make more space between you and another car, how to carefully brake to a stop. You can thank your inner GPS and pattern recognition for that feat. *Pattern recognition* is the term used to describe the brain process that matches a visual observation (although it can be tactile, auditory, or olfactory) with associated data in your memory. In order to make instantaneous decisions in our lives, we identify patterns and then make the association to know what correlates. It entails some exquisitely complex networking between your visual optics and your brain's processing at the speed of a race car. Consider when you navigate the supermarket for your weekly groceries and have something entirely else on your mind as you pull items off the shelf and drop them into your cart. Again, you can thank your pattern recognition skills for that accomplishment. It's a doable form of mental multitasking, and it is essential to life—not to mention key to getting things done.

We humans are creatures of habit, but it's not just the activities we perform consciously (or semiconsciously) that are powered by habits; our brains govern basic processes such as breathing, digesting, and pumping blood without our having to "think" about it. Imagine how difficult it would be to eat breakfast while talking to someone and having to consciously calculate your bites, chews, and swallows. The downside is that habits become so rooted in our lives that they are hard to break or change. They are as much shapers of our lives as we are shapers of our habits.

Habits are patterns of thought. The rhythms we follow in our thinking processes have everything to do with whether we can remember critical information, forget what's not important, speedily filter incoming data, tap creative areas in our brains, and free up mental energy to engage in complex abstract thinking that requires focus and concentration. Put simply, habits provide the bedrock to our overall cognition. They allow us to then explore outside of what we already know and spark new ideas, innovate, and advance ourselves. And when we find patterns in our thoughts, work, decisions, and daily duties, we can develop new habits to streamline our lives. We can sharpen our cognition, including our memory. Pattern recognition, in fact, is not unique to humans. It's a skill found throughout the animal kingdom, giving many species a sense of time and space; navigational skills to find food, water, and mates, and then get home again without incident (sometimes across impressively vast distances); and the ability to communicate using speech, which for us means spinning letters into words and stringing words into sentences to create language.

Patterns exist everywhere we look: in art, traffic signals, social interactions, computer programs, mathematics, bodily rhythms such as the ebb and flow of hormones and other biochemicals around the twenty-four-hour solar day, and nature in general. If you pick up any *National Geographic* magazine, you'll see the most spectacular photographs of patterns found in animals, landscapes, rock formations, flowers, stars, and sand. Take a walk for ten minutes and come back with at least ten patterns you spotted—the arrangement of trees and plants or whatever organic landmarks are in the environment, for example. This is a terrifically simple exercise for improving your cognition in minutes, as data are showing that this skill set is critical to fight declining cognitive function.

Adam Gazzaley at the University of California, San Francisco designed a video game, *NeuroRacer*, to enhance the cognitive abilities of older adults through physical activity and pattern recognition. In a study published in 2013 as the cover story of *Nature* magazine, he demonstrated that doing two tasks at once was associated with improvements in function in other areas, including memory and the ability to focus attention in subjects in their sixties, seventies, and eighties.[2] It's worth mentioning that many studies have historically cast doubt that memory training helps people improve cognitive functioning, but it's important to note that as scientists continue to debate what kinds of games or brainteasers can help improve cognition (and help prevent cognitive decline), there's really no downside to these fun challenges. You are not necessarily going to suddenly get smarter or improve the kind of intelligence that helps you reason and solve problems, but you might strengthen your ability to hold information and juggle different or competing thoughts and data in your mind.[3] Memory training is not the same as multitasking. It is simply being able to update and maintain information on multiple tasks, especially as you perform basic double-duty endeavors or switch between complex tasks. When you do your nature walk to note patterns, that's a form of real-world multitasking as you walk and think. Same goes for when you drive and talk (hands-free) on a cell phone. Or cook dinner, entertain guests, and corral a toddler somewhat simultaneously (without going insane).

If I give you a sequence of numbers such as 123, 234, 345 . . . can you tell me what comes next? If 456 comes to mind, you're right, and it probably happened within a fraction of a second. That's what's called a hierarchical serial pattern, and the ability to recognize it emerges in infancy, and it's not special to humans; it's used throughout the mammalian world. This ability to almost instantly recognize simple patterns helps a mammal adapt to and make sense of the world around it, as well as respond to stimuli (or how else would it find its trusty sources of food and water?). Pigeons, in fact, are able to solve this challenge as well as humans can, and even outperform us in some mathematical coups.

Most of us don't notice patterns unless we're challenged to find them or we become trained at distinguishing certain patterns in our work. I use a type of pattern recognition every day to get a sense of my patients' personalities and the biology of their cancers, and to strategize the most appropriate therapy course to proceed with. When I look under a microscope at a biopsy of a cancer, I can see the normal tissue, which looks like the neatly organized cornfields when you fly across the country and get a bird's-eye view: the pattern is tidy, structured, and orderly. And I can also see the invading cancer, which looks as if someone impolitely intruded and messed up the fields. I glimpse chaos and disorder—a pattern of disarray and destruction. But the results are not binary; there are gradations. Classically, the more disorganized the cells (the least like the normal tissue counterpart), the more aggressive the cancer is (see figure 1). This is the reason I try to look at every patient's sample under the microscope. Over many years of practice, my brain has gained a special kind of pattern recognition, and I can predict the outcomes of my patients. I can peer down at a sample and "know" or get a gut feeling that this cancer will be more or less aggressive than originally billed, and this guides my discussion with the patient about our next steps.

This is not just from textbook learning; it's also experiential over the course of many years. It's the same skill that, for example, allows the professional ballplayer to detect pitches early; the chess master to predict the best move; the birder to discriminate between two different bird species by their callings or chirpings; the sommelier to taste subtle differences among wines; and the art collector to instantly spot a counterfeit painting. And while you and I may not be able to identify a fake Monet, I bet we'd be able to differentiate a Monet and a Picasso—again, through pattern recognition. Many of our gut feelings, in fact, spring from our responses to pattern recognition, but we don't pay enough attention to those feelings. Those feelings are real; they represent the brain making conclusions based on an amalgam of prior experiences. Evolution has selected the best at this in the animal world because the ones who could not recognize danger well didn't survive. As humans, we have been taught to squelch this trait, but there is an important lesson here we can learn from nature: to trust our instincts.

I first learned the craft of pattern recognition in my field from training under one of my favorite mentors at Memorial Sloan Kettering Cancer Center in New York, the late David Golde. David

Figure 1

Examples of benign (left) and malignant (right) breast specimens stained and enlarged at different magnifications.

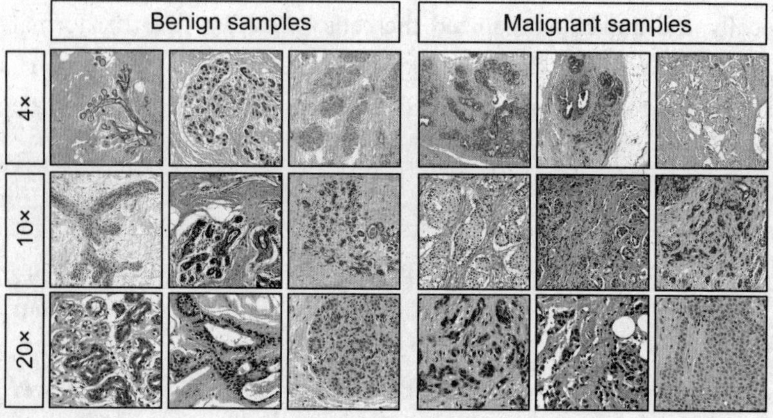

Source: Richard M. Levenson et al., "Pigeons (*Columba livia*) as Trainable Observers of Pathology and Radiology Breast Cancer Images," *PLoS One* 10, no. 11 (November 2015): e0141357.

was a world-renowned giant in medicine and a much beloved teacher, scientist, and physician. He taught me the importance of taking meticulous notes (and that the grammar and word choice in these notes mattered). Before every patient we visited together, we looked under the microscope at the person's peripheral blood smear, which could tell us, among other things, the state of their bone marrow and what their immune cells were doing, and we always peered at their cancer biopsies under the same microscope. The observations I made with him in his clinic and the accumulation of data that occurred under his tutelage ultimately became the foundation for my pattern recognition.

I should mention that a 2015 study (from which figure 1 is taken) showed that pigeons can spot cancer as well as human experts can, when they are trained.[4] Their bird's-eye view can pick the cancerous patterns.

Bird's-Eye View

After a short drive from Santa Monica to Westwood, I was able to visit Aaron Blaisdell's underground lab at UCLA's Brain Research Institute. It houses a closet-like room full of caged pigeons, each of which has a clever name—for example, Goodall, Vonnegut (see figure 2), Darwin, and Cousteau. It's where he studies their cognitive function and how they perceive and think about the world. Blaisdell conducted the experiment to show that pigeons can solve the 123, 234, 345 . . . problem. The complicated and elaborate experiment involved training the birds to learn rules about numbers and then use pecks to a touch screen to document their numerical feats. He found that pigeons possess an amazing neural processing speed: "When they peck at a seed to pick up, they can open their mouths to exactly the size of the seed—no bigger or smaller," he says. Unlike our two eyes relatively close together to bring our three-dimensional world into focus easily, pigeons' eyes are on the opposing sides of their heads. To compensate for this disadvantage, they have two foveae in each eye—the small pit in the retina with the clearest vision—compared with our single one: one fovea on the side of each eye to scan the world for threats and another in the center of each eye for zooming in on things at close range (like those seeds).

Blaisdell's work includes examining how pigeons use spatial pattern learning to simplify their visual world. Pigeons create spatial maps of the 3D world around them to navigate and orient themselves, as well as avoid threats. One of the most underappreciated talents humans share with pigeons is an extraordinary ability to create similar spatial maps in our heads and bring together maps acquired on separate occasions to make a cohesive picture. We (and pigeons) can even derive spatial relationships between things never seen before. Consider the last time you walked through the living room of a friend or a family member's new home and took visual note of the furniture placement and various items on a coffee table. You come back later and notice that someone has moved a chair. When you return at a much later date, you'll see that a new piece of furniture is there. Your mind has created visual maps—snapshots—every time you've entered this room. Each snapshot was a fraction of the data your brain collected at the moment, but enough to have a general sense of change when you come back to the room. If your brain remembered every single detail of the room, it would actually be much harder to assess if a chair had been moved. Your brain has made what's called spatial inferences with every new entrance as you reflect back on the memory of your previous visit and integrate that information into your present view. All of this is a clear sign of cognition in action. Imagine what would happen if your experience of the room felt totally different every time, as if you had never been there before. You'd become confused, disoriented, and maybe frightened, worrying that you've got dementia.

We make important inferences all day long to accomplish everyday tasks, and not just with space. Time inferences are another great example. If you know that bus B arrives roughly thirty minutes after bus A, then you know how long you have to wait for bus B if someone tells you bus A left twenty minutes ago. Your mind instantly makes that inference (and quite mindlessly, I'll add). This is important to understand with neurodegenerative diseases swiftly on the rise with an aging population: if we can understand the ways our minds work to keep us sharp at tracking our movements, environment, and the passage of time, we may be better able to treat and manage those difficult diagnoses. Discussion about a disease like Alzheimer's, for instance, often revolves solely around memory problems, but there's a lot more going on in this complex malady that involves spatial maps in the brain and general timekeeping. And while it may seem odd to study pigeons and their exquisite navigational skills to help us learn about our own cognition, birds can provide excellent study cases. It turns out a birdbrain is anything but stupid: birds are avian Einsteins.

Figure 2

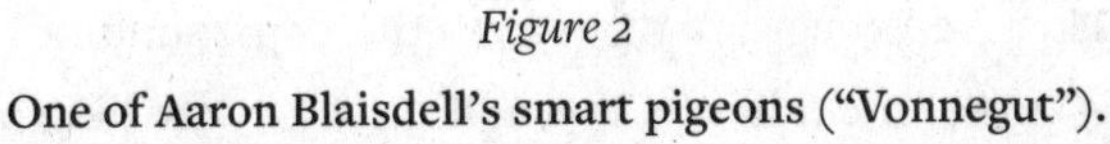

One of Aaron Blaisdell's smart pigeons ("Vonnegut").

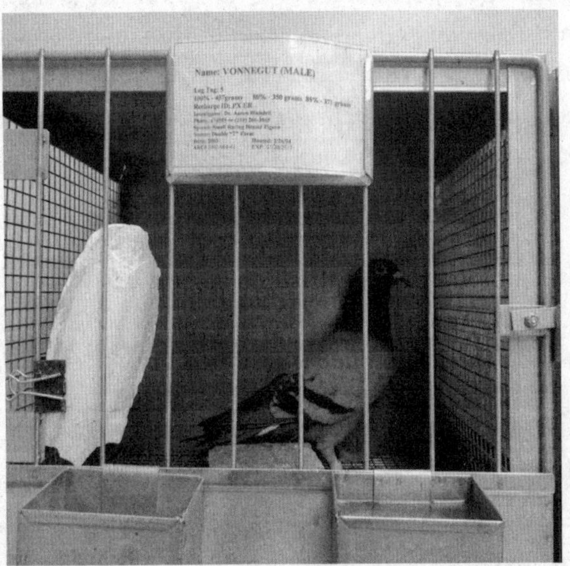

"'Birdbrain' Is a Compliment"

The term *bird-witted* arose in the seventeenth century to refer to a flighty person—someone who couldn't pay attention. By the early twentieth century, *birdbrained* was slang for someone who lacked intelligence, presumably because he or she had a small (birdlike) brain.* A bird's brain, however, is relatively large compared with its body size, and studies of pigeons show them able to discriminate cubist from impressionistic paintings. Blaisdell has a veritable love for his brilliant birds. A self-described naturalist who calls animals "nature's robots," he uses words like *endearing*, *cute*, and *humble* to describe

*In 2005, an international consortium, the Avian Brain Nomenclature Consortium, of twenty-nine neuroscientists proposed a renaming of a bird brain's anatomic structures to portray birds as more in line with mammals in their cognitive prowess. They wanted to see the outdated "birdbrain" term put to bed.

pigeons. "Most people ignore pigeons in their surroundings; they are background noise," he tells me. But to him, "They are like the clowns at the circus—goofy creatures doing their thing off to the side."*

Pigeons have an average life span of three to five years, though can sometimes make it above ten years if they can evade the clutches of a falcon or hawk.†[5] Humans have been domesticating pigeons for thousands of years for a variety of reasons—from having them as sport pets to race and admire their aerial acrobatics to employing them in communication. The common city pigeon (*Columba livia*), also known as the rock pigeon, is the first bird that was domesticated (and there's no such thing as a true wild or feral *C. livia*). If you're wondering why so many pigeons end up on city streets, it's because we brought them to our urban centers over the centuries and because pigeons happen to love concrete and hard surfaces. They evolved on the rocky ledges and cliffs of the Mediterranean Sea's shores. The group of birds known as the Columbiformes encompasses more than three hundred species of pigeons and doves. Throughout human history, pigeons have been critical to our existence as a source of food and functioning as utility players in our society.[6] It was a pigeon that delivered the results of the first Olympics in 776 BC and a pigeon that first brought news of Napoleon's defeat at Waterloo over twenty-five hundred years later. As a city dweller my entire life, I never gave pigeons much thought. But since my recent schooling on these "rats with wings" (an unfortunate nickname Woody Allen gave them in the 1980 film *Stardust Memories*), I will never look at a street

*Blaisdell happens to be allergic to pigeons. When he handles them with bare hands and comes into contact with an allergen in the bird's skin or feathers, his asthma is activated and then he develops flu-like symptoms.

†On the longevity scale, many other birds besides pigeons win that race. Many species of cranes, hummingbirds, barn owls, and bald eagles will outlive a pigeon. But the blue-fronted Amazon parrot can live up to sixty-six years in captivity, and there are anecdotal reports of some living as long as ninety years old. That's a life span equivalent to hundreds of years for humans. See endnote 5 in this chapter for more information.

pigeon—with its perpetually bobbing head and awkward prance, as if it doesn't know where it's going or wants to go—the same again.

They can find their way back home from thirteen hundred miles away—and accomplish that feat even if they've been moved to the starting point in total isolation, with no way to access clues as to where they are from sight, smell, or the earth's magnetic field (which turns out to be key to their navigational genius). Scientists can try to confuse them by rotating their cages around while in transport so the pigeons can't keep track of the direction they're traveling in, yet those pigeons mysteriously find their way back using the shortest route. We still don't know exactly how they do this, but what we do know is that the pigeon's piloting prowess has been appreciated and exploited for thousands of years.

At one point, more than one-quarter of all the birds living in the United States may have been passenger pigeons, which were famous for flocking in such great numbers together over North America that they'd darken the daytime sky to a night-like hue for hours at a time. Their "clouds," however, made them easy targets for hunting. Although it's rare for an entire species to be wiped off the planet in a matter of decades, passenger pigeons began to go extinct at the turn of the twentieth century. New research points the finger at human intervention—overhunting, habitat loss—as well as possibly some genetic diversity issues. The passenger pigeons were unique in that they not only banded together in dense flocks and lived in groups of billions, but also collaborated in finding food and rearing their young. Once their populations dwindled dramatically, they could no longer succeed.

Carrier and homing pigeons are still with us, the result of many years of selective breeding. "Racing Homer" is the official name for homing pigeons, which were bred for their speed and ability to always return home and used for sport over three thousand years ago. One of the most famous conquerors in history, the Mongolian ruler-warrior Genghis Khan, used them to communicate across his vast empire. Homing pigeons have played vital roles in many wars throughout history—no battery or electrical power needed, just food and water. They can provide relatively secure communication on the battlefield and replace radio when necessary. On October 4, 1918, during World War I, a US battalion of 194 men found themselves stranded and trapped behind German lines while under brutal attack. Confusion and chaos also had them under siege by friendly fire. Enter Cher Ami to the rescue—a fitting name: "dear friend" in French. This pigeon was their only hope. Desperate to stop the friendly fire lest they all be killed, the soldiers wrote a message asking their forces to cease fire, attached it to Cher Ami, and released him. Soon after, the Germans shot him out of the sky. Cher Ami was severely injured; he lost an eye and a leg, and a bullet had blown through his breast. But miraculously, he managed to take off again and wing his way twenty-five miles back to headquarters. The French army awarded him the Croix de Guerre, a medal of honor similar to the Purple Heart in the American military.[7]

During World War II, the United States had 200,000 homing pigeons at the ready. Today the Chinese military has a cadre of homing pigeons in case all of their fancy high-tech machinery fails in a war. And some of these pigeons, especially the quick ones, which can reach speeds of up to 100 miles per hour, don't come cheap. In 2013, the world's fastest racing pigeon was sold for nearly half a million dollars. In 2020, this was eclipsed by a pigeon named New Kim who sold for a whopping $1.9 million.[8]

Pigeon breeding was a common hobby in Victorian England—a craze that didn't discriminate, crossing class lines and attracting royalty and miners alike. Through creative breeding, some pretty strange birds were "created" by these enthusiasts. For Darwin, a huge pigeon fan who began pigeon breeding in 1856, it was less of a hobby and more of an experiment in learning about the breeding process; it quickly became an obsession. He owned a diverse flock, was a member of London pigeon clubs, and cozied up to famous breeders. In

1859, when he began to pass around an early draft of what would later become *On the Origin of Species*, one of his readers called the manuscript "a wild & foolish piece of imagination." He gave the practical advice to Darwin that he should instead write a short book on pigeons because, he said, "everybody is interested in pigeons." A book like this, he continued, would "be reviewed in every journal in the kingdom and soon be on every table."*

Around the same time, an enterprising journalist named Paul Julius Freiherr von Reuter founded a news service using carrier pigeons to send stock market prices from Brussels to Germany, which had the effect of linking Berlin and Paris when telegraphy was still evolving. Being able to get faster from point A to point B than the post train, pigeons gave Reuter quicker access to the important financial news from the Paris stock exchange. Eventually pigeons were replaced by a direct telegraph link, and Reuter would go on to expand his business into a global empire known as Reuters News Agency that today still bears his name and transmits information by computer around the clock to more than 150 countries.

But here's a question I have yet to answer: How do certain pigeons find their way home? What is at the heart of their navigational wizardry? And how can we learn from it to treat dementias as we age?

Homeward Bound

When you think about how you "know" where you are in the world—in time and space—many things come to mind. You have your senses—sight, hearing, touch, and smell—and a vestibular system

*A passion for pigeons has influenced many of the greats in history. John O'Neill in his book *Prodigal Genius: The Extraordinary Life of Nikola Tesla* described how Tesla used to care for injured wild pigeons in his New York City hotel room. He had a favorite one about which he wrote: "I loved that pigeon, I loved her as a man loves a woman and she loved me. That pigeon was the joy of my life. If she needed me, nothing else mattered. As long as I had her, there was a purpose in my life."

that perceives your body in relation to gravity, movement, and balance. Our vestibular system's hub lies in our inner ear, where the vestibular sensory organ is located symmetrically on either side of the head. Inside each end organ are tiny hair cells, which detect both linear and angular acceleration. Our vestibular system was one of the first sensory systems to emerge in evolution, and you'll remember from chapter 1 that it still shows signs of having evolved from our early ancestors in fish. If you've ever experienced sudden dizziness (vertigo) or the sensation that you're spinning and about to fall, chances are you have a problem with the sensory signals in your inner ear. We're still learning how the brain interprets and processes balance-related information; research currently underway will improve the design of cochlear implants to better help those with vertigo and balance disorders.

You also have a sense called proprioception, which enables your brain to know the relative position of your body parts and the strength of effort being used in each of your movements. Also referred to as kinesthesia, it's what some deem the "sixth sense." It's important because it lets you know exactly how you're positioned in space and allows you to plan your movements. The proprioception system comprises specialized nerve endings, or sensory receptors, in your muscles, skin, ligaments, tendons, and joints that collectively communicate your overall positioning to your brain. Sensations from central signals related to motor output are also key to this system. Examples of using your proprioception in practice include being able to walk a straight line with your eyes closed, maneuver through a narrow space, and apply the correct amount of pressure with your fingers to write with a pencil. Proprioception can deteriorate with age, leading people not only to become vulnerable to falls but also to increasingly lose the ability to perform basic functional activities that rely on this system working properly and that in turn triggers degenerative joint disease. One of the best ways to prevent deterioration of this vital system is to exercise, which keeps the system strong.

In addition to these senses that help you know where you are in the world, you have complex cognitive processes taking place to pull up your memory and experiences too. And then there's pattern recognition, an amalgam of all these elements. You visually see, you mentally take note, you recall from the past and bring facts and knowledge up to the present, you think and rationalize, you make decisions, you move, you see more . . . and so on. When you "know" how to get home, all of these factors come into play to help you navigate the spatial map in your head, as a pigeon would.

Homing pigeons have other processes that help them build remarkable memories of their environment. In addition to using visual cues or landmarks as we do, it's likely they also use the sense of smell and the position and angle of the sun. They can, as it were, tell time just as our bodies can using the twenty-four-hour solar day to dictate our hormonal cycles and circadian rhythms, though neither pigeons nor we are consciously aware of these powers that work behind the scenes. More recently, scientists have determined that homing pigeons also leverage the power of magnetoreception: the ability to detect and use the earth's magnetic field for navigation.[9] A concentration of iron particles in their beaks has been theorized to facilitate such an achievement, while cells in a pigeon's brain then record detailed information about the magnetic field to serve as a kind of biological compass. But critics of this idea say these particles are related to iron storage (iron is a major component of hemoglobin, which is necessary to carry oxygen in the blood), not magnetic sensing. Another theory suggests proteins called cryptochromes in the retinas of their eyes produce an electrical signal that varies depending on the strength of the local magnetic field, which scientists have suggested amazingly could allow "birds to 'see' Earth's magnetic field."[10] And yet a fourth theory puts the spotlight on tiny iron particles known as cuticulosomes in their inner ears, although apparently the magnetic properties of the cuticulosomes are not strong enough to sense the earth's magnetic field.

It's thought that Earth's magnetic field is part of why our planet is habitable, as it acts as a shield to deflect solar wind that might otherwise eat away at the atmosphere (and fry life from the sun's radiation). It is powered by the solidification of Earth's liquid iron core, the cooling and crystallization of which whip up the surrounding liquid iron, fomenting powerful electric currents. The earth's rotation on its axis causes these electric currents to form a magnetic field that extends around the planet tilted eleven degrees from the spin axis, as well as far out into space. At the earth's surface, the magnetic field forms two poles generated by electric currents that arise from the motion of convection currents, which are caused by heat escaping from the core. The convention currents stem from a mixture of molten iron and nickel in Earth's outer core. NASA researchers have observed that "the invisible lines of the magnetic field travel in a closed, continuous loop, flowing into Earth at the north magnetic pole and out at the south magnetic pole." Magnetic minerals in ancient undisturbed volcanic and sedimentary rocks, lake and marine sediments, lava flows, and archeological artifacts can reveal the magnetic field's strength and directions, when magnetic pole reversals occurred, and more.[11] Scientists are actively constructing a history of how the field has changed over geologic time. Research into what life on Earth can detect and how to leverage the field's powers has only recently begun.

Many organisms we share the planet with—from bacteria, bees, and snails to lobsters, rainbow trout, salmon, sea turtles, frogs, and dogs—appear to be able to detect Earth's magnetic field. Dogs prefer to orient themselves along the north–south axis of Earth's magnetic field when they defecate. But humans? Do we have a magnetic seventh sense? And if we can unknowingly sense magnetic fields, do those fields affect our behavior?[12]

In 2019, a team at the California Institute of Technology ignited a storm when it published a paper suggesting that we can sense Earth's magnetic field.[13] Using electroencephalography (EEG), according to Kelly Servick in *Science*, biophysicist Joe Kirschvink and his team "recorded brain activity from electrodes on the scalp to search for some response to changes in a highly controlled magnetic field equal in strength to Earth's."[14] They conducted their experiment two floors underground in a room with magnetically shielded walls to control everything. This allowed the researchers to expose subjects to custom magnetic fields generated by an array of electrical coils, while the EEG machine recorded brain waves. And they indeed recorded effects—a certain pattern of brain waves—and showed EEG changes in a particular wave (called the alpha wave) to the magnetic field, but only in less than a third of the participants, which means obviously we are all different. Whether it is a genetic difference or a learned difference isn't clear, but the data are intriguing.[15] We are far from understanding how magnetoreception is possible if it does exist in some of us—and by extension, what its benefits are, if any.

Servick's *Science* article went on to explain, "The mechanism of magnetoreception is only settled for certain bacteria, which harbor magnetite crystals that align with Earth's magnetic field. Bird beaks and fish snouts also contain magnetite, as does the human brain. Gilder and his colleagues recently found that it is most concentrated in lower, evolutionarily ancient regions—the brain stem and cerebellum. But no one has identified the proposed sensory cells that contain magnetite." A lot more research has to go into establishing a human magnetosensory system before we can address important questions: If we are able to subconsciously process geomagnetic stimuli, what does it do for us? And what else can it do in creatures other than act as an internal compass? Can exposure to magnets have negative consequences? Can magnets in aviation headsets impair pilots' natural sense of direction? Does the strong magnetic field generated by magnetic resonance imaging (MRI) machines change our magnetite?[16]

Adding another wrinkle is the newly minted theory of low-frequency infrasound, which is possibly the fifth method homing pigeons use to steer themselves in the right direction. When homing pigeons get confused and disoriented, they disappear in the wrong direction or scatter randomly rather than flying straight home. Scientists have proposed that disruptions in their ability to "hear" home by following ultralow-frequency sounds is what confuses them. *Infrasound* refers to sound waves coming from the oceans and ground that propagate at such low frequencies that we humans cannot detect them, but we know they are audible to pigeons. Just as we use our eyes to visually recognize the landscape near our houses, pigeons may use these sounds to image the terrain surrounding their lofts. But if weather conditions and terrain in certain areas interrupt the infrasound that pigeons rely on, this could help explain why some lose their bearings and fly the wrong way. What if we could one day dial into these sound waves and let artificial intelligence (AI) leverage their power? We could potentially develop tools more powerful than GPS devices to help us avoid ever getting lost. In the relative near term, AI will help decode animal-to-animal communication. The advances in this field are impressive; imagine having a Siri-like device that can interpret what an animal is saying to you . . .

According to Blaisdell, no one mechanism guides pigeons home; they rely on the most useful strategy available depending on where they are and where they need to go.

And that brings us to those bobbing heads, where this conversation gets really interesting. I recommend sitting on a park bench sometime and considering the following paradox: the rapid jerk of pigeons' heads is what allows them to momentarily fixate their eyes on objects to build a steady scene of their surroundings. Vision and motion don't go well together, so all animals need a way to stabilize the world around them, or it would be a dizzying blur. We have neuromuscular connections between our eyes and the part of our brain that tracks movement to facilitate instinctual slight twitches of the eye. Pigeons, however, leverage their long, flexible necks to motion-track, so they aren't really bobbing at all. What they are doing is darting their heads to lock their gaze in place on an object and then letting their body catch up to them. It takes the photoreceptors in their eyes (recall those foveae) about twenty milliseconds to capture a steady image of their environment. Then they repeat the action: darting their head forward, locking their eyesight onto something new, and bringing the rest of their body forward. Scientists figured this out decades ago by filming pigeons and analyzing their movements frame by frame; when pigeons are placed in a setting where their surroundings are stationary, they don't move their heads when they walk.

The more we can understand how animals track their movements and stabilize the constantly moving world around them, the better we may get at treating challenging conditions related to motion such as vertigo or problems with coordination. As I noted, we use a combination of our eyes, inner ears, and brains to be our GPS, and so any problems with these parts—abnormal eye movements, fluid in the inner ear, infection of the vestibular nerve, brain trauma in its balance center—can turn our world into a disorienting labyrinth so that finding home becomes impossible. Studies are currently developing new therapies for vestibular problems in humans based on what we've learned from other animals. Electrical implants, for example, that have been shown to steady balance disorders in chinchillas are in human clinical trials led by Johns Hopkins University.[17]

The Monty Hall Dilemma

Pigeons' surprising visual sophistication covers wide territory, literally. They can not only navigate as if they have built-in computer apps to show them the way, but also even perform better on certain tests of pattern recognition than we humans can. How so? The surprising answer is that they don't overthink what they see. Blaisdell shared with me that his pigeons have taught him to not overthink problems and to avoid biases—two common flaws we'd do well to work on. He relayed a story that epitomizes the drawbacks of such flaws: we can lose sight of the bigger picture.

Here's an experiment to illustrate what's called the Monty Hall dilemma. Picture yourself on a game show where you're presented with three doors. The host (who knows what is behind each door) tells you that a shiny new car sits behind one of them. The other two doors disguise mangy goats. You get to pick one of the doors and take whatever is behind it home (you're dreaming of that new car). You make your pick and then the host opens a door to one of the other two rooms, revealing a smelly goat looking at you. The host then asks if you want to stay with your original pick or switch to the remaining door. Which door do you choose? This is what's called the Monty Hall dilemma, so named after the presenter of a show called *Let's Make a Deal* that began in the 1960s and involved similar choices. It's a classic brainteaser that plays on probabilities.

The vast majority of people will stick with their original picks assuming it doesn't make a difference because their odds are 50/50. If that line of thinking sounds right, you've failed a now infamous puzzle. Your odds of winning the car *double* if you swap doors. This sounds like a cheap and lousy bar trick, but this dilemma long befuddled even acclaimed mathematicians, who refused to accept the explanation for the new odds until they were shown proof from computer simulations that revealed the incontrovertible truth: swapping every time is the best strategy. But the Monty Hall dilemma rarely fools a pigeon.

Science writer Ed Yong beautifully described the pigeon Monty Hall experiment for *Discover Magazine* in 2010.[18] At Whitman College in Washington State, psychology professor Walter Herbranson and his research assistant at the time, Julia Schroeder, showed that over the course of a month, pigeons can learn to make a better decision after some training and switch from their initial decision choices almost every time. You see, the odds of the car being behind each one of the remaining two doors are not 50/50. At the start of the game, you had a one-in-three chance of picking the door with the car. You also had a two-in-three chance of selecting a door with a goat. But the host doesn't want to reveal the car, so when he opens a door, he'll always pick a goat door. The fact that he chose not to open the other door suggests that door may well be hiding the car. The host's action increases the odds to two-thirds that you'll win by switching.

Herbranson and Schroeder worked with half a dozen pigeons and tweaked the game show format to allow the birds to use their beaks to indicate their choice. The team presented each pigeon with three lit keys as analogous doors, one of which could be pecked for food (the food being analogous to the beautiful new car). All three keys switched off at the first peck. But after a brief moment, two lights flicked back on, including the bird's first choice. The computer, which played the role of Monty Hall, had chosen one of the unpecked keys to deactivate. If the pigeon tapped the correct, winning, key of the remaining two, the bird earned a reward in the form of some food. On the first day of the experiment, the pigeons switched choices on only a third of the trials. A month later, however, all six birds swapped almost every time, earning their food pellet. The food prize reinforced the pigeons' behavior. When Herbranson and Schroeder switched the problem around, reversing the odds so the pigeons were rewarded more when they stuck to their initial choices, they picked up on the new probabilities and executed the right tactic after another month of training. Humans aren't so savvy. We're not as good at making educated guesses. In the words of Herbranson and Schroeder, who published their findings in 2010, "Most humans fail spectacularly when faced with the MHD."[19] We can't overcome our intuitive impulses.

Herbranson and Schroeder recruited thirteen college students and presented them with a similar setup to the pigeons'. The students were not given much instruction other than being told to win as many points as possible. They had to employ trial and error to figure out what was going on with the three keys, lit or not. Over the course of a month, they had two hundred attempts at guessing the winning key. In the beginning, they were just as likely to switch their first choices than to stay. But by the last attempt, they were still switching only two-thirds of the time. Put simply, the pigeons outperformed the college students, or the pigeons learned and the college students didn't.

Why aren't we better at addressing this problem? Herbranson and Schroeder think we can be victims of our own intelligence. When we face a problem like this, we try to think it through and use logic rather than trial and error to figure out the best solution. Such an approach would usually be acceptable, but here's the stumbling block: we're no good at problems involving conditional probability (i.e., "If X happens, what are the odds of Y happening?"). Try as we might at reasoning, we are most likely going to arrive at the wrong answer—and stubbornly stick to it. Pigeons, in contrast, rely on experience to work out probabilities. Their approach is much simpler and observational, and it's iterative. They will seemingly have an open mind and use the strategy that appears to be paying off the most. And they don't fall prey to what's called "probability matching."

As Ed Yong wrote, "If the odds of winning by switching are two in three, we'll switch on two out of three occasions even though that's a worse strategy than always switching."*[20] We will make predictions in a manner that "matches" the relevant outcome probabilities, even though that choice may ultimately be irrational.† The students in

*Ed Yong's most recent work, *An Immense World: How Animal Senses Reveal the Hidden Realms Around Us*, is an important book to check out.

†As Derek Koehler and Greta James described in a 2014 article in *Psychology of Learning and Motivation*, "Consider a simple computer game in which, on each trial, either a green or a red light appears. Your task is to predict which color will appear, and you will be paid a small amount of money for each correct prediction. What should you do, assuming your goal is to earn as much money as possible? Much of the challenge in this task arises from uncertainty regarding the process that determines whether the green or the red light appears on each trial. Does one light appear more frequently than the other? Is there a predictable pattern in the sequence of red and green outcomes? Does the probability of the green light illuminating change over the course of the game?" It turns out that in experiments with humans, we tend to make predictions that match the outcome probabilities. For example, if the green light is illuminated on 75 percent of trials and the red light on the remaining 25 percent, people are inclined to predict green on 75 percent of the trials and red on the remaining 25 percent. And that phenomenon is called probability matching. It's also known as the "matching law" or

Herbranson and Schroeder's experiments did exactly that—ruining their odds of winning. The pigeons, however, always switched. They don't probability match in their decision-making. Pigeons prevail because they don't overthink the problem. They follow the intelligence that their experiences give them, whereas we humans can become cognitively distracted by thoughts and so don't pay enough attention to what we're experiencing. We think too much!

Ironically, the youngest students perform best at this brainteaser. Eighth graders are more likely to figure out the benefits of switching than university students. (In fairness and in irony, those eighth graders have the advantage of not having taken advanced math yet.) Education, at least in this scenario, may be an actual hindrance. Herbranson and Schroeder write, "Pigeons might not possess the cognitive framework for a classical probability-based analysis of a complicated problem like the MHD, but it is certainly not far-fetched to suppose that pigeons can accumulate empirical probabilities by observing the outcomes of numerous trials and adjusting their subsequent behavior accordingly."[21]

The lesson is that sometimes it pays not to overthink things too much. Instead, trust your instincts—and perhaps take a pigeon to Vegas. (Casinos count on us to think like humans, prone to errors as well as biases. If someone counted cards and knew the correct statistics on each hand and made decisions based on these numbers, over time he or she would beat the house, which is precisely why card counting is grounds for denying service to people at casinos.) Avoiding the urge to overthink a problem is especially important when the issue is counterintuitive or causes cognitive dissonance, which is when you have two beliefs about the same thing at once that contradict each other. And that's exactly what the Monty Hall dilemma causes.

Herrnstein's Law and has been studied by economists and psychologists alike over the years and still isn't fully understood.

In the future, artificial intelligence will help us improve our decision-making by removing these distracting biases and errors in thinking. If I fed a computer, for example, the information on all of my cases I have seen throughout the years, it should be just as good as or better than I am at determining which courses of treatment to follow for patients. To be sure, artificial intelligence won't replace our brains, but it can become a useful tool to boost our thinking and ability to make better decisions quickly, easily, and with ideal outcomes—whether you're choosing a cancer therapy or helping your kid decide where to apply to college.

Creature Cheat Sheet

Three lessons from these studies on the pigeon can add to our productivity and quality of life.

First, *boost your perceptual intuition by paying close attention to patterns in your world.* By tuning in to these patterns daily, you can build better memories in general, speed up your brain's processing, and increase the chances that you'll make good decisions (and find your way home). Try going outside for ten minutes every day and come back with at least ten patterns you spotted. You may feel silly at first, but exercises like this make a difference in long-term cognitive function.

In addition, create new patterns by doing things like rearranging the furniture in your living room, using your nondominant hand to perform habitual tasks like eating or brushing your teeth, switching the arm on which you wear your watch, and driving a different way to work every day without using GPS. That last suggestion is not trivial. Getting lost is often among the first signs of cognitive decline—more so than the memory problems that crop up later. If you grew up in an urban environment with a predictable grid-like network to your surrounding streets, you might struggle to navigate in a rural area or unpredictable, unfamiliar setting. Your childhood surroundings have influenced not only your health and well-being but also your ability to get around later in life. So challenge yourself. When you have a destination to reach, pay attention to every step of the way without help. A small but worrisome study showed that people who use their car's GPS guidance system more often may have higher rates of cognitive decline as they age.[22]

Second, *take a step back when making important decisions because your humanness can be a hindrance.* Your gut response is tremendously important, especially when you need to make quick, semisubconscious decisions. But realize that it's not always driven only by pure data—and your memories can change with time and be influenced by your emotions, altering your recollection of past experiences. I have learned to sleep on important decisions. A new day gives new perspective, allowing us to think a bit more like the pigeon—with less emotion and more logic or rules based on what we've learned repeatedly to be the "right" answer (even when our memories may fail us or give us wrong intelligence, over time the "right" memories should dominate). When an important decision is at hand, write down the possibilities and the underlying premises behind each available choice (the pros and cons). This will help to remove the bias (the cognitive dissonance) that is in all of us and may yield a more appropriate decision. When you stop to think more deeply, you'll likely face those hidden biases, bringing them from your unconscious to the forefront of your consciousness to work through as you problem solve.

Third, *when you have an encounter you want to remember, jot down the basic details rather than minutiae*. After hearing this tip during my UCLA visit, I've been trying it and have found it's made a surprisingly big difference. Making simple summary notes from each encounter or meeting I have helps me remember events much better—and I'm able to learn much better from these events. I just jot down a few key words or make visual notice of a few things.

The more we expand and stimulate our brain, the better chance we have at a long and healthy life. This stimulation doesn't have to be picking up a new language, mastering pointillism, or reading about the theory of relativity. Novel and engaging experiences can work wonders, and challenging yourself every day can have important benefits. This can entail any number of things that may seem mundane but are anything but when you pay extra attention. You can start by exploring a new activity you've always wanted to try but thought you'd be bad at or that would make you uncomfortable. And when you can, take the long way home. Notice the nuances in the longer route filled with different patterns and landmarks. Take note the way a homing pigeon would.

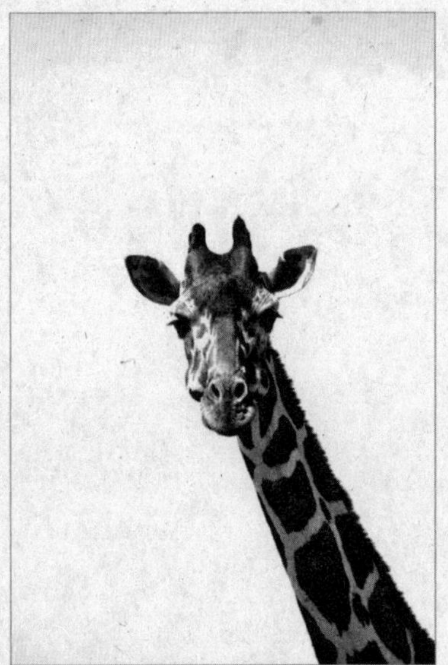

A beautiful giraffe I photographed at
Maasai Mara National Reserve, Kenya.

4

The Giraffe Paradox

What Long Necks and Gravity Teach Us about Ending Heart Disease

> *Nature is the source of all true knowledge. She has her own logic, her own laws, she has no effect without cause nor invention without necessity.*
>
> —LEONARDO DA VINCI

When you think of Leonardo da Vinci, my bet is at least one or two things come to mind: the *Mona Lisa* for sure and maybe his legendary *Vitruvian Man* drawing too. Those were two of his most masterful works of art that you can picture immediately even if you've never seen them in real life. But I also think of this consummate polymath's genius in science and technology. He predicted the modern use of helicopters, parachutes, calculators, and robots (among other current marvels), and his probing the mysteries of the human body have led to theories only now gaining proper appreciation. His greatest offering to humanity may not have been his artistry but his musings in medicine that informed his painting techniques.

More than five hundred years ago, at the height of his fame as a painter, when he was in his midfifties, Leonardo contributed to medicine in ways that were not fully validated until the twenty-first century. In 1508, the same year Michelangelo began his brushwork on the Sistine Chapel, Leonardo used his own deft, curious hands to dissect a cadaver and document, for the first time, the process of atherosclerosis, which results when plaque-like substances build up in the walls of arteries to the point they become inflexible, stiff, and thick.

This cadaver could not have entered Leonardo's life any timelier. Leonardo's interest in anatomy was initially inspired by an anatomist, Professor Marcantonio della Torre, who commissioned Leonardo to provide the illustrations for his text on the subject. As part of his preparation for this work, Leonardo began to dissect human corpses at several hospitals, starting in Florence with the Hospital of Santa Maria Nuova. (Now over 730 years old, the hospital is as busy today as it was in the thirteenth century.) He'd go there at night seeking specimens and to learn about physiology from the doctors. It was on one of these excursions that Leonardo met a dying man who claimed to be more than one hundred years old. Whether that was true, we'll never know, but for the artist, who proceeded to put his talents with pen and scalpel to work upon the man's peaceful death hours later, it was an opportunity with enormous historical importance. This man would become one of Leonardo's best models for many of the body's inner workings, particularly those of the heart, vessels, and muscles. Leonardo would go on to record many of his anatomical studies in the following years, acting as an artistic pathologist of sorts. Nearly twenty years before, he'd drawn *Vitruvian Man*, his concept of the ideal human body proportions, which would become the basis for my institute's logo. Note the symbology in the drop of blood and roots of a tree.*

*Walter Isaacson, author of one of the latest biographies of Leonardo da Vinci (titled simply *Leonardo da Vinci* and published in 2017), once got upset with me when I said "da Vinci," because it refers only to where he was from; he should be called Leonardo. I had wanted to give homage to the multidisciplinary scientist in the logo for our newly formed institute. Walter was the one who suggested *Vitruvian Man*.

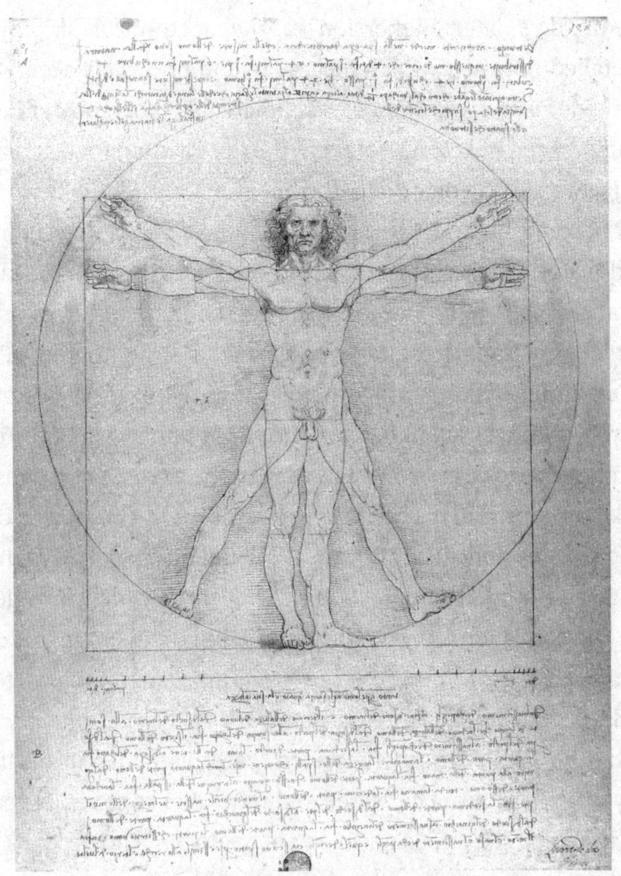

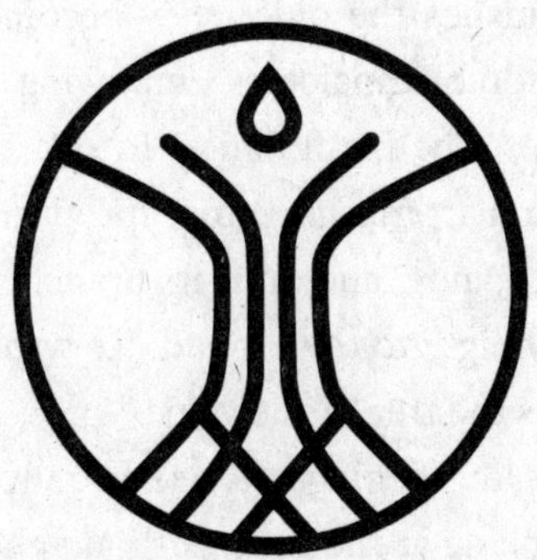

Leonardo da Vinci's *Vitruvian Man* (above)
and the Ellison Institute logo (below).

Leonardo's later immersion in the anatomical arts produced 240 detailed drawings, which include two impressively accurate studies of the fetus in the womb. In his remarkable biography of Leonardo da Vinci, Walter Isaacson wrote that the dead centenarian and his early investigations led Leonardo to document matters of the heart in what would become his most lasting medical legacy. He determined that the old man's demise occurred "from weakness through the failure of blood and of the artery that feeds the heart and the other lower member, which [he] found to be very dry, shrunken, and withered." The man had died either with or from atherosclerotic disease, as described by Leonardo, "brought about by the continuous narrowing of the passage of the mesenteric vessels by thickening of the coats of these vessels."[1]

Like any thorough scientist, Leonardo used the power of comparison to draw conclusions. A two-year-old boy had died at the same hospital and landed under Leonardo's hands, which unveiled that the boy's vessels looked very different. Unlike the old man's clogged roadways, the boy's blood vessels were supple and unobstructed. Not only did Leonardo chronicle coronary artery disease and atherosclerosis, but he also rightfully theorized that it was a factor of time: the older you are, the more cluttered and inflexible your vessels become. His written conclusion drew on an apt analogy: "The network of vessels behaves in man as in oranges, in which the peel becomes tougher and the pulp diminishes the older they become."[2] Leonardo liked using simple, memorable analogies employing scenes from nature or machinery to describe his findings. In one of his drawings that showed the heart and arteries next to a sprouting seed, for example, he labeled the seed a "nut" and drew its branches stretching upward and its roots stretching into the ground. He wrote: "The heart is the nut which generates the tree of the veins."[3]

Leonardo got a lot of things preternaturally correct, debunking the established thinking at the time. Although he never fully understood that the blood in the body circulates and he subscribed to the incorrect theory that the heart warms the blood—a notion that had been around since the second-century Greek physician Galen—he showed that the heart is simply a muscle at the center of the blood system. Blood was not, as previously thought, made in the liver. Leonardo described how the human heart was four chambered and that the palpable pulse in the wrist coincided with the contraction of the left ventricle of the heart. He then tied blood flows in the body to the opening and closing of the cardiac valves. And then he made the observation that arteries that develop plaque over time can yield health risks. That was quite a lot of observations for one man in the history of the study of this disease.[4] Centuries later, I'm still surprised in the autopsies I perform by the sheer prevalence of atherosclerotic disease. Most people have it, although not all are symptomatic and it does not cause a problem in many—a clue to explore further to understand who gets heart disease and why.*

What is amazing is that these critical observations by Leonardo, including his drawings, did not find the light of day until after he died, and his notes weren't studied until over two hundred and fifty years after his demise. Had they been published sooner, they undoubtedly would have made a major contribution to medical science and propelled us faster in our technological evolution. It took hundreds of years for anatomists to accept Leonardo's ideas on how the aortic heart valve works, closing and opening to let blood flow around the heart. Not until the work of researchers at Oxford University in 2014, who conducted experiments using MRI technology on live humans, did Leonardo earn the vindication he deserved centuries ago.[5]

In another recent nod to Leonardo's spectacular work, an inter-

*I've written before about the Maasai people in Kenya and Tanzania who live primarily off raw milk and raw blood and occasionally meat from their cattle. They have a low incidence of the diseases typically attributed to a diet high in saturated fat and cholesterol, such as heart disease and cancer. Although they do have atherosclerotic disease visible on autopsy, they have a compensatory widening of the arteries, so the disease didn't cause a problem in their lifetime.

national team of researchers in 2020, led by the Cold Spring Harbor Laboratory in New York and UK-based scientists, finally put to rest another question that Leonardo raised centuries ago, this one about the complex mesh of muscle fibers lining the inside of the heart, called trabeculae.[6] The first person to draw the trabeculae was Leonardo. His rendering showed them as "snowflake-like fractal patterns." While trabeculae make up 13 percent of the mass of the heart's left ventricle, they were long assumed to be just a remnant of embryonic development. In the sixteenth century, Leonardo took a guess that the purpose of the web network of trabeculae is to warm the blood as it flows through the heart.[7]

We know differently today. The scientists at Cold Spring Harbor Laboratory took the study of trabeculae to a new level. They examined 25,000 cardiac MRI scans from the UK Biobank data and showed that the trabeculae affect heart function and, later in life, risk of heart failure.[8] Reports by the European Bioinformatics Institute, which was part of the study, used a smart visual analogy: just as dimples on a golf ball reduce air resistance that makes the ball travel farther, in the heart, the trabeculae facilitate an ideal propulsion of oxygen-rich blood. The study also details six regions in our DNA that affect how the unique patterns in these muscle fibers develop; different fractal patterns may affect a person's risk of developing heart disease. What's more, the researchers discovered that two of these genetic regions also regulate the branching of nerve cells, suggesting "a similar mechanism may be at work in the developing brain."[9] Their research continues.

Many of Leonardo's conclusions continue to be elusive to most people, doctors and even cardiologists included. We can send people to outer space but still cannot grasp some of our own inner spaces. If you were to tell people on the street the heart warmed the blood, you'd probably be surprised at how many people would believe you if you argued the point convincingly enough; words like *heartwarming* and *warmhearted* are easily misleading. Fewer would be misled about the microgravity effects of outer space. These two phenomena—the cardiovascular system and our own solar system—share a story never told. And it may, just may, inform how we deal with heart disease in the future.

We are still learning about how the heart and blood flow work, and there is still much more unknown that will enable better understanding and future treatments. Today, more than half a millennium after Leonardo's death, heart disease is still the number one cause of death worldwide.* And in our search for solutions and new ways of thinking about the disease, we would do well to turn our heads upward to the sky—into space, but also to some towering creatures on Earth: giraffes.

The Heart of It

Heart disease and stroke have remained the world's leading causes of death over the past two decades. Although at times confused by many people, *heart attack* and *cardiac arrest* are two different conditions with very different physiology. A heart attack happens when an artery delivering oxygen-rich blood to the heart is blocked and that section of the heart begins to die; the heart does not stop beating, but the longer the artery remains clogged, the greater the damage will be, which can quickly lead to the individual's death. During cardiac arrest, the heart suffers an electrical malfunction that causes an irregular heartbeat (arrhythmia), which disrupts proper pumping action to the point that it stops beating entirely. The American Heart Association offers an easy way to remember the difference: "a heart attack is a 'circulation' problem and a sudden cardiac arrest is an 'electrical' problem." The cardiac arrest can be due to a heart attack, as the dying cardiac tissue can cause electrical disturbances in the

*Leonardo may have died from a series of strokes—an ironic fate given his own meditations about old age and vascular health.

heart. As the heart fails to pump blood properly to the brain, lungs, and other organs, death becomes imminent. Whereas symptoms of a heart attack can arise slowly over time, such as days or weeks before the actual event occurs, cardiac arrest happens suddenly and often without warning. Within seconds, a person can lose consciousness, a pulse, and soon their life.

Strokes are like heart attacks in the brain; they occur when there's a loss of blood to part of the brain due to a blood clot (blockage) or broken blood vessels in the brain. And like the heart, as the brain is starved of life-giving blood, it becomes damaged and begins to die. All three of these life-threatening problems share many of the same set of risk factors: high blood pressure, smoking, diabetes, high cholesterol, and atherosclerosis (the buildup of fatty material and plaque inside the coronary arteries). Older age and family history also play into the risk, but we know that lifestyle has much to do with whether your heart will give out sooner than it should. (The term *heart failure* is used to describe a general condition characterized by a heart being unable to pump effectively and efficiently to meet the body's needs. The heart hasn't stopped working completely, but it's not pumping as it should. A number of things can cause heart failure, from infections and kidney disease to conditions that damage the heart muscle, like a heart attack or coronary artery disease.)

More people need new hearts each year than there are (dead) donors to supply them. As public health measures have reduced the number of violent deaths and especially fatal car accidents (thanks to seat belt laws and better airbags), there are fewer hearts to go around. During the pandemic, when stay-at-home orders kept people safely off the roads, organ transplants across the country fell dramatically—the opposite of the silver lining in a dark cloud. Parenthetically, self-driving cars should reduce organ transplants even more, as an estimated 94 percent of motor-vehicle accidents involve some kind of driver error.[10] Still, it remains to be seen if computer errors in self-driving cars may become a new source of accidents, albeit likely causing dramatically fewer than the number caused by human errors.

Heart disease has bedeviled people for millennia. Although it has long been assumed to be an ailment of modern humans attributed to contemporary lifestyles, it's not as new as we once thought. A 2013 *Lancet* article used whole-body CT scans of mummies from four ancient societies—Egypt, Peru, the Puebloan of the Southwest, and the Unangan of the Aleutian Islands—to demonstrate atherosclerotic disease was present in those times.[11] The technology allowed the investigators to see the coronaries of the mummies without using any scalpels or scissors. The scientists found probable or definite atherosclerosis in more than a third of the 137 mummies scanned, whose time period spanned more than four thousand years. Though we don't know what these mummies actually died from and whether their arteries were to blame, the authors were still able to conclude that the disease was common in premodern humans, eons before we had fast food, sedentary lifestyles, and problems with obesity.

But it was not nearly as widespread as it became in the twentieth century. In 1900, heart disease was the fourth most common cause of death, trailing infectious diseases such as pneumonia and tuberculosis. Three decades later, heart disease became the prevailing cause of death and continued to increase until the mid-1960s. This rise in the first part of the twentieth century has been blamed on a confluence of factors: A 2014 study in the *American Journal of Medicine* pointed out that "Americans were living longer due to a decrease in deaths from infectious disease." Additionally, there were changes in our diets, including increased consumption of processed foods that contain more saturated fat, added sugar, and refined flour. The study also observed a general decrease in Americans' physical activity, in part due to more access to cars as transportation devices. And by 1965, 42 percent of Americans were smokers, up from less than 5 percent in 1900.[12]

The connection between smoking and heart disease may not

seem obvious, but cigarette smoke contains chemicals that cause the blood to thicken and form clots. Nicotine alone will damage the lining of blood vessels, increase blood pressure and heart rate, and cause less oxygen to be delivered to the heart—a problem compounded by the inhalation of carbon monoxide while smoking, which also blocks oxygen delivery. Over time, the constant constriction by nicotine of the blood vessels results in vessels that are stiff. Constricted, stiff blood vessels lead to a decrease in the amount of oxygen and nutrients cells receive. Tobacco is still a major issue in the United States, with 20 percent of cardiac deaths directly related to smoking. Approximately thirty-five thousand nonsmokers die from heart disease each year as a result of exposure to secondhand tobacco smoke.[13]

We were ready for another shift in habits, however, in the latter part of the century, with greater awareness of the adverse effects of smoking and high cholesterol. Historians have suggested that Franklin Delano Roosevelt's death from a stroke in April 1945 spurred public awareness for cardiovascular disease.* Coronary heart disease deaths decreased from 466 per 100,000 people in 1965 to 345 in 1980, a 26 percent relative decrease. From 1980 to 2008, the decrease was a colossal 64 percent: from 345 to 123 per 100,000 individuals. In that time period, we got better not only at treating sick hearts but also at preventing heart disease entirely as we learned more about what causes the affliction.

Lub and Dub

The work a heart puts out over a lifetime, one hundred thousand beats per day (give or take) to pump seventy gallons of blood every

*He was already clearly unwell, audibly wheezing and unable to complete sentences, at the Yalta Conference in Crimea two months before his death, where he met with Joseph Stalin and Winston Churchill to discuss how post–World War II Europe should be organized. Within twenty years of the conference, all three men had died from strokes.

twenty-four hours, is remarkable. The blood in your body travels twelve thousand miles in a day, four times the distance across the United States from coast to coast. Amazingly, it takes less than a minute—fifty seconds—for blood to do a full lap in the body.

Sitting about four feet above your feet, the heart has to overcome the effects of gravity to bring blood back up—over and over again with every beat every second or so. One squeeze of a tennis ball is approximately equal to the amount of energy your heart expends for one pump of blood through your body (in specific terms, this is about 2 watts of energy).[14]

The heart is the first sign of life in a fetus as the first functional organ to develop. It starts beating spontaneously four to five weeks after conception, when a doctor may still refer to the fetus as an embryo. By the tenth week, the heart is fully developed, and it'll continue to beat nonstop for many decades.

Two main phases of the heart's beat correlate with the blood flowing in and out of the heart's chambers through the valves as they open and close. When the heart contracts to push blood out into the body, that's called the *systole* (from the ancient Greek word meaning to contract)—the pressure in your arteries when your heart beats. When the heart relaxes to refill, that's the *diastole* (from the ancient Greek word meaning to dilate)—the pressure in your arteries when your heart rests between beats. The difference between the two phases is blood pressure, and the numbers associated with a blood pressure reading (e.g., 120/80) reflect the highest and lowest pressures your blood vessels experience with each heartbeat. The top number (120 in the example) is the systolic pressure, and the bottom (80) is the diastolic. Technically, the numbers measure how many millimeters of mercury are pushing up a calibrated tube (so, also technically, blood pressure is recorded as "mmHg").

Not many of us appreciate the constant task of keeping blood balanced throughout the body to serve every tissue and organ system. Think about the forces involved to support and counter your actions—walking, running, standing, squatting, dancing, doing a cartwheel or headstand if you're so inclined. During every maneuver, you've got gravity in the mix pulling on you (and your blood). Gravity is more than a force; it's also "a signal that tells the body how to act." The muscles employed to fight gravity by engaging (flexing), such as those in the calves and spine, help you to maintain posture. These muscles can easily lose around 20 percent of their mass if you don't use them—another reason to move around frequently (muscle mass can vanish, or atrophy, at a rate as high as 5 percent a week when not using it).[15]

The body manages blood distribution in the face of gravity with flap-like, flexible valves in your veins that stop blood from flowing backward; without the action of these one-way valves, you wouldn't get the blood back up toward the heart. Your leg muscles also act as pumps when they contract, helping to facilitate the blood to return up to the heart. The muscle movements happen naturally as you walk, stand, and move about (another reason to stay in motion to promote healthy circulation), and when you're not moving, demands on the circulatory system are greatly reduced, but you can see how prolonged sitting increases risk for poor, insufficient blood flow and pooling of blood in the lower extremities ("venous insufficiency," which affects more than forty million people in the United States).

Blood pressure varies across the body as a whole throughout the day, depending on what you're doing, and settles down at night when you're asleep. One of the reasons heart attacks peak in incidence during the early morning hours is related to our lower blood pressure during that time, which means that clots or plaques can form. When you're lying down, the blood pressure is the same (about 90 mmHg) throughout the length of your body. But when you stand, the blood pressure decreases above the heart and increases below due to the force of gravity. There's a less than 20 percent difference between blood pressure at your shoulders and at the ankles if you're healthy.

For a long time, even into much of the last century, we thought that high blood pressure (hypertension) was advantageous because it indicates strong blood flow, and strong blood flow appeared to mean a strong heart. But we know otherwise now: perpetually high blood pressure raises the risk for cardiovascular problems including heart attack and stroke. Today, normal blood pressure is anything less than 120/80 mmHg; elevated is 120–129/80; and high blood pressure (hypertension stage 1) is 130–139/80–89 mmHg. High blood pressure requires treatment if it stays in stage 1 or greater and immediate medical attention if the readings exceed 180/120 mmHg. The top contributors to hypertension are poor diet (too much salt, not enough fruits and vegetables), being overweight, smoking, lack of exercise, drinking too much alcohol, and for some, too much caffeine, and not getting restful sleep. Age also is a major factor, as being over the age of sixty-five increases risk pretty significantly. In fact, by age seventy, more than three-quarters of US adults have hypertension. As we age, there is a reduction in elastic tissue in our arteries, causing them to become stiffer and less compliant, which leads to increases in blood pressure. This isn't an individual's "fault" much of the time, but interventions with medications can offer significant benefits for long-term health, including slowing cognitive decline.

Hypertension is a silent killer and the leading single cause of disability worldwide—that is, if you're a human but not if you're a giraffe. Welcome to the giraffe paradox.

Sky-High Heads and Sky-High Blood Pressure

When my family went on safari in 2014, one of the highlights was horseback riding in Kenya on the open plain with giraffes, their elegant stride enabling them to playfully run ahead. In 1758, Swedish zoologist Carl Linnaeus named all giraffes as one species, *giraffa camelopardalais*. *Giraffa* was from the Arabic *zarafah* (meaning one who walks swiftly) and *camelopardalais* was because the ancient Greeks believed it looked like a camel (*kamelos*) with a leopard's spots (*pardalis* is Greek for "leopard"). These majestic, somewhat absurd-looking animals are the tallest mammals in the world. With graceful eyes and mild demeanors, they come across as gentle and as mute as the swaying foliage on which they munch. Giraffes communicate with each other at a frequency below our detection, sort of a hum, an infrasonic sound.[16] Occasionally there is a whistle, particularly when a mother is calling to young giraffes. They also use their eyes for communication, possessing some of the largest eyes in land mammals. Amazing vision helps the giraffe survive the wilds of the plains.* Not only can they see in color and over distances vast enough to spot a moving human a mile away, but also their peripheral vision is so wide-angled that they essentially can see behind themselves.[17] Their sense of touch isn't shabby either. And their dark blue-black tongues? That's due to the pigment melanin that protects their tongues from the sun's UV radiation as they munch on tall branches.

The next time you can look closely at a giraffe, note its skintight hide and take in the beauty and uniqueness of its ochered flagstone fur. Like our fingerprints, no two arrays of polygon-shaped patches are the same. The polygons are larger on the body than on the face and limbs, and the underbelly usually has no pattern at all. Each giraffe has his or her own pattern that helps it to camouflage from predators in trees and woodland.

Giraffes have been called the "forgotten megafauna," understudied and underappreciated, especially when compared to their more famous African counterparts—elephants, chimps, rhinos, and gorillas. But that is changing now that field scientists are focusing on this wonderful animal, which affords us the opportunity to learn

*The eyes are not only poetic windows to the soul; they are also windows into the health of the blood vessels. When the eye doctor pierces a bright light into your eyes, he or she is evaluating the state of your blood vessels back in the retina, which can show vascular conditions and signs of problems from diabetes to blood pressure issues. Indeed, eye doctors can often spot early signs of looming heart attacks, strokes, and other serious health problems far in advance of any other obvious symptoms.

from some of their extraordinary physiological wits. Giraffes sport the highest-known blood pressure of any animal—twice our average (280/180 mmHg)—but they don't suffer from any negative consequences. They don't develop heart disease or other organ damage often seen in hypertensive patients, and fluids never pool in their long, spindly legs. Even their wide eyes are unaffected by elevated blood pressure, whereas we experience visual disturbances when our blood pressure goes up. What's their secret?

I asked Alan Hargens that question in his compact, boxy office filled with mementos from a long and storied career. He's a pioneer in studying gravity's effects on the cardiovascular and musculoskeletal systems of humans and animals. Before moving to UC San Diego, where he is director of the Orthopedic Clinical Physiology Lab, he was chief of the Space Physiology Branch and Space Station and project scientist at NASA's Ames Research Center. Translation: he was a space doctor during the apex of NASA's programs in the 1980s and 1990s when the shuttle era was in its heyday. His work at NASA, which focused on exercise devices to maintain astronaut health in space, ultimately offered insights into helping the postsurgical rehabilitation of orthopedic patients and improving the performance of athletes.

Space is an environment like no other. At zero gravity, muscles atrophy quickly because the body perceives it does not need them. In fact, the lack of gravity also results in blood pressure being the same throughout the body—about an even 100 mmHg with no head-to-toe gradient. Without a blood pressure gradient in space, faces can get puffy and astronauts' legs become thinner as fluid distribution changes.[18] Space changes our senses of taste and smell, as the retention of fluids in the head can have the same effect as congestion from a cold.[19] Spacecraft are noisy vehicles, with noise levels of 65 dB to 75 dB—somewhere between an air conditioner and a vacuum cleaner.[20] The presence of loud noise suppresses how we perceive the saltiness and sweetness of foods. You've probably experienced a version of this while on an airplane where the craft's drumming noise overwhelms the brain and, as a result, your sense of taste. If you wear noise-canceling headphones on the plane, however, you can taste better and will gravitate toward the salty snacks. Try the experiment. It's pretty wild how well it works.[21]

Weightlessness remodels the brain and eyes as fluid moves around the body differently, changing the pressure in the eyes and around the brain. It increases blood flow in the absence of antagonizing gravity. And if you put baby animals and plants on the moon, they'd probably grow six times taller than they would on Earth as they adapt to one-sixth the gravitational pull that would otherwise limit the expansion of the spine's length. The problem with the equalization of blood pressure throughout the body, however, is that the brain thinks there's too much blood. On Earth, blood pressure in the brain is 60 to 80 mmHg, not 100 mmHg. While in space, astronauts can lose over 20 percent of their blood volume over a few days as errant messages from the brain dial things back. With less blood to pump, the heart can also atrophy.[22] This is not an issue while the astronauts are in space, but they have to readjust over the course of a few days to weeks (depending on how long they were in space) when they return to Earth and its gravitational forces.

In the mid-1980s, Hargens turned to giraffes to understand their adaptive mechanisms to gravitational pressure changes. They provide an excellent animal model to inform space medicine and, in turn, all kinds of medicine relevant for us. The main cause of disease and failure of kidneys in humans is hypertension, which causes the arteries around the kidneys to narrow, harden, and weaken. Eventually, damaged arteries don't filter blood well and are unable to deliver enough blood to the kidney tissue. But giraffe kidneys go unscathed despite their dramatically high blood pressure. Their renal capsule, a tough layer of fibrous tissue that envelops the kidneys, is strong enough to withstand it. What's most interesting, however, is that giraffes are not born with hypertension. They develop it as they grow and their necks begin extending. That's the reason giraffes evolved to have such high blood pressure in the first place: to get blood all the way up those long necks.*

With a giraffe's neck being about six feet long, it has been assumed that a very large heart would be needed to push the blood into its head and support its high blood pressure. But the giraffe's heart isn't as big as was thought. A heart the size needed (in comparison with the beating power of a human heart) couldn't fit into the chest of the giraffe. The giraffe's heart is slightly over 0.5 meters (around 1.6 feet) long and generally weighs more than 20 pounds, which in relationship to our heart is huge, but compared with the size of the giraffe, it is actually pretty small. The giraffe makes up for the relatively small size of its heart by the thickness of its left ventricle, the major blood pump of the heart, which is almost twice that of an average human's.[23] There is a calculated relationship between the length of the giraffe neck and the left ventricular thickness: for every 15 centimeters in length of the neck, the left ventricle is half a centimeter thicker.

This is the key point: in humans, thickening of heart muscles causes stiffening, or fibrosis, that can eventually lead to heart failure, but a giraffe's heart can withstand the thickening without any fibrosis because of mutations in its genome that we lack.[24] Researchers who analyzed the giraffe genome in 2016 found several giraffe-specific gene variants related to cardiovascular development and maintenance of blood pressure and circulation.[25] In 2021, a research group led by UCLA cardiologist Barbara Natterson-Horowitz also

*How did the giraffe get its long neck? Maybe, like me, you read in school that antelopes could have evolved into giraffes by stretching their necks to reach the higher leaves on a tree, with the "stretchiest" giraffes passing slightly longer necks to their offspring. But other possible origins remain a topic of debate. Another idea is that long necks help male giraffes use their heads to bash rivals, suggesting that long-necked males are sexually selected. And then there's the thermoregulation idea offered in 2017, which has stirred much curiosity: perhaps giraffes evolved long necks to keep cool, so they can point their heads and necks toward the sun and expose less of their skin as it becomes shadowed.

reported giraffe-specific variants in genes involved in fibrosis.[26] Such variants give them an advantage to sustain high blood pressure at no cost to their cardiovascular health.

What can we take away from this knowledge? We can't change our genes to mimic those of a giraffe, but since the animals are a model of perfection for cardiovascular wellness, the more we can understand the genetic and molecular magic underpinning their distinct traits, the more biomedical scientists may be able to find novel approaches to treating diseases of the heart. Scientists have already started to perform gene-editing experiments on mice to make the rodents gain giraffe-type genetic traits that make them impressively resistant to hypertension. (They also gain higher bone mineral density, another gene-driven adaptation in the giraffe to assist their high stature.) So, yes, it's not science fiction to imagine a day we can safely tweak our genes to render ourselves hypertension-proof or that scientists will develop drugs so the human body can mimic the genes of the giraffe.

Clearly we have not evolved yet to live with chronic high blood pressure, and until we do, we should avoid the condition at all costs. This means keeping tabs on your blood pressure regularly and recording your numbers, especially if it has been abnormally high or low in the past. You can do this easily at home with a kit bought online or at your local pharmacy. Start by checking it for a few days in a row at different times to note highs and lows related to your activities; find patterns, and then keep monthly or bimonthly checks on it. And avoid the triggers of hypertension: smoking, excess weight, physical inactivity, poor sleep, too much alcohol, too much dietary sodium and refined sugars, and even too much stress.

You can also lower your cardio risks by keeping excellent oral hygiene because of the connection between gum health and risk for heart disease. While the two may not sound related, scientists believe that the heart can be negatively affected by proteins in the blood that respond to inflammation, and chronic gum disease produces ongoing inflammation. What's more, you don't want certain bacteria that live in your mouth—particularly if you have gum disease—to make their way into the bloodstream and reach the heart. Giraffes have their own dental hygienists at the ready: little oxpecker birds love to feed on bits of food stuck between the giraffes' teeth, so it's like getting a deep clean and floss all at once. We'd do well to follow their dental lead (don't forget to floss daily).

There is one unique adaptation the giraffe has perfected that we can easily mimic, and it has to do with how a thirsty giraffe prevents a serious head rush when dipping down into a puddle of fresh water. To quench thirst, the giraffe splays its front legs and lowers its head, but its high blood pressure could send blood surging into the brain from this pressure and the animal could collapse from a stroke. Going the other way could also be hazardous, as raising its head would cause pressure to drop precipitously and the giraffe to faint (fainting happens when there is reduced blood circulation to the brain, causing loss of consciousness).[27] In 2020, Christian Aalkjær, a cardiovascular physiologist at Aarhus University in Denmark, reported on the results of a study he performed to study giraffe blood flows to its head. He put giraffes to sleep with anesthesia and made a contraption that would raise and lower their heads with ropes and pulleys while they slept.[28] He demonstrated that blood pools in the big veins of the neck when the head is down, which reduces the amount of blood that returns to the heart; thus, the heart generates less pressure with each beat, as there is less blood volume. As the head is lifted back up, all the blood in the neck veins suddenly *returns* to the heart. The heart then goes into overdrive with a strong, high-pressure pumping action to drive blood back to the raised head. It's an exquisitely choreographed interplay like an analog switchboard gone fully digital thanks to evolution.

All of this reflexive buffering to changes in blood pressure is controlled without the giraffe consciously thinking about it. Thick blood vessel walls stop leakage and continuously contract and relax as the volume of blood changes due to the giraffe's activities. This system regulates proper circulatory distribution. Tough collagen fibers also help with keeping the blood in the right place, as these fibers are inflexible and don't stretch or leak with increased blood flow, similar to the way compression socks work in humans to aid blood flow in shifting gravity. These fibers thicken with age and as a giraffe's neck continues to grow. These adjustments continually support the maintenance of their blood pressure without the bad effects we see in humans with elevated blood pressure.[29]

And what about those spindly legs? How do they stay so lithe? In humans, as blood pressure goes up, and as we stand all day, blood pools in our legs and we can be swollen at the ankles. Given the height and blood pressure of giraffes, you might expect their ankles to show it, but they don't. Their biohack again shares parallels with space medicine. It helps to "wear" skintight antigravity-like pants, so to speak.

Skintight Pants

High blood pressure can trigger tissues to retain fluids in a bid to maintain adequate blood volume—a condition called edema—as the high pressure forces water out of blood vessels and into the surrounding tissues. This usually happens first in the lower parts of the body; as gravity brings the water to the lowest point, swelling is first seen in the ankles (many first notice this when they see marks on their ankles from their socks). You don't ever see giraffes with cankles (wide, thick ankles that are indistinguishable from the lower calf), as their bodies have a couple of ways to solve this problem. The arteries that are closest to the ankles have extra thick walls and their skin at this point is remarkably tight, so there is no space for any fluid to collect.[30] The skin that covers their legs is also extremely tough, and if you feel their legs, you will see it is tightly bound, not loose, because an inner layer of fascia (like glue) adheres to the muscles and doesn't allow room for blood to collect. "They have natural antigravity suits in their legs," Hargens tells me. Being without gravity can pose issues to the astronaut's circulatory system over time. Because that system is not being used to fight gravity to return blood to the heart (as on Earth), the blood vessels and surrounding musculature weaken considerably. If the astronaut spends a long period in space, this can cause an issue on the return to gravity.

Giraffes have evolved a solution to this problem. The amazing sight of a two-hundred-plus-pound newborn giraffe standing moments within an hour after birth, helped in part by the veins in the legs that elastically inflate immediately, gave NASA's medical and science team an idea. They developed a device that would create negative pressure on the lower half of the astronaut's body, with an airtight seal and vacuum pressure. The NASA space gravity suits worn six to eight hours a day (the same amount of time approximately we spend on our feet) fight the lessened gravity of the weightlessness in space. The interval activation of this device keeps the veins in the lower extremities of the astronauts in shape while in zero gravity.

While most of us don't have access to space suits like giraffe skin, we can use TED (thrombo-embolus deterrent, or antiembolism) stockings, a graded pressure stocking (fit to your leg size at a pharmacy) that can promote increased blood flow velocity and also decrease blood clots in the legs, which happen when blood pools or with long periods of inactivity. I wear them on long flights to prevent blood clot complications; I put them on just prior to the flight and remove them on landing.

Clean Your Brain Lying Supine

You're not likely to catch a giraffe sleeping. Giraffes in the wild don't get much sleep, and much of the time their rest happens while standing up.[31] Although I know a few people who claim they can sleep while sitting upright (at their desks no less), this is not ideal. We have evolved optimal positions for good sleep: our hearts and brains must rest at nearly the same physical level to achieve deep sleep, hence the need to lie flat.

Relative to the rest of the body, a head tilt too far up or down by just a few degrees can have surprisingly big effects on our physiology. For example, lying down in a position where your head is tilted back six degrees below the body—in what's called head-down tilt (HDT) position that mimics the effects of weightlessness—reduces blood flow (perfusion) to the brain and leads to jugular vein congestion. Such a backup means the glymphatic system, by which the brain clears metabolic waste products, comes to a halt. As we saw in chapter 2, this system is responsible for removing toxic metabolic waste products that build up during our waking hours as part of the brain's normal metabolism, including the dangerous beta-amyloid protein that has been associated with Alzheimer's disease. Space doctors today use HDT on people in laboratory settings to mimic spaceflight and study the challenges of weightless sleep, as astronauts' sleep is often disturbed.

Sleeping with your head elevated has also been shown to significantly decrease glymphatic action in the brain, which may have long-term implications for cognitive decline and risk for Alzheimer's disease. But don't panic if you enjoy a lot of pillows beneath your head at night: you're not going to compromise your brain's housecleaning by a slight lift. Sleep deprivation and poor sleep will do more to undermine the glymphatic system than extra feathers. But ideally, supine is superior. Sleep is medicine, but position matters.

The Heart as an Endocrine Organ

With the current prevalence of hypertension reaching epidemic proportions, with more than a billion people globally walking around with elevated blood pressure, one can only hope that we humans do not have to evolve into giraffes. Approximately 20 percent of the entire US population is hypertensive at any given time, and the majority of the population develops some degree of hypertension with increasing age. Given the downstream effects that raised blood pressure causes in the body, it remains the leading cause of death globally, accounting for 10.4 million deaths per year, half a million of them in the United States. We are not so cleverly designed as the noble giraffe.

After Roosevelt's untimely demise and well into the latter part of the twentieth century, as awareness about hypertension exploded, so did our understanding of how to treat the condition with medications that take into account the importance of hormones. Although the hormonal basis for the development of hypertension is far from simple, it is gradually being figured out. Recent developments have helped firmly establish the heart as an endocrine (hormonal) organ, and this is probably not unique to us humans. Scientists are finding that the mammalian heart is linked to a cavalcade of important hormones related to its health, blood pressure control, and even kidney function—giraffes included. But giraffes remain the exception to the rule that hypertension is bad. An important difference between the giraffe's physiology and ours is that giraffes evolved to have high blood pressure to accommodate their elongated necks and survive, whereas we do not gain a survival benefit from it. Quite the contrary, our hypertension puts us in danger. We are not giraffes, and so we must protect our hearts and circulatory systems lest we experience heartbreak.

Creature Cheat Sheet

The cleaner we keep our arteries throughout our lifetimes, the better. We don't need giraffes or space doctors or even *Mona Lisa*'s master to tell us that. Monitor your blood pressure regularly (once a month or so, at various times during the day) and aim to keep it at 120/80 mmHg or lower. You can find patterns in your levels if you track it more closely throughout the day and match your numbers to your activities (and levels of stress). This can give you good information about how your behaviors and mindset factor into your physical being. If you cannot gain control of a healthy blood pressure, medications will help and significantly lower your risk for serious conditions related to chronic hypertension, including premature aging and death.

The keys to keeping blood pressure in check are clear: maintain cardiovascular fitness and leanness, don't smoke, sleep soundly in as flat a position as possible, maintain dental hygiene, and move frequently throughout the day—jacking your heart rate up 50 percent above your resting baseline for at least fifteen minutes daily. When you can't get up for long periods of time, say, when traversing an ocean on an airplane, imitate the giraffe's built-in technology and wear compression socks even if you don't think you have a circulatory problem (and think about those noise-canceling headphones to enjoy the journey and your meals). For those with chronic high blood pressure, drugs are critical to help bring those numbers into better balance. And the next time your vision blurs, make an appointment with the ophthalmologist. A look behind the eyes might be just what the doctor ordered.

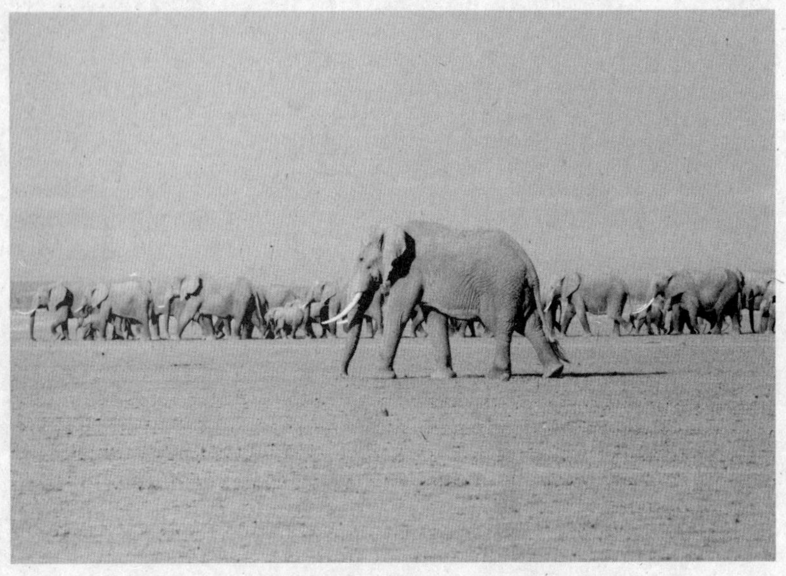

A herd of elephants roaming in Africa.

5

"Yo, Elephant Man"

A Cure for Cancer and a Call to Protect Our DNA

> *Nature's great masterpiece, an elephant; the only harmless great thing.*
>
> —JOHN DONNE

Days before the inauguration of President Donald Trump in January 2017, I was in Davos, Switzerland, for the World Economic Forum when Vice President Joe Biden called out to me in a crowded hallway: "Yo, Elephant Man!" Contrary to what you might be thinking, that was not an insult (though he had forgotten my name). Biden was not referring to the unfortunate story of the nineteenth-century Englishman, Joseph Merrick, who was born with a rare genetic disorder that severely and progressively disfigured him starting at the age of five, leading to the cruel nickname. I am "the elephant man" for a story about real elephants that I had told the prior year at the same event; a "war on cancer" meeting had been hastily organized at the behest of President Obama, who'd placed Biden in charge of a cancer moonshot initiative at the State of the Union address days prior. Biden was not the only one in the room intrigued by my story. You see, elephants have an innate genetic oddity: they evade developing cancer. But before we get to the cancer story, let's get to know these gentle giants that have been roaming the planet since about fifty-six million years ago, when they originated in Africa from ancestors the size of pigs.

Elephants belong to the order Proboscidea (Greek for "having a nose")—in reference to their trunks. The name *elephant* is from the Greek word *elephas*, referring to ivory and not the animal, and later became the name of the animal. Elephants are the largest land mammals in the world and don't have any natural predators, but they are terrified of ants and bees. And for good reason: if you had a trunk that was highly sensitive and full of nerve endings, imagine getting a swarm of ants or bees inside it. Like humans, elephants can live to be over seventy and sometimes eighty years old.* To keep up with their size, they can eat up to three hundred pounds of food a day, sometimes spending as much as sixteen to eighteen hours chomping down grasses, small plants, fruit, twigs, tree bark, and bushes (they are not picky eaters, but they are herbivores).

Elephants are a keystone species, meaning they create and maintain their own ecosystems. Keystone species help define an entire ecosystem and often ensure the survival of other species in the same shared environment. In fact, many plant and animal species are dependent on elephants in their habitat to live, and were it not for the presence and activities of the elephants, these other living creatures would cease to exist. One way elephants contribute to the ecosystem is by digging watering holes during periods of drought that help hydrate smaller animals. And elephants transport seedlings in their dung to spur new plant growth, as well as help control the tree population

*Pachyderms may avoid cancer, but they don't avoid bad teeth. Their lives can hinge on dental health. Elephants die mostly from old age when their teeth wear out and they cannot eat. This is true of many animals in the wild. According to the CDC, nearly one in five adults aged sixty-five or older in the United States have lost all their teeth, which can affect nutrition. Those who have no teeth or have dentures tend to prefer soft and easily chewed foods and can miss out on nutrient bombs such as fresh fruits and vegetables.

to support the grasses that feed them. As they tramp across the land, they thin out young trees by stepping on or eating them.[1] Keystone species live throughout the tree of life, from deep in the sea to the tallest of mountains and include fungi, bacteria, and other microbes, in addition to species of plants and animals.

When I was on safari in Africa with my family, we were entertained by a teenage elephant that seemed to be as entertained by us as we him. He would take a few steps toward our Jeep, away from his family pack, throw his trunk, and sound off, playfully communicating with us before falling back in line with his relatives. It's astonishing to watch these behemoth creatures move, eat, play, and tend to their babies. One of the things I admire most about them is that at the watering hole, they are respectful of other animals, a lesson we humans would do well to learn. These pensive, highly intelligent animals embody compassion, loyalty, teamwork, kindness, family, and individuality. And they are more like us than you probably realize. It's no surprise that some of our most beloved fictional characters are elephants: Disney's Dumbo, Dr. Seuss's Horton, and Jean de Brunhoff's Babar from the series of books dating back to the 1930s.

Empathy, Memory, and Respect

The San Diego Zoo Safari Park is one of the largest tourist attractions in San Diego County and a terrific place to see elephants. The park was installed in 1962 as a breeding ground for wild and endangered animals, but its popularity eventually compelled the county to open it up to the public. Today more than two million people visit the park annually, which houses over twenty-six hundred animals from more than three hundred species from six continents, as well as thirty-five hundred varieties of plants. The park has the world's largest veterinary hospital and a loyal following: some of the people I met there had been working in the zoo for more than three decades. The animals are their family.

Mindy Albright, one of the main elephant caretakers, shared the delights of working with an animal that gets to know its keepers, one of the indications of an elephant's incredible memory. Not only can they remember people and other elephants from previous years, but they can also remember paths to food and water they have visited in the past.[2]

Elephants are highly intelligent. They are right up there with dolphins, apes, and us. Most mammals are born with brains weighing about 90 percent of what their brain's ultimate weight will be. However, elephant and human brains develop significantly after birth. We are born with about 25 percent of our adult brain weight; elephants are born with about 35 percent.[3] Such continued brain growth outside the womb leaves adult humans and elephants with larger brains (as a proportion of total body size) than other mammals, including other primates, which may well account for our intelligence.

In 2006, researchers at Emory University in Atlanta reported that elephants belong to an exclusive group of animals that can recognize their reflections in a mirror.[4] That says a lot. Because elephants have the ability to recognize themselves in mirrors, it means that they acknowledge themselves as individuals rather than as just part of the herd. Because of this "self-awareness," elephants seem to show empathy and support for one another, working collaboratively and cooperatively with their fellow pachyderms. We know from human studies that more self-awareness makes for more cognitive empathy, so it's not hard to note similarities with elephants. Although it's hard to prove that anecdotal observations of elephant empathy are in fact real examples of empathic displays on par with those of humans, researchers who spend a great deal of time watching herds of elephants in the wild have found that they routinely help one another when in need. This is especially true among the females when there's a baby in distress. If a baby falls, all the females will run over to the baby to see if she or he is okay. Responses to distress calls from infants are common across many species in the mammalian kingdom, but elephants take SOS calls to the next level.[5] Apparently, it takes a herd to raise a child. Cynthia Moss, an elephant researcher whose 1988 book *Elephant Memories* was nominated for the National Book Award, once saw a baby elephant fall into a watering hole. The mother and her sister could not lift her out, so other elephants in the pack dug a ramp to lift the baby out of the hole.

In 2014, elephant intelligence researcher Joshua Plotnick of Hunter College and primatologist Frans de Waal, who studies animal behavior at Emory University where Plotnick used to work, published the first empirical evidence of elephants consoling others in distress using vocalizations and physical touches with their trunks.[6] Their observational study focused on a group of twenty-six captive Asian elephants spread over about thirty acres at an elephant camp in northern Thailand over the course of nearly a year. Other research has revealed that elephants can even take a great interest in the bones of their deceased, perhaps a sign of grieving for the dead. In 2016, a student studying elephants in Africa caught this behavior on camera; as she watched, three different elephant families came to pay tribute to the dead matriarch and repeatedly walked past the body.[7]

Elephants have strong familial bonds that they maintain for life. They travel in matriarchal family groups called herds, which are led by the oldest (and usually largest) female. Experience is respected, as things the matriarch learned many years earlier might be helpful for the herd's survival today. If there's a drought, the matriarch might lead the herd to a watering hole she visited at some time in her past, even if this was many years before, or she might usher her family away from an area that is showing signs of decline (quite different from our own society, in which elderly wisdom is all too often not prized). In human studies dating back to the 1980s, scientists have shown again and again that the need to feel valued—to matter and belong—is a basic one across all ages and particularly so among the elderly who are more likely to face marginalization in our society.[8] Elephants show us that respecting elders goes a long way to protecting everyone—giving everyone a survival advantage.

An example of this matriarchal benefit comes from a 2008 study by the Wildlife Conservation Society and the Zoological Society of London.[9] The study looked at three herds of elephants in 1993 during the worst drought in Tanzania's Tarangire National Park in thirty-five years. During a nine-month period, sixteen of eighty-one elephant calves in the study died, a mortality rate of 20 percent—much greater than the typical 2 percent mortality rate of calves during nondrought years. The researchers documented a striking difference between the calves that perished and those that survived: age of the leading mother. Two of the groups left the park, presumably because their respective matriarchs—aged forty-five and thirty-eight years—remembered the warning signs from droughts past and sensed danger ahead. They suffered lower mortality rates than the group that remained, which suffered 63 percent of the mortality for the year. In their conclusions, the researchers pointed out that the matriarchs in the herds that moved out of the park likely recalled the drought of 1958–1961, when they were little ones themselves, whereas the group that remained in Tarangire had no individuals old enough to remember the historic event. Other studies have found that herds led by matriarchs over age thirty-five have better survival rates.[10]

It's astonishing to think that elephants can be so wise and so empathetic when they have no obvious language. But they do have their own way to communicate that we humans cannot easily hear or detect and then interpret (they use distinct sounds at high and low frequencies, as well as employ tactile signals through touching). If I could tune in to this channel, I'd ask a few questions. Chief among them: How'd you get to be so good at avoiding cancer?

How to Not Get Cancer

Elephants' gigantic bodies carry up to one hundred times more cells than ours do, which you would think would make them much more prone to cancer. Cancer is unregulated cell division that initiates in one cell that acquires a mutation in a gene involved in cell growth. The more cells you have, the more likely it is that any one of those cells goes rogue, turning into a tumor. Broadly speaking, taller people have a statistically higher risk of developing cancer, with some studies showing that the risk goes up by about 10 percent for every four-inch increase in height.[11]* But variations and variables abound, and risk for some cancers, such as pancreatic, esophageal, stomach, and mouth, do not seem to increase with height. It's important to keep in mind that even if you're very tall and carry a slightly increased risk for certain cancers as a result, your underlying genes, environment, and other lifestyle factors will weigh much more heavily into your overall lifetime risk.

Elephants somehow dodged this statistical bullet entirely in what has become one of cancer's great conundrums, called Peto's paradox. Sir Richard Peto is an Oxford University medical statistician and epidemiologist whose work in the 1970s pointed to the link between smoking and cancer. He first wrote about the paradox that today bears his name in 1975 when he noted that on a cell-for-cell basis, humans are much less susceptible to cancer than mice: "A man has 1000 times as many cells as a mouse . . . and we usually live at least 30 times as long as mice."[12] When you take into consideration the mere cell count difference between a mouse and human, you'd think

*So, does that mean heavier people are more prone to cancer too? Yes, but not so much because extra weight, or obesity, means larger organs with more cells. Obesity is a risk factor for cancer for a whole host of reasons, from how excess fat tissue influences metabolism and hormonal signaling that in turn affect how and when cells die, to how that visceral fat around vital organs stokes the fires of inflammation.

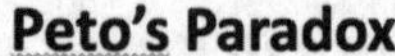

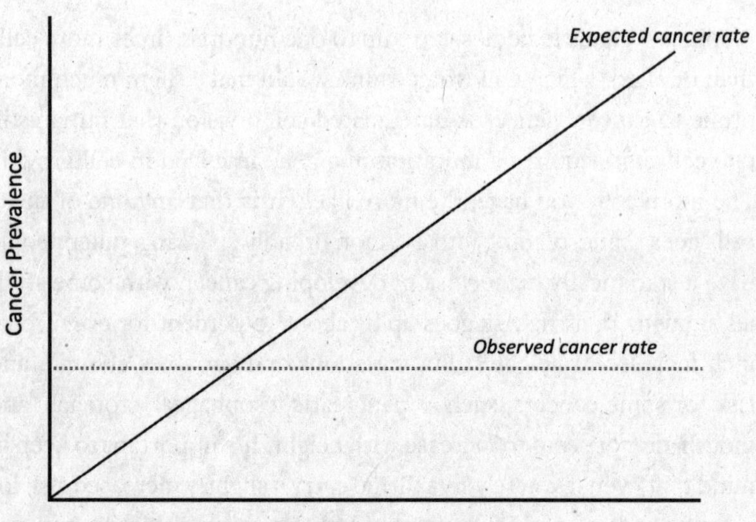

Cancer is defined as a disease of uncontrolled cell growth and division, and the risk of developing cancer should theoretically increase with the number of cell divisions during the lifetime of an organism. Hence, the expected cancer rate for very large and/or long-lived species should be much higher than for smaller and short-lived ones. The solid black line is the expected linear relationship between cancer rate and body mass x life span. The dotted line represents the observation in nature that there is no relationship between cancer risk and body mass x life span. For instance, lifetime cancer risk in humans (39.5 percent of developing cancer, 19.5 percent chance of dying from cancer) is not dramatically different from mice (life span of only 2–3 years and average weight of less than an ounce). In contrast, cancer risk was estimated to be less than 5 percent in elephants (life span of 50–70 years and weight of up to 15,000 pounds). Cancer rates in whales (blue whale life span of 80–90 years and average weight of 290,000 to 330,000 pounds) are not known, but these models predict that 100 percent of the blue whales should have cancer by age ninety, which has not been what has been observed in nature. Adapted from M. Tollis, A. M. Boddy, and C. C. Maley, "Peto's Paradox: How Has Evolution Solved the Problem of Cancer Prevention?," *BMC Biology* 15, no. 1 (July 2017): 60.

we'd be more vulnerable to cancer (and, by extension, premature death), but we're not. While the concept of "more cells, more cancer" makes intuitive sense, the data don't support it across species. The increased cancer incidence in mice compared with humans clearly makes the statement that there is more to cancer than the number of cells in an organism. Peto went on to suggest that evolutionary considerations were likely responsible for varying per cell carcinogenesis (cancer formation) rates across species. In relation to elephants, we are like the mice—prone to cancer even though we carry far fewer cells.

Baby elephants come out of the womb weighing in at a whopping three hundred pounds and grow to more than ten thousand pounds in fewer than ten years. Such a rate of explosive cellular division would seemingly make them highly vulnerable to the disease from birth. If elephants weren't prepared for cancer, they'd go extinct. But nature has solved this potential problem for them.

Almost 25 percent of us will die of cancer. (A human's lifetime risk of cancer is between 33 and 50 percent—roughly 43 percent for men and 38 percent for women—but today, 75 to 89 percent of people diagnosed with cancer survive.) By the time humans reach adulthood, their cells will have divided and DNA been copied about *thirty trillion times*, and each of these events could result in a cancer-causing mutation. Cell division is a carefully controlled process involving hundreds of genes, some encouraging cell proliferation and others suppressing it. Other genes signal when damaged cells should undergo apoptosis, or programmed cell death. When a normal cell becomes cancerous, enough mutations have accumulated in the genes that control cellular growth that the damaged cell is no longer able to destroy itself. By some measures, most cancer cells have sixty or more mutations, including on both copies of the genes within a cell normally responsible for apoptosis (also known as tumor suppressor genes). These cells divide more rapidly than their healthy "parents," becoming less dependent on signals from other cells that would help with controlling their growth and death. So although cancerous cells possess multiple abnormalities that would otherwise make them prime targets for apoptosis, they are clever enough to evade programmed cell death. They go rogue.

Although some genetic mutations that can lead to cancer may be inherited from a sperm cell or an egg, in what's called a germline mutation, most mutations are acquired in life from things like exposure to tobacco, radiation, viruses, or merely age. Some people erroneously think extra vitamins and supplements will fill holes in our diets and protect us from developing cancer as we age. Yet those extra nutrients can actually work against us, disrupting our systems and increasing our risk of disease, cancer (and heart disease) included. Too much of anything can be hazardous, and when it comes to vitamins and supplements, many of their active ingredients have strong effects on the body that at large doses can be harmful and entail serious side effects, with no benefit. So what should you do? Take the advice I've already doled out: get your vitamins and minerals from real food. No megadosing. Wild animals don't supplement, and even the size of an elephant can be sustained through real food.

Mighty elephants' cells rarely go rogue, and so their cancer risk is a fraction of ours. An elephant's lifetime risk of cancer is less than 5 percent, and fewer than 5 percent of all elephants will die of the malady. Scientists have known this for decades, ever since Sir Richard Peto began his investigations in the 1970s, but only recently have we begun to crack the code, so to speak, to understand the elephant's anticancer profile.

Elephants have a robust cancer defense system that is based on a protein called p53. ("53" is the protein's molecular weight as measured in kilodaltons.) This anticancer molecule and the tumor-suppressing gene that encodes it—TP (for tumor protein) 53—has gotten a lot of attention in the past thirty or so years, especially since *Science* magazine declared it Molecule of the Year in December 1993.[13] When it was discovered in 1979, it was initially thought to be an oncogene—a gene that turned cancer *on*. Not until a decade later did we begin to understand its anticancer effects. Like a county sheriff, p53 protein is called or activated within cells' nuclei when there's trouble: damaged DNA. The activated protein attaches directly to the DNA, essentially arresting the cell to determine whether the DNA will be repaired or the cell undergoes apoptosis. If the DNA is fixable, p53 activates other genes to repair the damage before the cell can divide again. And if the DNA is not restorable, which can happen when there are too many or too complex mutations, p53 prevents the cell from dividing and orders (signals) it to self-destruct. More recently, researchers have found that another key element to this anticancer machinery is a so-called zombie gene that's normally nonfunctioning in mammals but becomes activated in elephants by p53 when there are damaged cells that could be precursors to cancer cells. The gene, called LIF6, awakens to make a protein that dashes to the damaged cells' mitochondria, or energy center, and assassinates the cells by poking holes in them.

Tumor protein 53 (TP53) is the most popular gene studied today.[14] On average, around two papers are published every day describing new details of its basic biology. The gene for p53 (the gene is called TP53 and the protein it encodes is p53) resides on chromosome 17. This gene is mutated in roughly half of all human cancers. In patient after patient, the cancer pathology report I get says that TP53 is mutated. There is a syndrome (I describe it shortly) where the defective gene isn't just in the tumor; it is also in the underlying genomic sequence of the individual (called germline DNA) that is passed on to the next generation. Children who inherit the defective copies of the TP53 gene from a parent have a high likelihood of developing cancer—approximately 73 percent in men and close to 100 percent in women.[15] Here's the other thing: we humans have only two copies of the TP53 gene, one from Mom and another from Dad. Lots of other animals that avoid cancer entirely have more functional copies of TP53—like having extra pairs of running shoes when your worn-out ones go bad before you've finished the race. Elephants have

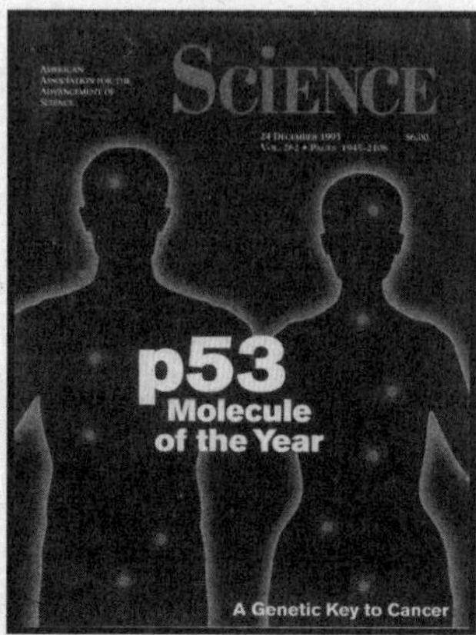

Cover of *Science* magazine, December 24, 1993, declaring p53 the "Molecule of the Year."

at least twenty copies of TP53, a biological bonus that's the secret to their cancer-free status. They possess dramatically more tumor-suppressing powers than humans, and it turns out that elephants' p53 only kills bad cells; it won't even leave them to be repaired.

Interestingly, studies have found that most of the TP53 genes in elephants are retrogenes, meaning that elephants originally had only two TP53 genes and that these extra genes were selected for over a long period of elephant evolution. It's thought that elephants gained more TP53 genes coincidentally as they evolved from smaller ancestors.

How does knowing this help us? Next time you're at a zoo watching an elephant, take a look at those veins in its floppy ears. That maroon blood coursing through them may one day be a source for generating new anticancer therapies. Unfortunately, the obvious solution—forcing more p53 production in humans—hasn't worked. Arnie Levine, one of the discoverers of p53 while at Princeton University, told me that he once tried overexpressing the gene by putting extra copies into the mouse genome in a laboratory setting, but the animals died before they were born. And forcing more activity out of the gene may trigger other problems because the gene is also linked in humans to neurodegenerative diseases. There's a complexity here to consider, which will likely vary depending on species' unique physiology. A balance must be struck in its regulation—when it should be turned on versus off.

Nevertheless, there's a clue here that we must explore further. The LIF6 discovery has ignited interest in developing drugs that get cancerous cells to turn on their existing zombie copies of the LIF gene. One passionate scientist already thinks he might be onto something.

Out for Elephant Blood

Cancer is deeply personal for Joshua Schiffman. Growing up in Providence, Rhode Island, he was fifteen years old when his father, an oncologist at Brown University, palpated Schiffman's enlarged lymph nodes in his neck and knew what lay ahead. Schiffman's illness was diagnosed as stage 2 Hodgkin's disease, a type of blood cancer—one not too different from the cancer that had afflicted the family dog, Frank, a German shepherd. The summer of 1989 became one of "R and R," as he puts it: rest and radiation. After working in the morning, Schiffman's dad would pick him up at lunchtime and drive the fifty miles to Boston Children's Hospital for radiation, after which they'd drive back home and Schiffman would spend his evenings vomiting (the radiation hit an area of the brain where the nausea response is triggered)—and then do it all over again the next day.[16]

It was a time for good father-son bonding for sure, but Schiffman jokes today as a father himself that it must have been annoying for his dad to listen to him in the car ask twenty questions every hour. Schiffman was cured, and cancer medicine has since become his area of specialty. Although he spent a blink thinking about being a Hollywood screenwriter, his father's persuasions soon had him in Brown's eight-year combined baccalaureate-MD program. This was not a common education. Brown's program in liberal medical education emphasizes a humanistic approach to medicine, with classes taught by poets and playwrights.

After graduation, Schiffman felt pulled to go west and found himself at Stanford University, where he became interested in palliative care for children, caring for them near the end of their lives. One weekend, a four-year-old girl came into the hospital where he was on call. Two years earlier, she'd survived a brain tumor with surgery. Now, her father had just died from brain cancer, and her uncle (the dad's brother) had also died of the disease. This was a big clue that some underlying genetics were at work, and Schiffman's curiosity was sparked.[17]

I first spoke with Schiffman years ago when he was beginning his efforts to design a new cancer therapeutic based on the natural cancer resistance of elephants. By then he'd moved to Salt Lake City, where he'd taken a job at the University of Utah to continue his work in pediatric oncology. He wanted to know why some kids seemed to be born with a predisposition to cancer, as if they'd inherited some unlucky gene. He increasingly trained his expertise on Li-Fraumeni syndrome, a rare genetic disorder (that we mentioned a few pages back) where a person has only a single normal copy of the TP53 gene. Of all the genetic predispositions to cancer to study, arguably none is as extreme as Li-Fraumeni syndrome, which gives people with the syndrome as close to a 100 percent chance of developing cancer as you can get. Utah was an ideal destination partly because Schiffman loved the "big spaces and openness to ideas," but mostly because the Mormon community's genealogy culture provided a built-in cohort to study. One family in particular, the Thompsons, passed the mutation down through multiple generations, living with fatal cancer diagnoses or the threat of them.[18] One can only imagine the agony of harboring a strong desire to have children with the knowledge that any one of your children could become a certain cancer victim.

Schiffman is a father to three kids of his own and as spry as cancer is wily. His cluttered, unglamorous office is testament to his dedication: there are disordered piles of papers behind him that he needs to read, and two kids' drawings that look as if they were hastily taped to the wall. Voluble and intense, with a childlike passion, the sort of person who sees the glass as half full, he's either immersed in his research, teaching, collaborating, and ministering to sick children, or taking his own brood to the zoo to see the elephants. His appreciation for elephants came in the summer of 2012, twenty-three years after his own touch with near death. He was in Bar Harbor, Maine, for a conference about evolutionary medicine and comparative oncology, the study of cancer across different species. He was hoping to learn how to translate what we know about cancer in dogs to cancer in humans. He had no idea what he was in for.

One of the presenters was Carlo C. Maley, who at the time was an associate professor at Arizona State researching cancer and evolution (and who is now the director of the Arizona Cancer Evolution Center). When Maley got up to lecture and announced he was going to talk about elephants, Schiffman nearly bolted for the door. What could an elephant teach him about cancer? A lot, it turned out. It was there that Schiffman first learned about Peto's paradox. Elephants spend about twenty-two months in the womb, an extensive time attributed to their need for more brain development so as to gain complex cognitive skills immediately usable at birth to survive in their environment. And females can keep reproducing until their old age: after fifty. As Schiffman explained to me, elephants that are able to suppress cancer can continue to have children until a late age and then pass on this ability to the next generation. Most humans develop cancer in late middle age, after they classically have had children, but at a point when cancer-causing mutations have amassed over time and can overwhelm tumor-suppressing genes. This is why, in Schiffman's words, "cancer is a disease of aging."[19] Mother Nature is not so protective of you once you've fulfilled her wishes of procreating and parenting.

After Maley's talk, Schiffman asked him about the prospects of getting his hands on some elephant blood to study in the lab. Maley's response: "Josh, if you can do that, I'll tell you what: we'll put your name on the paper." Schiffman's paper would be years in the making.

A few weeks after the event in Bar Harbor, Schiffman went to Hogle Zoo on the edge of Salt Lake City with his three young children. His request to obtain some elephant blood was first met with a threat to call security, but eventually he befriended the elephants' caretakers and gained approval. From the zookeeper's perspective, if people realized that elephants possessed the cure for cancer, they'd take greater care to save them. (An estimated one hundred African elephants are killed each day by poachers seeking ivory, meat, and body parts as trophies.)[20] Since 2012, the procedure has always been the same: the zookeeper at Hogle draws elephant blood from a big, prominent vein behind their ears into large test tubes, which then travel the short distance in Igloo coolers to Schiffman's lab. The elephants receive a lot of praise and treats during the blood draw; they've gotten used to it, as have their keepers. Once the blood samples are in the lab, Schiffman's researchers conduct a series of biochemical reactions with reagents and centrifuges to pull the cells apart, trying to understand what makes elephants resistant to cancer under the magic of their p53 genes. Schiffman has also partnered with the Ringling Bros. and Barnum & Bailey Center for Elephant Conservation in Polk City, Florida, home to the largest herd of Asian elephants in North America, which will give him a treasure trove of new genetic data.

Schiffman thinks medicine could eventually arrive at a compound that replicates the p53-rich nature of elephants or even find a way to insert elephant p53 into people. In order to translate his laboratory finding to patients, he cofounded a company, PEEL Therapeutics ("Peel" not surprisingly means elephant in Hebrew), with a nanotechnology team based in Israel to find suitable drug delivery systems for his synthetic elephant p53, known as eP53. Can they create an anticancer delivery system via a pill or an injection? So far, eP53 has been successfully encapsulated in tiny, ultrafine nanoparticles that are 1/1,000th the size of a single human hair; in petri dishes, the compound has been demonstrated to kill cancer cells within twenty-four hours. Will it work in humans? Will we one day be mixing nanoparticles into a morning shake for an anticancer breakfast? Will our dogs get some in their kibble?

One point that elephant studies emphasize is that the initiation of cancer requires a DNA change. And so until these new medicines become available, we have to strive to decrease any possibility of DNA alterations that could spell trouble. This includes obvious cancer-busting habits: Stay out of the sun during peak hours of the day, as higher-energy UV rays often have enough energy to remove electrons and molecules from atoms in the skin, which damages DNA and triggers mutations. Avoid inflammation. When an inflammatory process starts in the body, chemicals including cytokines, histamine, and prostaglandins are released by the damaged tissue to help spur the healing process. If this continues for too long, these highly reactive molecules can cause DNA damage. Inflammation itself also stimulates cells to divide. This is why, for example, people with chronic inflammatory diseases, such as ulcerative colitis and Crohn's disease, have an increased risk of colon cancer. People who are overweight also live with a higher risk for cancer because excess fat tissue is itself inflammatory, as fat tissue contains adipokines, a special type of cytokine. Any metabolic disorder, in fact, regardless of weight—from high blood pressure or cholesterol to insulin resistance and diabetes—will increase one's risk for cancer due to the heightened inflammation that occurs when the body's metabolic status is abnormal. In an unhealthy environment, cells begin to behave differently. Even toxic levels of psychological stress can do damage through the increased production of hormones like cortisol. So yes, how you *think*—and respond to stressors in your life—factors into your risk for cancer. While it's hard to consider intangible thoughts concretizing into cancer, we're finally documenting this trail from the invisible to the visible. Our behavior *does* matter.

An elephant has fault tolerance built in with its TP53 duplications, which ensures that even if one or two copies of TP53 become damaged, the animal has enough others to compensate. *Fault tolerance*, a term borrowed from the computer and electronics world, refers to redundancies built into a system, so that if one part fails, the system can continue to operate properly. A single glitch won't cause the entire thing to crash. The human immune system is a huge player in our own biological fault tolerance, capable of preventing infections from approximately 10,000,000,000,000,000 (10^{16}) foreign sources. That's ten quadrillion potential threats. Unfortunately, cancer is also extremely fault tolerant. Every time I treat a case of metastatic cancer, the tumor cells figure out a work-around to the pathway I am targeting. None of the targeted therapies developed so far are curative in the metastatic setting. (That is one terrifying whopper of a statement.)

I'm heartened, however, to know that researchers like Joshua Schiffman are seeking out inventive ways to help us protect ourselves. In 2021, a group of scientists at the Wellcome Sanger Institute in Cambridge, England, reported on some captivating genetic studies that looked at how ordinary healthy cells of the esophagus gain mutations with age that would seem likely to lead to cancer.[21] By middle age, more than half of the cells lining the esophagus contain mutations, an alarmingly high percentage, but esophageal cancer remains rare; it's only the fourteenth most common cancer in adults of more than one hundred types. It turns out the cells that carry these mutations (known as mutant clones) are actually outcompeting early tumors so they never grow into cancer. The high density of mutant clones in the esophagus makes for a competitive environment in which cancer cells can't find space to survive. In other words, clones of cells with "advantageous" mutations act as police; they have a tumor-suppressive role in the environment that is independent of the body's immune system. This research goes to show that the survival of early tumors may not depend solely on the mutations they carry, but also on the mutations within the neighboring normal tissue.[22] Once again, this reinforces the power of the environment to support, stall, or halt the development of bad cancers. It's astonishing to think we can gain protection from cancer, a disease of mutations, from other mutations. Such a finding may one day allow us to use mutant clones in the war on cancer—in addition to any medicines we can develop from elephant blood.

Schiffman's elephant blood almost didn't make headlines. When he and Carlo Maley, who remain close collaborators, submitted their seminal paper with a consortium of scientists to describe how TP53 works in elephants, it was rejected by some of the most prestigious publications before it was finally accepted and published in the *Journal of the American Medical Association* in 2015.*[23] At each rejection, Schiffman never doubted the purpose of his mission. Schiffman told *Newsweek*, "Nature's figured it out. The elephants have already done it. The whales have already done it."[24] Bowhead whales also live up to Peto's paradox, sometimes living in arctic waters for two hundred years, cancer-free. As Schiffman said: "Why can't we?"[25]

Spatial Intelligence and Forgetting

It may take years for us to realize how we can turn an elephant's robust fault tolerance and anticancer biology into medicine we can use, but it shouldn't take years to learn from elephants' memory skills. I don't know anyone who doesn't worry about losing their mind to

*It's common for academic papers under peer review to face multiple rounds of editorial feedback and skepticism before being accepted by a prestigious medical journal. And it can take time before a new idea in scientific circles gains enough traction and support to further inspire research and more studies. In the words of one of the great p53 researchers, Moshe Oren, "Nowadays, p53 is like a Dreamliner airplane, riding the high skies of cancer research with dignity and pride."

what is now the most common form of dementia in the elderly, Alzheimer's disease, which rivals cancer as our most dreaded ailment. We'll be revisiting this ailment in chapter 9 when we address intelligence through the eyes of some sea creatures, but it's worth highlighting here that elephants have much to teach us about one particular aspect of memory: spatial awareness.

Spatial awareness is not about eyesight acuity per se; if it were, then elephants would not be good models because their vision is not that sharp. In 2015, scientists figured out that elephants' excellent spatial memory is what allows them to track down water resources across large distances of the savanna; they can choose the shortest distances to quench their thirst even when they are thirty miles away.[26] Spatial awareness is being aware of objects in our environment and our relationship to them; for example, you drive on the right side of the highway in the United States and doing otherwise feels awkward. Are we cognizant of people's personal space so we don't get uncomfortably close? Is our coordination good enough to catch objects with ease? Can we walk and drive without the help of apps? Do we struggle with reading, writing, and basic math? These three skills actually require a lot of spatial awareness—for grasping sentence structure, grammar, geometry, and number arrangement.

Although multiple areas of the brain are involved in our spatial awareness, the right side—the hub for controlling artistic endeavors, creativity, and imagination—dominates. This also means that some of the best ways to improve our spatial intelligence are fun: find a new creative hobby such as drawing, painting, photography, or learning a musical instrument; play games that get you thinking creatively or have a visual-memory component (e.g., puzzles, chess, even some video games that involve moving objects); and engage in physical activities that force your body to move through space and navigate accordingly, from vinyasa yoga to jogging or cycling.

And let's not forget to forget. Perhaps that's another way elephants have such strong memory power: they don't try to remember everything the way we do. The brain is ill-equipped to handle an abundance of data. People who win memory contests often attribute their extraordinary recall abilities to forgetfulness—to discarding unnecessary data so they can retain what's important. While we used to think that forgetting was a passive process that served no useful purpose, research in the past decades proves otherwise: it's an active mechanism constantly at work in the brain to keep it poised to learn new things and store more memories. As novelist Henry Miller once stated, "My 'forgettery' has been just as important to my success as my memory."

Training our brains to forget starts with actively not paying attention to anything that doesn't serve us well or gets in the way of our goals. We can consciously decide not to dwell on past disappointments, weakening the neural connections around these memories, and to instead engage in life with verve. When we maintain high levels of social interaction, our brains lose focus on the memories that make us feel lonely and depressed because we're so busy making new memories. Again, our elephant friends, with their sociality and dynamic interactions within the herd, show us the way.

There's much science to back up the importance of forgetting in not only supporting mental health but also strengthening our memory skills and charging our mental flexibility, which is necessary for creative thinking and imagination. There's even a group of neurons in the brain specifically responsible for helping us to forget. They're called melanin-concentrating hormone (MCH) neurons, and they're most active at night during REM sleep when the brain is reorganizing itself to streamline memories and prepare for the next day of incoming data. These MCH neurons start firing electrical signals in the brain's memory hub—the hippocampus—to disrupt other neurons that help consolidate memory. Part of the reason so many of us don't remember our dreams may be due to the action of these MCH neurons. The discovery of how these unique memory-policing neurons operate came only in 2019 from a team of neuroscientists in Japan who documented the phenomenon in mice.[27] They surmise that these neurons function in a similar way across many species in the animal kingdom. Other neural reactions are no doubt at play in our memories as well. We know, for instance, that the neurotransmitter dopamine is involved in forming and forgetting memories. Maybe such insights can one day inform treatments for things like dementia, anxiety, or even erasing traumatic memories.

Jane Goodall certainly doesn't want to remember her first encounter with a chimpanzee chowing down on baby monkey brains. For a vegetarian like Jane, as you're soon to learn, meat-eating chimps are the proverbial elephant in the room. But we can learn a lot about diet from our hominid relatives and come to understand how to eat better ourselves.

Creature Cheat Sheet

Elephants are models for us in many ways, from how they interact positively with one another and work together for the collective good, especially during moments of distress, to how they look up to their elders for memorialized wisdom based on past insights for survival. They also tap into their spatial intelligence to help encode those important memories. And their cancer-proof blood may one day help us find new solutions to better understand and then beat the disease. Until we have our own built-in anticancer system like elephants, we must do whatever we can to protect our DNA from mutations: avoid dangerous exposures (e.g., UV radiation including that from the sun, excessive vitamins, and other supplements) and keep inflammation under control, a key concept we'll further explore later on—it's the elephant in the room on all things related to longevity. And when it comes to preserving our memories, we can't lose sight of the power of forgetting. To forget is to open the door to new possibilities.

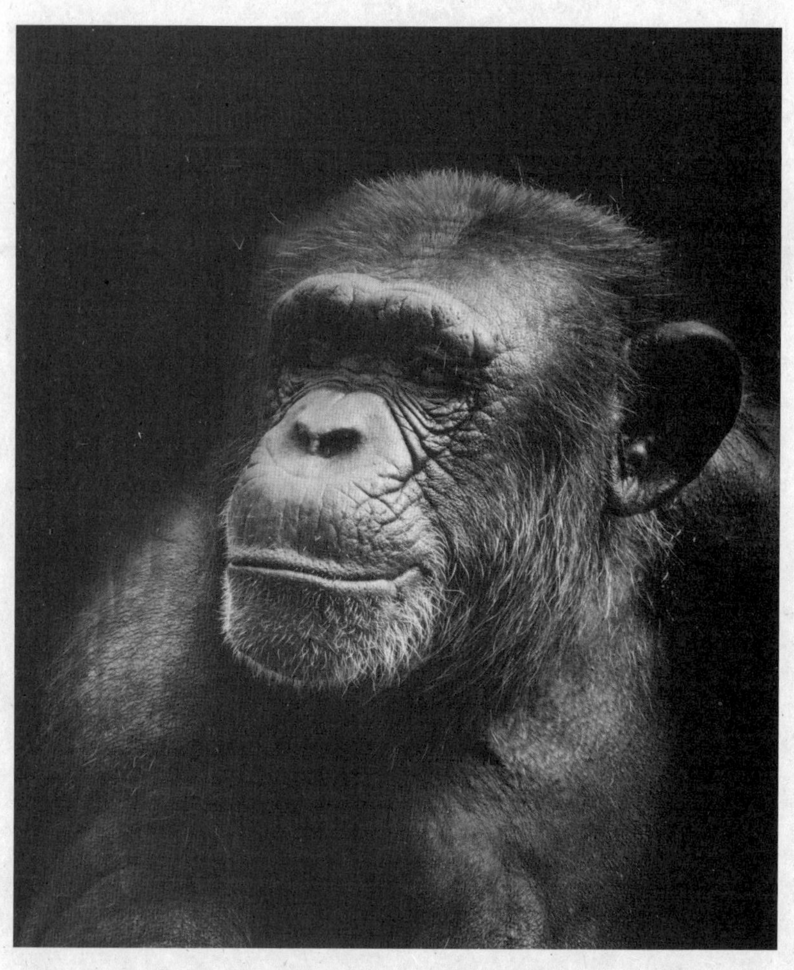

6

Carnivorous Males and Permissive Moms

Cues from Our Cousins on Eating Meat, Sharing, and Caring for Children

> *One of my best days was when I . . . offered [chimp David Greybeard] fruit on my outstretched hand, and he turned his head away. I put my hand closer—and he took the fruit, dropped it, and gently squeezed my hand, which is a chimp reassurance gesture. . . . We communicated perfectly in a language that predates words.*
>
> —JANE GOODALL

Each week I invariably receive a request to read a forthcoming book and endorse a particular diet or other fad. In the past decade, we've all encountered a dizzying array of eating plans with promises to make us thinner, happier, and healthier: paleo, low-fat, low-carb, vegan, keto, fasting, flexitarian, carnivore, raw, macrobiotic, ancestral, shepherd's, to name a few. And then there are the diets attributed to a person or brand such as WW (formerly Weight Watchers), Dubrow, Gundry, South Beach, Atkins, Noom, Dukan, Whole30, DASH (Dietary Approaches to Stop Hypertension), MIND

(Mediterranean-DASH Intervention for Neurodegenerative Delay), OPTAVIA . . . the list goes on. I am often asked which diet is best. You might be surprised by my answer: "The one that works for you and your body and allows you to enjoy a diverse but consistent variety of wholesome foods." Is sugar toxic? Not when consumed in moderation. Are the benefits of the ketogenic diet proven? Not for everyone. Is red meat so bad for our health that we should all go vegetarian lest we get cancer and heart disease and die young? I'll answer that by sharing that I love a juicy burger once in a while and I eat steak about once a week. Grass fed.

No long-term randomized studies on diets can truly be done, as diet is hard to enforce. The Mediterranean-style diet has long been shown to be a healthy choice, but it's merely a basic framework for eating that can be tailored to most cultural cuisines. Almost all of the large studies have been questionnaire based, which has its own issues (trusting participants to respond accurately). And so it's easy to cherry-pick the science to make bold claims, some of which can be absurd. Vegan advocates cite studies showing that plant-centric plates improve a man's virility; carnivores point to studies showing that meat-free diets reduce metabolism and double the risk for broken bones. It's an endless war.

The truth is we have evolved to metabolize animal protein, unlike all nonhuman primates such as chimpanzees that are frugivorous for the most part, meaning they eat mostly raw fruits, succulent fruit-like vegetables, roots, shoots, nuts, and seeds (but wait until you hear about what happens when the adult males come across a tree full of monkeys). This relatively recent meat-eating adaptation has had staggering outcomes: it allowed us to develop big brains, intellectually surpass our hominid relatives, and even shape human social behavior. No joke: sliced meat has been more beneficial to our evolution and sophistication than sliced bread.

My search to understand more about our diet in relation to one of our closest relatives, and their lower risk for disease, took me to see a primatologist who has spent most of his career observing the mammals in their native habitat. I soon learned that there's a lot more to this complex story than whether we should choose the T-bone or tofu.

A Cancer Doctor and Primatologist Meet

About a twenty-minute drive east of my former lab on USC's campus near downtown Los Angeles sits South Pasadena. It has a lazy small-town feel to it with a tidy business district whose main intersection shares the comings and goings of a modern light-rail transit system. Mom-and-pop retail shops and outdoor cafés pepper the streets that are lined by beautiful native California trees against which people leave their bicycles leaning as they meet with friends over coffee or lunch. No wonder South Pasadena is a popular stand-in for midwestern and northeastern towns in movies; scenes from films as diverse as *American Pie*, *Halloween*, and *Gone with the Wind* were shot on location in the area. Part of the original Route 66 runs through town, eventually emptying out to the Pacific several miles west. It's an area rich in history—from serving as a gateway to travel and commerce for aboriginal peoples to being where Mexican colonial rule ended in California in 1847. It became one of the first suburbs of sprawling Los Angeles. And it is here where I met Craig Stanford for lunch on a quintessential Southern California day, sunny and bright, to ask him a few questions that had been perplexing me.

In the late 1980s, when Stanford was finishing his doctoral research in Bangladesh, following a group of capped langur monkeys while living in a "ramshackle cabin" on stilts at the edge of a rice paddy, he began to think about his options for postdoctoral study (after his PhD was finished). A colleague pushed him to write to famed Jane Goodall, who was at the height of her career. Not expecting a reply, Stanford was delightfully surprised to find an invitation to go work with her in Gombe National Park to study predator-prey dynamics of chimps and the animals they sometimes hunt when given the opportunity. Stanford's way in with Jane was the carnivore in him. A typical hunt by wild chimps is brutal and savage in nature, but Stanford didn't mind watching meat-eating chimps, whereas Jane is an avid vegetarian and couldn't bear the fieldwork necessary to document the chimp diet. As Jane has written, "Farm animals are far more aware and intelligent than we ever imagined and, despite having been bred as domestic slaves, they are individual beings in their own right. As such, they deserve our respect. And our help. Who will plead for them if we are silent?"[1]

Today Stanford is professor of biological sciences and anthropology at USC. He is also a research associate in the herpetology (think reptiles and amphibians) section of the Los Angeles County Natural History Museum. We got along like old friends and after initial pleasantries, I got right to the first questions I wanted to ask: Why don't chimps get cancer? They are nearly 99 percent like us genetically yet don't suffer the same. And why are there no records of dementia?

What unfolded over the next two hours in lively conversation astounded me and got me thinking like never before. I look at things from a vanishingly small, finite, and molecular perspective—zooming in on cells and their dynamics in the nearby tissue environment. Stanford watches animals at a distance in open spaces whose three-dimensional expanse is practically infinite. Stanford even looks like someone who'd work outdoors. He's tall and broad-shouldered with a mop of thick dark hair and an aura of Indiana Jones. I couldn't imagine him confined to a lab.

To my surprise, he didn't have a good answer as to why chimps don't get cancer and why there are no records of dementia. These things apparently are not studied. In fact, chimpanzees in general are not well studied in the wild; at any given time, there are probably fewer than a hundred scientists actively engaged in chimpanzee field observation. But when new studies do emerge from this work, it's often front-page news because they provide clues to our own humanness. Stanford and his team have historically been most interested in the nature of aggression and communication, including sexual power plays and violent ambition.

Stanford's invitation to join Jane in Africa may have come about fortuitously, but it also involved more than her need for a carnivorous researcher. At the time, Jane had a field site in Tanzania at Gombe Stream National Park that had been off-limits to visitors for more than a decade. She was hoping to reestablish a camp there to study the predator-prey interactions between chimpanzees and the red colobus monkeys, whose flesh they devoured when the opportunity arose. Located in a former British colonial hunting reserve, Gombe is a small oblong patch of forest and hills, about ten miles long and two miles wide. Up against the shores of Lake Tanganyika, the camp is reachable only by boat from the harbor town of Kigoma.[2] This was where Jane's team conducted her pioneering work beginning in the 1960s, but it does have some darkness in its history.

In spring 1975, forty heavily armed rebel militia from neighboring Zaire (now the Democratic Republic of the Congo) traveled across Lake Tanganyika and kidnapped four of Jane's camp members in an intense midnight raid. Jane escaped capture, but three Stanford University students and her Dutch research assistant weren't as lucky. They were taken at gunpoint, dragged from their huts, beaten, and bound. A week into the ordeal, one of the hostages was released to deliver ransom letters demanding nearly half a million dollars, a cache of weapons, and the release of fellow rebels from Tanzanian jails. The Tanzanian government rejected the demands, and neither Stanford University nor the US government would pay the ransom. The families were left to gather enough money to end their nightmare.*

*This story never became front-page news in the United States, and the students themselves feared too much exposure to go public, so they made a pact to say nothing about their abduction. They broke their silence in 1997 when their captor, Laurent Kabila, seized control of Zaire—hoping the United States would hold him accountable for his terrorism. But their pleas fell on deaf ears. Much of the politics of the day remained

A year after Craig Stanford wrote to Jane, he reached Gombe with a permit from the Tanzanian government and a pint-sized budget. When he began his work there in the late 1980s, he didn't know much about chimpanzees other than that each member of a matriline had a name starting with the same letter. Soon enough, he'd come to know a lot about these animals—and Fifi, Frodo, Gremlin, and Goblin—as he immersed himself in their daily lives. We don't like to accept aggression—especially when it's extreme, like that of those militia raiders—as a natural human trait. But when you watch how chimps behave—how they prey, use meat as social currency, and engage in power plays—you can't help but see parallels. We'll first cover our meat-eating proclivities that we share with chimps and then see how our cousins can teach us how to be good role models for our children, which of course means showing them how to share, engage with others, and regulate their emotions.

Mastering Mastication

The next time you're slicing through a steak (or your preferred meat alternative), try to think about what it must have been like to acquire, prepare, and eat such a meal thousands of years ago, before cooking became common. We take our forks, knives, and grills for granted today, but for many animals, the act of chewing is one of life's most tedious endeavors. Our primate cousins, the chimps, spend as many as six hours a day grinding fruits and the occasional monkey between their teeth. This is possible thanks to big teeth and large jaws similar to the ones our early ancestors had. So what happened in our evolution?

First, kitchen tools had to find their way into our history. New science points to the development of primitive kitchen tools among our

---

swirling around the Cold War. When asked about it today, Jane recalls the hostage event on her watch as one of the lowest points in her celebrated career.

early ancestors long before we learned how to roast beef—as far back as more than 2.5 million years ago.[3] That's about two million years before cooking became common. *Two million.** These early ancestors, upright apes called hominins, fashioned simple stone tools to slice meat and pound root vegetables such as yams, beets, and potatoes, which had the effect of making it much easier to gain the calories they needed to survive.

A quick note about terminology: *hominids* refers to all modern and extinct great apes: humans, chimps, bonobos, gorillas, and orangutans; *hominins* refers to any species of early human that is more closely related to humans than chimpanzees. What separates the great apes from other primates, monkeys included, is that we have larger brains, larger bodies, and no tails. It's important to remember that we did not evolve from chimps, but we do share a recent common ancestor with them; chimps possess about 98.6 percent of our DNA. Now let's get back to those early ancestors of ours, who discovered how to slice raw meat. . . .

In 2016, a team of researchers from Harvard led by Daniel Lieberman and his colleague Katherine Zink conducted an experiment that may sound absurd at first.[4] They put raw-meat eating to the masticating test, taking a few dozen volunteers on something of a chewing contest.

The experiment involved the placement of electrodes on the outside of the jaws of the participants in the study so they could measure the amount of time and force required to chew certain foods, including meat and vegetables. The meat used was goat meat because it more resembled wild meat of the day (today's cows have been bred to have softer flesh). What they found was that the goat meat was remarkably difficult to eat. Lieberman tried to eat the goat meat

*Archaeological evidence shows that cooking first appeared 1 million years ago and was widespread by about 500,000 years ago. Clear evidence of habitual use of fire comes from caves in Israel dating back between 400,000 and 300,000 years and includes the repeated use of a single hearth in Qesem Cave and indications of roasting meat.

himself and commented in a *Science* article, "Eating raw goat is not pleasant, you chew and you chew and you chew and you chew and nothing happens."

The study went on to calculate that slicing the meat and pounding the vegetables, both of which make it easier to chew the food, would reduce the number of chews by 17 percent, which may not sound like a lot, but in the course of a year, that equates to 2.5 million chews! This enabled the hominids to evolve other facial traits, as before they were optimized only to chew. Now evolution could favor mouths and lips that were more maneuverable for speech, and balanced heads to help with movements like running and hunting.[5]

In a paper published in *Nature*, they posit that such a dramatic reduction in the number of chews per year facilitated early members of our genus *Homo* to evolve smaller teeth and jaws more suitable for the development of speech and language. Our delicate oral bone structure and smaller snouts, which made room for flexible lips, are unique to us humans and facilitate the pronunciation of about sixteen thousand words a day. By comparison, we perform an average of nine hundred chewing movements while eating—making talk a much more demanding skill. Having a slight overbite—with our upper teeth coming down over our lower mandible—rather than having an edge-to-edge bite allows for complex sounds like those with the letters *f* and *v*. Smaller, external noses on a more vertical face also made our heads better balanced for running and, by extension, hunting, leading us to add even more meat to our diets.[6]

But to understand our meat-eating metabolisms, we have to go back still further in time, for the consumption of meat paved the way for astonishing developments in our evolution.

Monkey Brains

Watching a band of chimpanzees undertake a hunt for meat is an unforgettable experience—an education in pure primal behavior. It's a well-calculated event similar to a militaristic takedown of a target. As opportunistic hunters, the male chimps begin innocently enough, seeking out fruits and vegetables, only to come across a tree filled with monkeys. While chimps eat other forms of meat such as bushpigs and baboons, monkeys are their filet mignon, especially baby and adolescent red colobus monkeys. Although colobus monkeys are primates like chimps and humans, they're distant relatives. So when a chimp eats a monkey, it's not a form of cannibalism, but it's violent.

"It's hand-to-hand combat with the monkeys," Stanford tells me. Their success rate is about 50 percent, which is high compared to other animals and likely attributable to the chimps' cleverness. The hunt can take up to an hour; they survey their prey, strike, and chaos ensues. Once a monkey is captured, they get it out of the tree. The meat is controlled by the alpha male, who sits down and bites into the carcass, usually starting with the brain and bone marrow. It's thought that the brain is gobbled up first because it's nutrient rich, with fat and long-chain fatty acids. Then the fat is chewed on.

This carnivorous behavior happens predominantly during the wet season, when food is plentiful and so it's fine to take the risk and hunt, as other sources of calories are more readily available if the hunt fails. During the dry season, when food is not as plentiful, chimps avoid the unnecessary energy expenditure. Stanford notes that he's seen significant improvements in chimpanzees' cognitive capacity when they are in meat-eating mode. He also tells me that the females drive the system for meat-eating binges when they are in heat. Apparently, wooing a female with a special meal is not specific to humans: male chimps who share their hunted monkey meat with females can double their chances of having sex with the female dinner partners, according to *National Geographic*.[7] Meat is a commodity among the chimps, a social currency for control and manipulation. Chimps are nearly Machiavellian in their sharing. They may fight, steal, and even barter sex for a piece of meat that's a fraction of the size of a steak. Sometimes long hunting binges—ten weeks—can ensue where the chimps will kill 10 percent of all the monkeys in the forest.

Meat is a nutrient-dense food—much denser in nutrients than fruits and vegetables. It is also harder to procure. (Fruits and vegetables don't run away.) Among primates, we humans are uncommon in how much meat we eat—on average, ten times as much meat as chimpanzees, who eat the most meat among wild apes. And unlike any other primates, humans have specialized throughout evolution in eating big-game animals (larger than ourselves) like reindeer and mammoths. Stanford has studied our meat-adaptive genes and how they slowed our aging process relative to other hominids.

A chimp's life span is shorter than that of a human. Chimps age faster and are more prone to cholesterol accumulation in blood vessels and vascular disease—especially when they are in captivity, where they are more sedentary compared with their wild counterparts. Heart failure is the leading cause of death in captive apes. I should point out, however, that although heart issues are common in both humans and chimps, the major causes of the ailment are different between the two species. We're more likely to develop atherosclerosis, a buildup of fatty plaques in our narrowed arteries that leads to heart attacks, whereas our closest relatives suffer from scarring of their heart tissue that gives rise to irregular heart rhythms and, eventually, sudden cardiac arrest. Scientists are still trying to figure out why chimps' hearts accumulate dangerous collagen, the source of the scarring, in a condition called myocardial fibrosis.* But

*This is the same condition that kills young athletes suddenly on the playing field. When we hear tragic news reports of an otherwise healthy teenaged soccer or track-and-field star collapsing and dying within minutes during strenuous activity, the cause is often arrhythmogenic right ventricular cardiomyopathy (ARVC), which is characterized by the same buildup of fatty and fibrous scar tissue on the heart.

although these animals experience heart issues a bit differently than we do, they are nonetheless a crucial model for understanding the evolution of human longevity.

Diet has changed remarkably during human evolution. All direct human ancestors are believed to have been largely herbivorous. But when humans began to evolve to eat fatty animal tissues, our genes changed so we could become more resistant to disease risks associated with eating meat. Meat is not only high in fat and cholesterol but also may contain parasites that can lead to mad cow disease, which is caused by abnormal infectious proteins (prions, derived from the words *protein* and *infection*) that destroy brain and nerve tissue. Mad cow disease probably goes back millions of years and would have potentially wiped our species off the planet if we didn't develop or select for genes to resist it.[8] This disease resistance in turn facilitated a longer life and supported a host of other behaviors that tapped the power of our growing brains, and set the stage for living longer in complex societies.

One gene in particular that emerged during the change in our diet toward eating meat is apolipoprotein E (APOE), and specifically the E2 variant, or allele, that has the ability to reduce the risks of vascular disease as well as Alzheimer's. Briefly, some genes have a variety of forms located at the same position on a chromosome; in the case of APOE, there are three forms: E2, E3, and E4. We inherit one form from each parent, and the combination determines our APOE genotype. The APOE gene is important for managing our cholesterol, as apolipoprotein E, the protein made by the APOE gene, helps transport the molecule.* Cholesterol often gets a bad rap, but we need a certain amount of it for survival; it serves many roles in the body, from comprising cellular membranes to making certain molecules

*The APOE gene is also involved in calculating our lifetime risk of Alzheimer's disease (depending on which combination of APOE genes we inherit from each of our parents).

such as hormones, fat-soluble vitamins, and bile acids for digestion. In the blood, apolipoprotein E guides different proteins containing cholesterol into the liver. In the brain, it chaperones cholesterol between neurons. Other genes evolved for us to metabolize fat.

So how can we explain the modern problem of cardiovascular disease, which remains a top cause of death, if we allegedly evolved to avoid it? USC professor Caleb Finch, the ARCO-William F. Kieschnick Chair in the Neurobiology of Aging, has said that "the shift to a diet rich in meat and fat occurred at a time when the human population was dominated by hunters and gatherers. The level of physical activity among these human ancestors was much higher than most of us have ever known. . . . Our ancestors only ate bird eggs in the spring when they were available, now we eat them year-round. They may have hunted one deer a season and eaten it over several months."[9]

The case against a meat-heavy diet was strengthened by a 2019 study published in the *Proceedings of the National Academy of Sciences* showing that the functional loss of a single gene in our evolution about two to three million years ago might be one of the reasons that too much meat can lead to atherosclerosis and cardiovascular disease.[10] The researchers, from the UC San Diego School of Medicine, were inspired to investigate why naturally occurring coronary heart attacks due to atherosclerosis are virtually nonexistent in other mammals and why even human vegetarians without any other obvious cardiovascular risk factors (e.g., smoking, hypertension, physical inactivity) are still very prone to heart attacks and strokes. The single gene was the CMAH gene (or more accurately described as the gene that encodes cytidine monophospho-N-acetylneuraminic acid hydroxylase), whose main function is to help the body produce the sugar molecule Neu5Gc (N-glycolylneuraminic acid). Humans can't make Neu5Gc because the gene encoding it is mutated, but most other mammals can make it. It appears to function to significantly reduce the accumulation of atherosclerotic plaque in our arteries. Evolutionary scientists hypothesize that a malaria parasite millions of years ago recognized the Neu5Gc, and by eliminating it, we were saved from the parasite (the proverbial door for entry was closed to the parasite), but the downside was that we became more susceptible to the heart attack–inducing atherosclerotic plaque, the fatty deposits in arteries.[11] Using genetically engineered mice whose CMAH gene has been switched off, the research team demonstrated stunning results: the mice that were engineered to be without CMAH (just as humans are without CMAH) had almost twice the atherosclerotic load than mice that had CMAH. And when the mutant mice were fed red meat (which contains Neu5Gc), the atherosclerotic load increased even more. The UCSD team hypothesized that perhaps in our diet, contact with Neu5Gc in foods like red meat sets off an immune reaction that can lead to continued inflammation of the blood vessels and, over time, progressive atherosclerotic disease in those with a diet high in Neu5Gc.[12]

There's a lesson here: eating meat is fine, but in moderation and with ample exercise. If you have heart disease in your family, keep extra-watchful eyes on your levels of cholesterol and other blood fats, blood pressure, and markers of inflammation like C-reactive protein and consider statins and baby aspirin if you're middle-aged or above, as these can help control inflammation. These drugs are not for everyone, but everyone should ask their doctor if they are at increased risk.

The chimpanzee's diet is only about 1 to 3 percent meat. Tell that to the paleo folks who eat meat daily. And for those who prefer a more vegan lifestyle, bear in mind that the fruits our ancestors came across were far from what we find in the grocery store today. They were likely to be surprisingly bitter and fibrous—what the chimps today eat in the wild. Stanford once had a go at eating a typical fruit "from the wild" so enjoyed by chimps, and he gagged. Unfortunately, a lot of vegetarians and vegans today think they are eating a healthy diet, not realizing that not only can they be missing nutrients and certain vitamins and minerals (like vitamin B12, calcium, and iron), but they also can end up consuming more processed foods high in sugar and inferior fats. And supplementing for lost nutrition is not a good solution: nutrients in foods are far superior to anything manufactured for a supplement. Just like you can't put broccoli in a pill and fill a bottle, you cannot supplement your way out of a bad diet. I realize I'm repeating myself from the previous chapter's advice, but cases of overdosing on supplements continue to increase. We would do well to obtain our nourishment from real foods, no matter which diet we follow. Remember what I also said in chapter 1: we should eat as close to nature as possible, which brings us to the meaning of a diverse diet.

Diversity without the Buffet

As you can imagine, the forest is a massive supermarket though without the food packaging and frozen section. Chimps eat an extremely diverse diet—hundreds of food species of plants, insects, nuts, and the occasional meat. By moving from plant to plant, they lower their risk for ingesting too much of any particular toxin. They spend much of their day seeking food and traveling long distances, sometimes up to the equivalent of half a marathon. Exactly what's on the menu depends on the time of year (wet versus dry season). But according to Stanford, they do seem to seek variety for its own sake, as do we humans—sometimes to our waistlines' detriment, as unlike our cousins, we don't have to travel far for a food fix. Our food habits are part of us, wired into us. But we can learn from these cousins many things that can help us make better decisions, mainly by understanding our impulses and desires. Cognitively, captive chimps have the same inability to control their impulses when confronted by a buffet of food that we do. And we have some elegant science to explain this phenomenon.

Studies show, for example, that the greater the variety of food choices in front of us, the longer it takes to feel full—what's known as sensory-specific satiety.[13] As Herman Pontzer, an evolutionary anthropologist at Duke, said to the *New York Times*, "It's the reason you always have room for dessert at a restaurant even when you're full. Even though you've had a savory meal and you can't eat one more bite of steak, you're still interested in the cheesecake because it's sweet and that button hasn't been worn out in your brain yet."[14] In primates, including humans, the activity of neurons in an area of the brain called the orbitofrontal cortex is related to sensory-specific satiety. These neurons dial down their responses to the food already eaten to satiety but show much less of a decrease in response to other foods. Throughout our evolution, this would have been advantageous to humans, as a varied diet would help ensure eating at least some of all the nutrients required for optimal performance[15]—hence, studies that demonstrate how unsatisfied we can be when faced with a wide variety of delectable foods. Chances are good you can consume up to 60 percent more when served multiple courses that contain different sensory qualities rather than a single sensory-dampening course. This is true whether you're lean or overweight, as studies also show that body mass index (BMI) does not affect sensory-specific satiety.

Chimps in the wild may eat a diverse array of foods, but they don't get obese like we do. The reason? Cooking—or processing. We are processing foods to the point they elude our brains' sensory circuitry that tells us we don't need to take another bite. I read Mark Schatzker's book *The Dorito Effect: The Surprising New Truth about Food and Flavor* a few years ago, in which he describes how we've tricked our brains to crave certain combinations of flavor that trigger pleasure centers and blunt satiety centers. These foods are called "hyperpalatable," and a 2019 study showed that over half of the foods that make up the American diet meet some criteria of this irresistibility.[16] These foods contain the perfect alchemy of mouthwatering sweetness, saltiness, and richness that breaks our natural appetite regulatory systems. These foods can stimulate the release of metabolic, stress, and appetite hormones, including insulin, cortisol, dopamine, leptin, and ghrelin, all of which play a role in cravings.

In the age of Doritos and their powerful, unnatural flavorings produced in a food lab that resembles a chemistry laboratory, fresh foods and grub with minimal added seasonings have fallen off the palatability curve altogether—a shame, because the real secret to a healthy diet is rather simple: eat what we evolved to eat. This includes fruits and vegetables (which we've admittedly changed pretty dramatically over the past few hundred years), with animal protein in moderation. The food needs to be eaten in the context that we evolved to eat it too. For example, we evolved to chew an apple and absorb the nutrients from the whole fruit and its fibrous skin, swallowing and slowly absorbing the food as it travels from the stomach through all of the intestines—not absorbing it all at once in the stomach, which can happen when the food is processed by a blender. And while you might think salami, bacon, sausage, or commercial burger meat is natural, aim for less-processed meats without high salts or other additives, and go for grass-fed real beef when possible.

Energizer Bunnies of the Animal Kingdom

Humans have other advantages over our primate relatives, like brains that are three times bigger than a chimp's. In 2016 scientists finally figured out that we have a higher metabolic rate too, burning calories at a much faster clip—27 percent faster to be precise—to keep up with our voracious brains.[17] The researchers also confirmed that we are fatter than other primates, giving us extra energy stores for times of scarcity; if you're going to burn fuel faster, you need a bigger backup supply. This study was eye-opening for those who like to figure out clues to our evolution—like why, for example, we do energy-expensive things like maintain big brains and produce more babies in shorter intervals than our ape relatives.

For a long time, we didn't think there were any differences in the rates at which different species burned calories. But now we know much more about the trade-offs between the energy demands of different body parts. Evolutionary anthropologist and professor emerita of the University College London Leslie Aiello and her colleagues "proposed that when our brains began to expand significantly about 1.6 million years ago, our direct ancestor, *Homo erectus*, evolved a smaller gut that absorbed less energy."[18] The energy that would have gone to support a larger gut spurred the evolution of our bigger-brained ancestors. Other researchers suggested that "humans reduced muscle mass to save energy, walked and ran more efficiently, or got extra calories faster by eating a higher-quality diet, cooking food to cut down on the energy spent in digestion, and sharing food."[19] However we managed it, it seems fitting that high among the finer things in life our large brains have permitted us to enjoy are the pleasures of a good meal. Toss in a few friends around the table for fellowship, and you've got yourself the perfect blend of good medicine for a longer life.

A Cure for Menopause?

Although chimps do remain fertile into old age and experience few of the neurodegenerative changes associated with old age in humans, they pay for that advantage in a shorter overall life. That's the trade-off. The females don't even go through menopause, which brings up the question of why human females evolved to end their fertility decades before death. The human female reproductive system does not age at the same rate as the rest of the body. Women stop menstruating when they still have thirty or more years left to live. The only other creatures we know of that can live decades after postreproductive life are some species of whales like belugas, short-finned pilots, narwhals, and killer whales.

Although chimps' fertility does decline between ages forty-five and fifty, female chimps as old as sixty have been known to give birth. Moreover, male chimps prefer older females, even ones that have gone bald. The fact the males are consistently more sexually interested in more mature females could be due to advanced age being a sign of genetic fitness or simply more life experience (and thus wisdom) to ensure the survival of their progeny. For animals that live in social units where the children stick around and don't mate beyond their group, however, it could be risky to have a mother able to reproduce until her death, as over time, her pod becomes increasingly full of her own offspring. This theory supports why female killer whales go through menopause but doesn't explain why humans do. Some have theorized that menopause enables women to provide for their grandchildren—what's called the "grandmother hypothesis"—but this remains hotly debated, with no clear way to study and confirm this.

Could menopause just be a fluke of nature—an evolutionary trait that has come along for the ride without providing any adaptive benefits? Perhaps we just haven't evolved yet to accommodate for how much longer we live now compared to millennia ago. After all, women live thirty years longer on average than they did just a century ago. And another thing to keep in mind, which certainly separates us from other species, is that it takes a long time to raise a human. Not only do we have long postmenopausal periods, we have long childhoods and adolescences too because it takes us a long time to mature, physiologically and mentally, to the point that we're capable of being independent. We can't even walk until around one year old (or older), and our brains are not fully developed until our midtwenties, even though they grow at a pretty dramatic rate. A three-millimeter (one-tenth of an inch) neural tube in a fetus will end up as a brain with more than one hundred billion neurons at the time of birth, meaning it must grow at an average rate of about 250,000 nerve cells every minute throughout the pregnancy. And that's just the start. New research points to the number of neurons in our cerebral cortex—the part of the brain most associated with higher cognition—not being maxed out until age twenty-five.[20] So mothers have to be around to supervise their offspring as they go off to work or college, vote, and maybe get married and have their own brood. They can't be busy having more kids.

For this reason alone, nature may never find an end to menopause such that women may one day give birth naturally as octogenarians. But we do need to get better at studying menopause, as many new health risks emerge once women are postmenopausal. The dramatic decline in the hormone estrogen has lasting health consequences for several decades—from heightened cancer risks to greater chances of developing Alzheimer's disease, heart disease, osteoporosis, and stroke, which means menopause and beyond deserve special attention.

I joked above about evolution needing to keep mothers to watch their twenty-somethings, but the responsibility for raising well-adjusted children shouldn't fall entirely to women. We've all heard the saying, "It takes a village to raise a child." As you're about to find out, we can take some cues from chimps in our child-rearing as well.

Be Permissive with Kids and Respect Your Elders

In the early 1990s, a meningitis outbreak gave Craig Stanford the opportunity to spend time in the Gombe forest alone with the chimps; he was the only one who met certain vaccination requirements. He recalls looking into the chimps' eyes and thinking he was peering into the minds of very intelligent beings—a little like aliens. *What the hell are they thinking?* he wondered. He likes to believe he can read their emotions. To him, they exhibit hunger, fear, guilt, embarrassment, and even shame. They laugh but don't cry.* The dynamic of the females in pursuit of their mates and their relationships with their children were of particular note to him. Contrary to what you might think, it's the females who choose their mates. They are highly promiscuous and will mate with, say, sixteen males in a small window of time, keeping quiet during sex so that other females don't find out and thus preventing any unwanted competition. By "small window of time," I'm talking about the interval during which they exhibit sexual swellings, lasting six to eighteen days. Like humans, chimps mate all year long, and the females get pregnant about once every five years (their menstrual cycles are also similar to those of women with a full cycle lasting about thirty-six days).

This seems at first against the Darwinian model of evolution, which states that the female will choose the most attractive and impressive male as a partner. But having multiple male partners is actually thought to be a protective and strategic behavior: each male will help to care for her offspring, not attack the progeny, as each thinks it may be his own. It sounds a bit shocking at first. But perhaps chimps can inspire us to open ourselves up to a new perspective on the meaning of family, one less reliant on blood and better suited to our modern trends of blended families and marriage equality. Chimps set an example for us, making great use of extended kinship and coparenting within the whole group. We ought to take a lesson from them, thinking less about giving only our children the most attention, and instead sharing that care with all the children in our communities. Be surrogate parents for others when appropriate and helpful. It does indeed take a village.

*Animal emotions have long been debated and difficult to study, but there's evidence that chimps can show pain, fear, distress, amusement, empathy, and even disgust through their facial expressions, behavior, and grunts or other vocalizations. But they don't cry (or blush) like we do. We don't know why other animals don't shed emotional tears like humans or why we evolved to weep—to literally eject liquid out of our eyes—as a sign of distress or hurt rather than some other reaction.

Motherhood among the chimps is another activity we can learn from. Unlike overprotective, helicoptering humans today, chimp mothers are permissive; they let their offspring play and fall down. Researchers can pick out the baby chimps who will become leaders: they are the ones whose mothers let them play but also keep an eye on them, so they have guidance. A chimp mother will intervene only when necessary to teach a lesson or prevent serious injury. That line between nurturing and independence dictates a chimpanzee's later ability to be a leader or follower. The same has been found in human studies on the long-term effects that various parenting styles have on children. Overprotective parents raise less confident kids who grow up with less self-esteem than they would have gained from parenting that gave them a sense of autonomy; this translates to fewer problem-solving skills and a lack of proper psychosocial development necessary to be a good leader. In studies on teenagers, the more overprotective their parents have been, the less the teens are perceived as having leadership potential by others and the less likely they are to be in leadership roles.[21]

The mother-child bond in chimps is exceptionally strong, especially for the mother-son dyad. Male chimps maintain their strong relationships with their mothers even as adults. Camera traps in recent years have captured mother chimps teaching their young how to fashion primitive tools for termite fishing. It takes a baby chimp about two years to use the tools. Baby chimps mimic one another extremely well and copy one another in their learning curve. And if a baby dies, the mother will carry her dead infant for a long time. As with the elephants, we still don't know for sure if this is a sign of grieving or just a lack of awareness of the baby's death.

Also like elephants, chimps respect their elders. Monkeys in general are seen to pay more attention to the voices of those older than them. It's thought that this is part of our primate heritage—a bid to gain some of our elders' wisdom. As reported in *New Scientist*, "Older monkeys play a key role in regulating the social network . . .

[they] know the forest better . . . they're better at spotting predators, and they're better at finding new food."[22] Senior monkeys also help youngsters forge friendships and climb the social ladder, taking the juveniles under their wing in social situations. That too is something to think about in our own social networks, which classically consist of our peers. We would do well to expand our networks to include people who live considerably different lives than we do. How many people do you interact with who have different habits, expertise, careers, customs, or circumstances? Who are much younger or, conversely, older than you? If you have children, make sure they spend time with grandparents or other older members of the community.

That was one of the great lessons Craig Stanford passed on to me: the role of older leaders. Our human elders are increasingly isolated and lonely. By some metrics, more than one-third of people aged forty-five and older feel lonely, and nearly one-fourth of those sixty-five and older are considered to be socially isolated, having few people to interact with regularly. The main culprits are not only living alone and losing loved ones but also having chronic illness, as well as hearing loss.

That last factor might surprise you, but one study from the VU University Medical Center in Amsterdam showed that for every decibel drop in auditory perception (the participants were aged eighteen to seventy), the odds of developing severe or very severe loneliness increase by 7 percent.[23] That might not seem like a lot, but the problem with hearing loss is that it's gradual and subtle over time, and the vast majority of people who suffer from hearing loss either don't know they have a problem or simply don't want to know. And yet the repercussions are enormous. As hearing loss intensifies, people disengage and behave in ways that favor isolation. Research shows that loneliness is also associated with high blood pressure, elevated stress hormones, and weakened immune systems.[24] A *JAMA Internal Medicine* study of subjects from the Health, Aging, and Body Composition Study showed that feelings of isolation independently raised the risk of dementia by 40 percent and the odds of early death by 26 percent. In this study, hearing loss wasn't addressed, but it has been previously shown that untreated hearing loss increased the risk of dementia by a staggering 50 percent and depression by 40 percent over a decade.[25] Untreated hearing loss also upped the risk of falling down by 30 percent.[26] Such numbers have moved scientists to declare loneliness as hazardous as smoking fifteen cigarettes a day. Keep your elders engaged, and be sure to help them get their hearing tested. It's an easy fix with a big upshot. And you may learn something from them. Nowadays, some hearing aids are available over the counter, so there's no excuse.

In the previous chapter, I mentioned that elderly wisdom is often not prized in modern society. One of the exceptions is in Japan, where the elderly population is held in high regard (one in four Japanese citizens is sixty-five years or older). There's even a national holiday to honor its seniors (Respect for the Aged Day, held on the third Monday of September each year), and this could be a factor in Japan's impressive number of centenarians in the world. If only more countries followed its example, especially now that the world's overall population is aging. By 2050, there will be roughly ninety million people aged sixty-five or older living in the United States, almost a doubling of older folks from today's numbers, and it will encompass about 20 percent of the total US population. Not only does this make it essential that we consider how to best safeguard and improve the health of older Americans, but also that we motivate the younger generations to rise to the occasion. It could start with a greater appreciation and respect for their hard-won wisdom and leadership, key to the health and happiness of everyone at every age.

Creature Cheat Sheet

Before I get to the "cheats" we can glean from the chimps, I must tell a quick story about an old friend whose teachings will help you remember the lessons here. If ever there was an elder in my life who influenced me greatly in my thinking and being, it was dear old Murray.

I met the late Murray Gell-Mann at a dinner party in July 2009 at the Aspen Ideas Festival. Murray was a famed physicist who had won the Nobel Prize in 1969 for his work on the theory of elemental particles, including postulating the existence of the quark. He was also a consummate mentor. "You always look at the mean of your data," he once told me. "Look at the outliers." He used to recite to audiences a poem that he had seen on the wall of a doughnut shop and is known as the optimist's creed:

As you ramble on through life, Brother,
Whatever be your goal,
Keep your eye upon the doughnut,
And not upon the hole.

Murray would tell you to keep your eye on the hole. The hole is the outlier you're probably overlooking, and this line of thinking led me to ask new and important questions, such as why we didn't build models in medicine like they did in his world to try to understand complex systems and why we try to understand cancer at all. Why don't we just try to control it?*

We humans are as much outliers in the animal kingdom as the chimps are among our other great apes, and we share more genetic

*Another thing I always loved about Murray that I noticed once, when he was onstage with me at the Aspen Ideas Festival for a conversation, is that he, one of the smartest people on Earth, had written in capital letters under his notes for each question: REMEMBER TO SMILE.

similarity with these primate relatives than with any other creature on Earth. By turning to our fellow outliers, we can find secrets to living better lives—secrets that have a lot to do with the power of moderation. Like the chimps, we can be aggressive and predatory but temper our behaviors; we can eat a diverse diet that includes some animal protein but need to take care that we control our impulses; we can enjoy meals with others as currency for connection; we can teach our youngsters to take some risk while still keeping a watchful eye on them; we can look up to and learn from our elders, keeping them engaged and connected; and we can enjoy a long post-childbearing period while helping younger generations, not only in our own families but also in our communities.

And as you're about to find out, it also helps to have good friends who will come to your rescue.

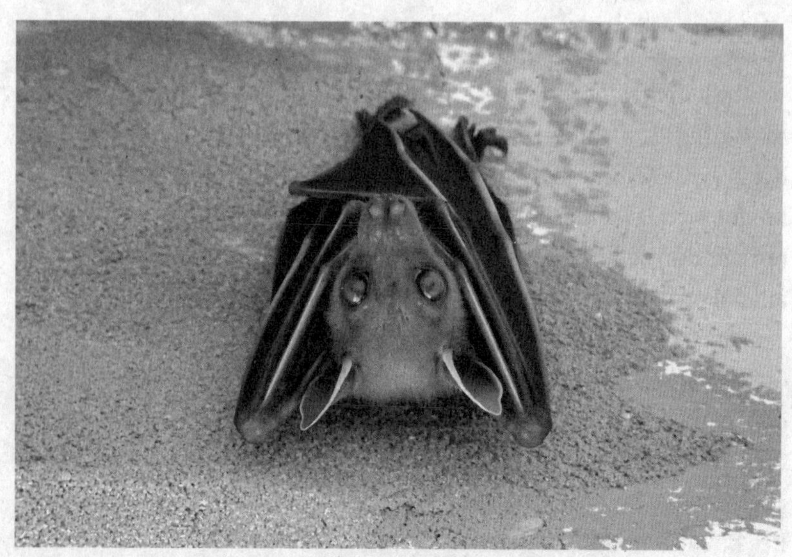

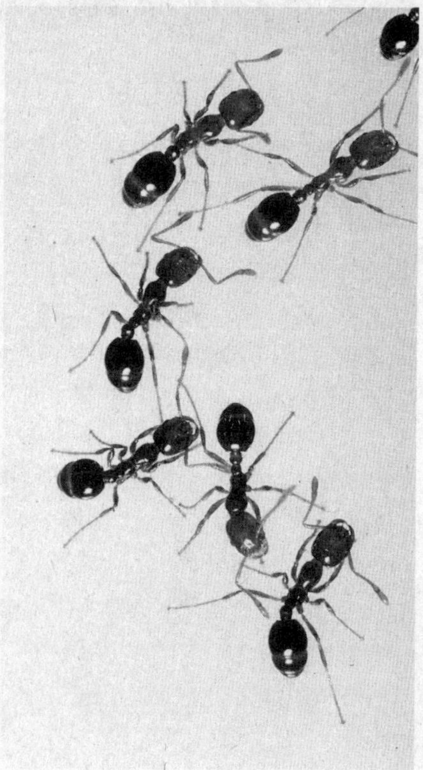

A bat (above) and some fire ants (below).

7

Team Effort and Social Immunity

Be Collaborative and Paramedical, and Take a Sick Day

> *Ants are so much like human beings as to be an embarrassment. They farm fungi, raise aphids as livestock, launch armies into wars, use chemical sprays to alarm and confuse enemies, capture slaves. . . . They do everything but watch television.*
>
> —LEWIS THOMAS

It is said that a butterfly that flaps its wings at just the right time in just the right place can cause a torrential storm thousands of miles away. The concept of this "butterfly effect" was first proposed by the late Edward Norton Lorenz in 1969.[1] Lorenz had established the theoretical basis of weather and climate predictability, spending his entire professional career at MIT. While he originally thought to employ the imagery of seagulls, he settled on the butterfly analogy to describe the fact that small events can have big effects. The new virus that caused the COVID-19 pandemic was a consummate example of this butterfly effect.

I marvel that viruses can be so crafty in their makeup and

machinations—so simple and primitive yet so powerful in their impact—able to kindle profound fear in people and hobble nations without any effort on the virus's part. A virus has no brain, no eyes, no mouth, no limbs, no lungs, no heart (and no emotions)—not anything we'd equate with actual life. Some argue that viruses don't deserve to be called microbes for this reason. A virus doesn't have a pulse or other typical vital signs. It doesn't even make decisions, and it mates with our cells without any exchange of fluid or cellular currency. It uses special proteins to attach to cells, delivers its data, and replicates itself. It doesn't even choose whom it infects. It's a crude microscopic copy machine. It may as well be a kind of robot.

We often think of viruses as villainous; the word connotes morbidity and mortality, destruction and death. But viruses, like many bacteria, can be beneficial to human health and agriculture. It is not known how many species of virus exist in the world, but it's estimated that the number is in the trillions.[2] We are aware of a few hundred thousand kinds of viruses; however, fewer than seven thousand have names and only about two hundred and fifty can infect human cells.[3] We aren't their only targets, of course. Viruses infect other animals and plants, from beans and blackberries to ticks and dogs. The virus uses the machinery of the target cells to enable it to replicate—make copies of itself. But some viruses, especially retroviruses, can integrate their genome into the host chromosome. HIV, the retrovirus that causes AIDS, is one such example. Today, our DNA contains relics of ancient viruses that have wormed their way into the human genome over millions of years. We owe many ancient viruses for our ability to read, write, think abstractly and creatively, and even form memories. The mammalian genes for syncytin, for instance, a protein essential in the establishment of the placenta, were incorporated into our DNA on several different occasions throughout our evolution. That's right: we owe part of our ability to have children to ancient viruses.

Viruses have shaped our DNA and, for that matter, our entire existence, for millennia. One fact that staggers me and anyone else I share it with is this: we have four times more viral genetic material inside our genome than our own genes. A choice few of these genetic parasites have helped us build immunity. Mammalian viruses can provide immunity against bad bacterial germs and even act as anticancerous agents. Nonsymptomatic (latent) herpesviruses, for example, arm natural killer cells, a special type of white blood cells charged with killing both tumor cells and cells that are infected with pathogenic (disease-causing) viruses. The latent herpesviruses equip natural killer cells with antigens that enable them to identify problematic cells. In the plant kingdom, certain viruses can render plants resistant to drought or help a plant manage its intake of nitrogen from the soil, making many viruses key to agriculture.

Contrary to what you might think, viruses are everywhere. They thrive in our oceans where, at last count, almost two hundred thousand different viral populations have been found from the surface to more than thirteen thousand feet deep.[4] And they flourish inside us, coating our gastrointestinal tracts (among many other organs), where they serve important roles—some of which we haven't begun to crack yet scientifically. Even our skin houses its own virome.

Some viruses, as we're now painfully aware, can be deceptively promiscuous. They are nature's James Bond villains—cunning hijackers, opportunists, and murderers. It took the genome of the human species roughly eight million years to evolve by 1 percent.[5] Many animal viruses, like the no-longer-so-new coronavirus, can evolve by more than 1 percent in the time it takes for the weather to change. It is their nature to evolve fast, thanks to their mere simplicity, whereas we're a lot more complex. Coronaviruses, single-stranded RNA molecules, accumulate mutations at a rate one million times faster than human DNA does. Such a breathtaking mutation rate gives these viruses the ability to survive against an immune response: they can quickly change their clothes, as it were, to swindle the immune system and enter our cells. Some of our most notorious infectious agents are RNA viruses.* In addition to the coronaviruses that give us colds and COVID, other RNA viruses transmit hepatitis C, Ebola, influenza, polio, measles, and HIV. In 2022, virologists documented more than five thousand new RNA viral species floating in our oceans.[6] Not all of these are infectious to animals; in fact, only a tiny fraction may be invasive to life. But the finding could reshape our understanding of how these submicroscopic infectious agents drive ecological processes in our oceans.

Infectious diseases prematurely kill more than seventeen million people every year.[7] One of the more alarming reports by the United Nations states that on average, a new infectious disease emerges in humans *every four months.*[8] One feature of the pandemics of late that makes them stand apart from those in previous centuries is that their provenances are decidedly wild. For thousands of years, we contracted most of our infectious diseases from domesticated animals. The common cold (rhinovirus) appears to have originated in camels, and many strains of influenza (flu) have originated in birds and pigs.[9] Now, however, our pandemics spring from close encounters of the wild kind. The dominant protein of the new coronavirus had approximately 96 percent similarity to the same protein from a virus isolated from a bat. How and exactly when the jump from bat to human happened and whether there was a creature in between remain unanswered questions.[10] But we can learn a lot about living with viruses from our batty friends.

*If you want to understand the difference between DNA and RNA, the power couple in all living organisms that sustain life and bear hereditary information, here's a brief explanation. RNA is single stranded, while DNA is double stranded and therefore more stable. Their chemical makeup or "ingredients" are also not identical. RNA nucleotides contain ribose sugars, while DNA contains deoxyribose; RNA uses predominantly uracil instead of the thymine present in DNA. But both DNA and RNA work together in a multitude of ways. In most organisms, DNA stores the genetic information in each cell and transmits it to offspring, while RNA is mainly involved in transferring the code to make proteins from the DNA to the cell's machinery. DNA resides classically in the nucleus of cells whereas RNA is usually found in the surrounding cytoplasm.

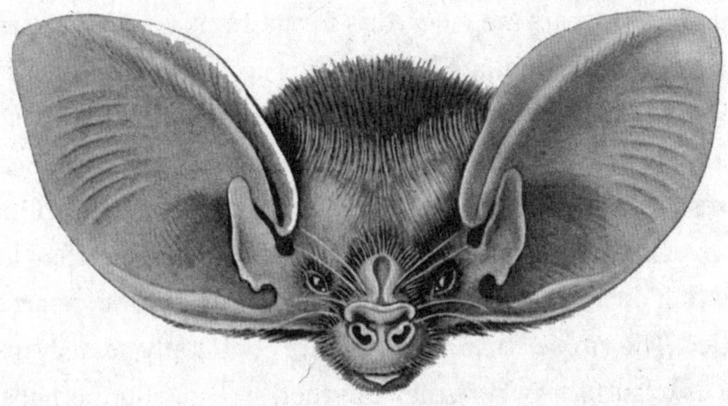

One of Ernst Haeckel's legendary illustrations of his vampire bats in *Kunstformen der Natur* (*Art Forms in Nature*), which was published in 1904.

Batty

Bats—order Chiroptera, which derives from Greek and literally means hand wing—have been around for a lot longer than we have: at least 65 million years versus about 6 million years ago for primitive humans. Over the 65 million years, bats have thrived and are found all over the earth.[11] One in four mammals on the planet is a bat, also sometimes known as a "flying fox" (and 50 percent of mammals are our friend the rodent, though to be clear, bats are not a form of rodents). In China, bats are traditionally symbols of good luck and happiness. As legend has it there, if a bat resides in a theater and appears during rehearsal, the play will be successful. We Westerners tend to malign bats. We view them as disease-riddled, bloodsucking flying menaces and associate them with horror stories, death, vampires, and haunted houses. Even our language steals from them to convey negative attributes: someone we say is batty or batshit is considered crazy or insane. Such notoriety may be partly why bats are one of the least-researched animals in history. But they may hold the clues to longevity and disease resistance.

While bats can carry thousands of viruses, they lead largely disease-free lives—seemingly unaffected by the viruses they bear. So far, we know that bats are reservoirs for more than sixty viruses that can infect people, including Ebola and rabies. Bats are one of the main players in the transmission of zoonotic viruses (infections spread from animals to humans). These creatures contain massive amounts of viruses and thus infectious materials that are spread prolifically, in part by the bat's ability to fly, as well as the fact that they live so close to humans and livestock everywhere in the world, apart from Antarctica. The viruses that bats carry are commonly passed through their feces to surfaces where they can then spread.[12] But perhaps bats are learning from their "mistakes": little brown bats, one of the most common species in the northeastern United States, used to hibernate in dense colonies. When an outbreak of a fungal infection that's particularly harmful to bats started to spread in 2006, the brown bats that survived changed their hibernation habits. This particular fungus attacks them in their sleep, so sleeping together in clusters for warmth was asking for trouble. Remarkably, 75 percent of little brown bats now hibernate alone. Scientists have also documented adaptive changes at the genetic level related to their hibernation, clear evidence of evolution at work.[13] The fungus has decimated populations of the little brown bat across North America, from southern Texas to the western edge of Newfoundland, but as some of the bats gain genetic resistance to the fungus, we may see a comeback.

I can only imagine how many people think that exterminating the bats in our world would help us prevent more zoonotic infections, but it turns out that bats serve many critical roles for the ecosystem. They are biological—and economical—pesticides; bats keep our insect population in check and are also involved in Earth's food chain through pollinating many fruit trees. For me, knowing that bats have many seemingly redundant DNA repair genes that probably play a role in preventing a disease like cancer (bats aren't known to get cancer) is an important observation that needs further study.[14] The genes that protect them likely came from evolving to fly, an energy-demanding capability that produces lots of free radicals—unstable toxic molecules that can damage DNA—that need to be managed.

New research suggests that the answer to how bats carry and survive so many viruses may also lie in how bats' evolutionary adaptations to flight changed their immune systems.[15] In mammals, the adaptation to true-powered flight has only been seen in bats.[16] Very simply, bat wings are basically an arm supporting a membrane.[17] Evolution enabled tweaks here and there in the arm to facilitate pretty impressive flight.

While at rest, bats are thought to have a temperature close to their surrounding environment. When in flight, bats' temperatures can rise to a range of 99 to 106 degrees Fahrenheit, and while these temperatures in mammals are generally a symptom of infection, research indicates that the bats' increase in temperature during flight may be a significant factor in modulating their immune systems and preventing infection (fever turns on certain immune system genes). This may prevent actual illnesses in them while still allowing them to transmit viruses and infections. Bat viruses adapted to be more tolerant of the fever response in their hosts, but this adaptation also left them less virulent to their hosts.[18]

Bat flight requires a tremendous amount of energy and leads to the death of some cells and leakage of pieces of DNA into the bat's circulation.[19] Such an event could invite an immune response because the DNA is not where it should be—in the nucleus of the cell. The bats (and some other mammals) have developed a system to identify these small pieces of DNA in the bloodstream and not think they are a piece of a foreign organism like a virus or bacteria.[20] It's called a DNA-sensing system. This dampened part of their immune response is precisely how they can live with all these viruses.

This is a huge clue for those of us who study human health. Inflammation lies at the heart of cancer, degenerative diseases, aging in general, and even how the immune system reacts to infection. Death from an infection is often the result of the body's own inflammatory response—friendly fire run amok. This was the case for a multitude of people who succumbed to COVID-19. The germ foments a lethal blaze in the immune system—what's called a cytokine storm. I mentioned cytokines briefly in chapter 5 within the context of cancer risk; cytokines are proteins (messenger molecules) secreted by cells in the body, one of whose major function is to control inflammatory processes. But when too many cytokines are released too quickly, a storm ensues in the immune system that can overwhelm the body and cause major life-threatening damage. The "Bat Pack"—a group of researchers from the Australian Centre for Disease Preparedness and the BGI Group—investigated the genes of a large fruit bat (the black flying fox) and a tiny insect-eating bat (David's myotis) and discovered, in findings published in 2012, that both species are indeed missing a gene segment that triggers the cytokine response to infection.[21]

This raises the question: Can we game our own system to suppress our cytokine response with new drugs that minimize inflammation? These drugs might be anti-inflammatories to calm the inflammatory process by blocking the effects of those pro-inflammatory substances, or they might be in the form of genetic therapy that targets certain gene segments. One of the ways we currently treat deadly infections, COVID-19 included, is to lessen the cytokine storm with drugs that have classically been used for autoimmune diseases such as rheumatoid arthritis, and with immune-suppressing steroids such as dexamethasone. This was one of the dramatic lessons learned from the COVID-19 pandemic, one that we should have seen earlier from how the bat deals with these viruses. The combination of anti-inflammatories and immune suppressants is the one-two punch to combat infections.

Mimicking bats' muted immune response could also prove crucial in treating other conditions rooted in inflammation, including cancer, degenerative diseases, and aging in general. Earlier I called chronic inflammation the "elephant in the room" because it lies at the center of virtually all of our most pernicious ailments—from diabetes, obesity, vascular diseases, and autoimmune challenges to dementias and even depression. And while it may be hard to grasp the connection between, say, cancer or depression and chronic inflammation, the common denominator is the adversarial environment that the inflammatory process engenders to trigger the development of these illnesses. As a reminder, just as chronic inflammation can damage DNA (and, hence, increase cancer risk), it can also wreak havoc on brain chemistry, which drives "changes in neurotransmitters and neurocircuits that lead to depressive symptoms," according to a review written in 2019 by Dr. Jennifer Felger.[22] In the heart, chronic inflammation promotes the growth of dangerous plaques, and when the storm hits hormonal signaling, that same chronic inflammation plays into every metabolic problem imaginable.

When the pandemic began in 2020, we made mistakes. We looked to scientific models to make predictions and define policy, but we soon realized that most models weren't accurate. We'd have to learn as we went, resorting to old-fashioned tactics like wearing masks and standing at least six feet apart in an attempt to curb the supply of human cells for the virus to find. Interestingly, to learn how we can better manage a germ's spread and prevent further pandemics, we may not want to look only at past pandemics, computer-generated models, and the lessons history can provide. The basics to outbreak control and the future of our species can be learned from a six-legged insect that scampers around at our feet. Look down. Look closely. Look really closely.

Of Ants and Men

We often forget that we're a young species compared with some other earthlings. Many animals (and plants) have been dealing with infectious disease longer than we have because they have been trying to survive on the planet since before we evolved. Bacteria were among the first inhabitants out of the earth's primordial soup, and they've developed clever ways to protect themselves, some of which we've learned to benefit from. For example, bacteria create antibiotics to ward off other bacteria competing for the same nutrients. Bacteria have been making antibiotics for billions of years probably, but it took us a long time to find them—and to learn they worked magic for our own bacterial infections. During the golden age of antibiotic discovery in the 1950s, 70 to 80 percent of all discovered antibiotics were derived from a single genus of bacteria: *Streptomyces*. All around us, animals are coming up with ways to prevent and treat infection, and some of the best mentors are right under our noses hoping to score a bread crumb from above.

Erik T. Frank is a myrmecologist: he cannot kill an ant (*murmēk* is Greek for "ant"). After all, he jokes, "Ants are mostly cleaning up what you left over." If bats dominate the mammalian dynasty in terms of sheer numbers, ants claim the prize in the insect world. They make up two-thirds of the biomass of all the insects.[23] And while we're at it, consider the following, highlighted by David Attenborough in his iconic book *Life on Earth*: "For every human being alive there are over a billion insects. Put together they would weigh perhaps seventy times as much as the average human being. Army ants march in columns through the South American countryside looking for prey. Sometimes a column comprises 150,000 individuals."[24] In 2022, it was revealed that Earth's ant population of twenty quadrillion outnumbers humans by 2.5 million times. Put another way, the total mass of ants on the planet outweighs all of the world's wild birds and mammals combined.

Although Frank originally studied international relations at the University of Exeter in southwest England, he moved into biology following a fascination with tropical species. He is now a biologist at the University of Würzburg in Germany in the Department of Animal Ecology and Tropical Biology, where he studies a peculiar rescue behavior among certain types of ants. Plenty of research had been done on ants' hunting behavior but not their medic behavior, so it was a whole new field to explore. And explore he did by the most fundamental of operations for a field biologist: he sat patiently in front of their nests and waited for their hunts to begin. Given his air of boyish youthfulness, I could instantly picture him in his element out there among his little subjects of intrigue.

Of the sixteen thousand species of ants, one in particular—the Matabeles native to sub-Saharan Africa—holds Frank's attention. These combat warrior ants are experts at battlefield triage. After they raid a termite colony for a meal, they go into rescue mode and carry their wounded home, where they take turns caring for their injured comrades. The heavily wounded ants are left on the battlefield for dead, and they play dead as a signal to others: *Go on; leave me alone to die*. Frank explains this behavior in a rather mercenary way: "Heavily injured ants—the ones that have many severed limbs and can't stand up on their own . . . are probably not going to recover and are not good for the colony." He compares the phenomenon to cells in the human body that self-destruct when they become useless or deranged, in a process that we call apoptosis (Greek for "falling off"). But it's extraordinary to think that it's the mortally wounded ants that initiate this process.

Frank was the first person to observe this phenomenon in the field in 2017. When he formally documented it in a 2018 academic paper, the work became a brief Internet sensation.[25] It marked the first time any scientist had seen a nonhuman animal systematically nurse fallen soldiers back to health. Frank hadn't been looking for this behavior initially. At the time, he was a PhD student making trips to the Ivory Coast with colleagues to observe wild colonies of Matabele ants that attack termite nests as often as four times a day. These ants march in columns stretching up to 164 feet away from their nest, or about half the distance up the Statue of Liberty. Their process for attacking a termite colony starts with neutralizing the soldiers and attacking the workers; they then steal the pile of eggs from inside the termite colony to take back to their colony as food. Although the ants and termites are similar in size, the ants are faster and their bites are ferocious. (Ten bites are enough to paralyze a human arm.) But their raids do not come without losses of their own.

Frank's chance glimpse at the triaging after a raid-like event happened one day when he accidentally drove his Land Cruiser over one of the ant columns. When he got out of the car and walked back (remorse brewing) to see the carnage, he noticed something extraordinary: the healthy ants were helping out only those that had lost one or two of their six legs. The ants in worse shape were ignored. This was the moment Frank realized that the ants' triage system is controlled by the patient, not the nurse. Injured Matabeles release compounds called pheromones to alert their healthy mates to the need for a rescue mission, but heavily injured Matabeles don't emit those SOS signals. What's more, mortally wounded ants actively thwart any efforts to be rescued by their friends. In one of his experiments, Frank painted the ants with panic pheromones, meaning they were forced to send an SOS signal, but when the troops arrived to help, the painted ants didn't allow themselves to be helped. They flailed around, making it too difficult for the rescuers to get close enough to help. The rescuers eventually were confused by the mixed signals and left the pheromone-coated ants alone.[26]

The ants that are rescued and taken back to the nest undergo astonishing medical treatment worthy of an ER scene. Frank used a camera placed into the nest together with infrared light to watch a group of ants surround the wounded comrade, and the "nurses" would take turns licking the wound a few minutes each.[27] This treatment apparently works: only 10 percent of ants whose wounds were licked died compared with 80 percent of those who didn't receive the licking therapy. Many creatures have antibacterial and antifungal compounds in their saliva as a protective mechanism, so maybe our next human antibiotic or antifungal will come from studying these

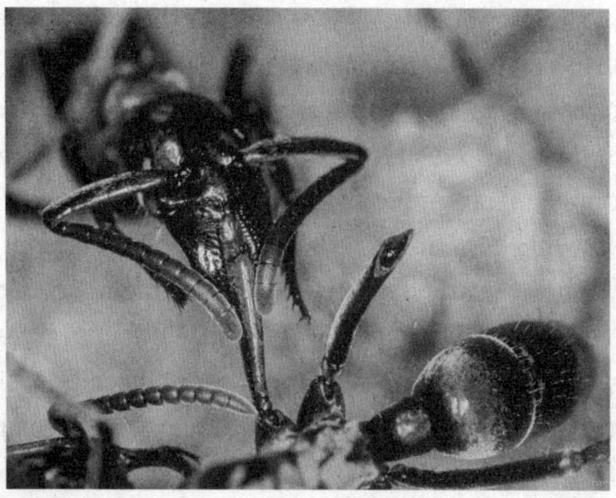

A Matabele ant acting as a medic to help his injured comrade.

ants.[28] Future research will figure that out and perhaps add to our own arsenal of antibiotics and antifungals.

We are in desperate need for new antimicrobials in a world becoming increasingly resistant to our current weaponry in the medicine cabinet. The ants' behavior is amazing, and I could sense the excitement from Frank's voice as he studied a real medical system inside an ant colony. Sensing my wonder, he was quick to inform me that this doesn't necessarily mean they are intelligent; this may be an ingrained behavior to optimize the size of the colony for the best functioning.* Although ants missing one or two legs are handicapped for life, they get used to running on their remaining legs in a single

*Ants don't have the same kind of intelligence as we do, but don't underestimate their braininess. Not even Darwin could refrain from calling out their smarts. In his *On the Origin of Species*, he writes: "It is certain that there may be extraordinary mental activity with an extremely small absolute mass of nervous matter: thus the wonderfully diversified instincts, mental powers, and affections of ants are notorious, yet their cerebral ganglia are not so large as the quarter of a small pin's head. Under this point of view, the brain of an ant is one of the most marvelous atoms of matter in the world, perhaps more so than the brain of a man."

day. And it's thought that roughly a third of the ants in a colony have lost a limb at one point.

What these ants show us is the power of an established health care system with a built-in support protocol for injured or unhealthy companions using a unique triage protocol for resources, favoring those that would benefit most. But ants also have lessons for us individually. They view the fight to keep fellow members of the colony alive as a fight for the survival of the entire community, something we'd do well to remember. In chapter 11, we'll see how similar, but more altruistic, behavior is key to breaking through painful situations and managing chronic pain. For now, let's appreciate the benefits of helping others when they are unable to stand on their own two feet. They may not ask for help or even think they need it, so it behooves those of us in the kingdom of the healthy to reach out and play our part. We should learn CPR and the basics of first aid and have a mobile supply kit available for emergencies (licking human wounds doesn't work very well, so topical antibiotics and bandages are well worth having around). And then one day, it'll be our turn to let others prop us up, lick our wounds, so to speak, and nurse us back to health.

Long Live the Queen!

Ants follow a division of labor and an accepted hierarchy that rivals any advanced civilization in humanity. And according to Frank, there is variability among the ants: "They have personalities." Younger ants do the hard labor: cleaning the nest and taking care of babies. As they age, they take on riskier tasks and go out and forage. The scout ants get the short end of the stick as the reconnaissance team: they are charged with looking for the termites but live only about a week, maybe a little longer depending on their species and environment. The worker ants, who are all female but sterile and so are ironically called "unproductive females," live between three and six months, while the queen,* who has the same underlying genome, can live up to eighty times longer—as long as thirty to forty years. In some species of ants, the queens live over five hundred times longer than males and fifty times longer than the workers. That makes ants, especially the queen, one of the longest-living insects in the world. (Frank says *queen* is a misleading term, as she doesn't lord over the other ants. "She's just an egg-laying machine," he notes, that pumps out hundreds of thousands of fertile eggs in a matter of days.) The life span of the queen has piqued the curiosity of scientists for decades. There's something to be said for long outliving your comrades that spring from the same genetic roots. Such a radical disparity in ant longevity has spurred lots of research to better understand the aging process. Who better to learn from than the queen?

Within days of hatching, ants can switch their internal programs, which influence their social roles, ability to learn the spectrum of tasks they perform, and longevity. They make these changes depending on the colony's needs. Imagine being able to physically change how your body is programmed all the way down to your DNA as you grow up and adapt to your environment and the needs of your community. This is not science fiction. In chapter 2, I briefly mentioned CRISPR, the gene-editing tool that's akin to having Microsoft Word's find-and-replace function for your biological genes. Let's take a moment to explore this further.

In December 2015, *Science* magazine announced its Breakthrough of the Year: CRISPR (also known as CRISPR/Cas9, pronounced "crisper," and short for "Clustered Regularly Interspaced Short Palindromic Repeats"). Broadly speaking, CRISPR is a guide molecule that can find the part of the genome a scientist is interested in with accuracy, and Cas9 is an enzyme that acts like molecular scissors to

*Researchers can study a colony of ants for many years. They paint the ants with different colors to be able to identify the individuals over the study period. We know the life expectancies of the various ants because we could follow them individually with this color system.

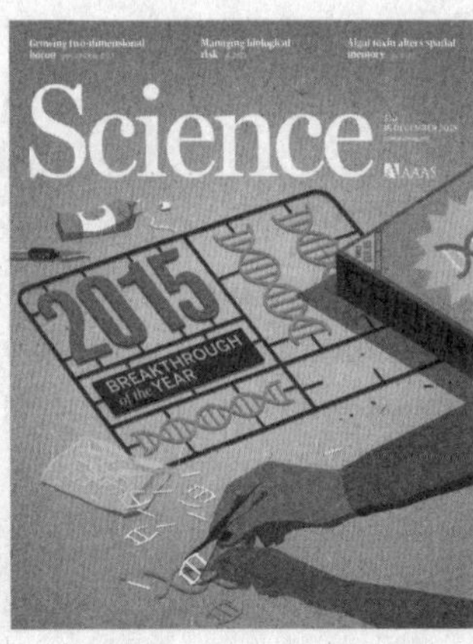

Cover of *Science* magazine in December 2015 when it declared CRISPR the "Breakthrough of the Year."

cut and paste the double-stranded DNA at whatever spot to create a genetic modification of exquisite precision. It can change a single letter in the three-billion-letter DNA alphabet I described earlier. So this amazing enzyme can be used to turn off genes but also to add or change genes for an improved or new function.

Those of us in medicine were already familiar with this dazzling new technology, whose origins date back to the late 1980s, but it took many advances in research over several decades to learn how exactly this technology works. CRISPR was identified in nature. It was used by single-celled organisms like bacteria to block viruses and other intruding DNA from harming the organism (by cutting up the DNA). When the components to these processes (CRISPR-derived RNA and various Cas proteins, including Cas9) are transferred into more complex organisms, they allow "editing" for the manipulation of genes. It was the yogurt company Danisco that first identified this antiviral machinery of bacteria (specifically *Streptococcus thermophilus* bacteria, which are commonly found in dairy cultures), but it would take until 2017 for us to get a real sense of what this process looked like.

That year, a team of researchers led by Mikihiro Shibata of

Kanazawa University and Hiroshi Nishimasu of the University of Tokyo published a paper in *Nature Communications* that visualized the dynamics of the CRISPR-Cas9 complex.[29] This came on the heels of two seminal research papers published in 2012 that helped transform bacterial CRISPR-Cas9 into a simple, programmable genome-editing tool.[30] In a paper that led to a Nobel Prize, Jennifer Doudna, Emmanuelle Charpentier, and Martin Jinek showed that the CRISPR/Cas9 system could be used to target any piece of DNA in the genome they wanted. The tool that scientists had been dreaming about was here.[31] Soon after, the research exploded, and hundreds of papers were published demonstrating that this worked on a range of organisms, from baker's yeast, zebra fish, fruit flies, and nematode worms to mice, monkeys, and human cells.

CRISPR is an incredible innovation and turns out to be relatively inexpensive to operate, as well as a versatile scientific tool. Before CRISPR, the cost of editing a gene could be prohibitive, not to mention slow going, taking potentially years. *Vox* recently reported that editing one gene with CRISPR could cost $75 and take only hours.[32] The new technology will bring sweeping changes to many industries, not just medical ones. In addition to changing the course of a disease or genetic defect in humans—from cystic fibrosis, type 1 diabetes, and sickle cell anemia to HIV, heart disease, and hearing loss—it promises to revolutionize farming and drug development. In the very near future, CRISPR-like systems will be used to create drought-tolerant crops and more nutritious plants (neither would be GMO, as no new genes are being introduced), as well as develop new ways to treat bacterial and viral infections. It may correct DNA errors to help eliminate some inherited diseases and is being developed to eliminate disease-causing mosquitoes among other things. But it's still in development, and although it's precise, it's not perfect. It can have off-target effects.[33]

Everything is connected, so when you change one thing over here in the genetic code, you could potentially change another thing over there that you didn't expect. And that can be devastating—and potentially fatal. This is why we shouldn't yet be using this technology on embryos when the children born could suffer lifelong consequences and pass that suffering on to future generations. We should initially try this technology in people with diseases where we can change a single letter and they can benefit today. Ethically, that's where the technology needs to be applied to start. And to clarify, when you use CRISPR on children and adults, you can change their DNA (and that DNA's behavior) *but not the DNA of their offspring*. Again, it's the editing of human embryos that's controversial and bears consequences for newborns and their descendants.

My hope is that alongside these astonishing technological advances and disruptions will come new rules to serve as a form of checks and balances. Science, technology, and culture must evolve together. Now that we potentially have the power to change evolution, our responsibilities have grown immensely and immeasurably greater. CRISPR systems could be used not just to change an organism, but to create a totally new species artificially (not through evolution, as has been done with new species to date). Do we want to be doing that? In chapter 8 we'll cover the power of epigenetics, which is another way to sway the behavior of our genes. But for now, let's get back to the queen ant. She still has things to teach.

A 2019 paper by German scientists pointed out the paradox with queen ants: they are both extremely long-lived and highly fertile.[34] In most organisms, the relationship between longevity and fertility is inversely related: the longer you live and rack up molecular damage to your body, the less likely you can successfully reproduce. But queen ants live long enough to mother hundreds of thousands, if not millions, of progenies that will tend to her—no questions asked. And therein lies a clue: queens are so well cared for by their broods that they don't have to invest so much energy in their immunity and resistance to environmental and physiological stress as they age. Queens don't have to forage, go to war, or even be touched by an infection that's threatening worker ants far from the lair. The queen is catered to in ways that allow her—and her genome—to focus solely on living long and laying eggs. Established older queens are famous for overproducing age-defying antioxidants to preserve their DNA—and for us, this is something else to think about: we must protect not only our immune function and resistance against environmental and physiological stress but also our DNA, particularly after our childbearing years. I've mentioned this lesson before, because DNA preservation is the linchpin to longevity. Mutational errors can open the door to diseases from autoimmune challenges to degenerative ailments, including cancer. This message is not an endorsement of synthetic shortcuts to antioxidant abundance through vitamins and supplements. Nearly all of the studies to date show an increased risk of cancer from taking these unnatural pills, which may interfere with the body's own production of antioxidants. The ideal way to ensure you've got good levels of antioxidants is to heed tried-and-true medicine: consume wholesome fruits and vegetables and prevent inflammation, which can be the initiating event leading to these DNA changes.

The ants are ahead of us in their pharmacology; they can produce their own antimicrobials and methods to tame inflammation, whereas we've had to develop ours from outside sources. The anti-inflammatory benefits of having lean body mass and potentially taking statins (compounds that inhibit a liver enzyme that plays a central role in the production of cholesterol) and aspirin are real and well-documented.* Virtually all chronic conditions have been linked to chronic inflammation, but a daily low-dose aspirin has been shown to significantly reduce the risk of developing certain malignant cancers, as well as to reduce the risk of cardiovascular disease. I like to call aspirin the cheapest fountain of youth around.

*Statins are the most commonly prescribed drugs to improve blood cholesterol levels in people who cannot optimize their cholesterol through diet alone, but statins are also powerful anti-inflammatories. Their positive effects on lowering risk for cardiovascular events could potentially be attributed to this feature.

What's truly unbelievable about queen ants, however, is that they do not inherit their crowns. Any female ant larva can become a queen, which is more good news for us because it reminds us that DNA does not always drive outcomes; we can control how our DNA behaves to some degree. The ants who become queens do so mainly due to their diet, one rich in protein that apparently primes a female baby ant for her throne (and to produce more eggs). There are, however, still some genetic forces at work here, as there are likely switches in the queen's DNA that signal to her the kind of diet she needs to fulfill her role. The ants seem to know who is who, and each one performs its role accordingly. More research is needed to understand all of the molecular mechanisms—and environmental forces—behind the strange phenomenon of ant royalty, including differences among species of ants, but one thing is certain: learning how ants age depending on their role may ultimately shed more light on aging in general, including in humans. The queen ant is a picture of youth through her long life, while her offspring, the workers, age and die at a pretty rapid pace. Work by scientists has shown that changing the ant's tasks or having them mate can significantly change the pace of their aging process.[35]

And what if a queen dies with no new queen ready to replace her? In addition to speeding up, slowing down, or even reversing aging in ants simply by having them mate or change their tasks, scientists can also employ molecular pressures to explore different outcomes. In 2021, researchers at the University of Pennsylvania found that a single slight tweak to the expression of a gene that activates a certain protein can turn a worker ant into a queen.[36] Once again, this is proof that multiple possible behaviors are written into the ant genome, with gene regulation affecting which behavior ultimately takes over. Ants' behavior is plastic, and so even though an ant is born into a fateful caste system, a given ant's future is not always written in stone. The same can be said for us: we have the power to change the activity of our genetic code, as well as to change our behavior.

Queens can also protect their DNA from the adverse effects of "jumping genes" whereby certain sections of DNA inactivate other genes that are important for healthy aging. The queen can mute these jumping genes. No doubt further study of jumping genes, which are new to the scientific roundtable, can help us grasp the secrets of our own genome and how we can control it to increase our own longevity.

Communication Is Key

Ants' pheromones are important for more than just battlefield Morse code. Chemical communication through pheromones occurs widely in the animal kingdom, especially within the context of sexual attraction. Each animal in nature, including humans, has a personal "smell" signature. And it turns out that opposites do attract in our own species: we tend to prefer body odors of others with genetic profiles that are different from our own. From an evolutionary perspective, this makes sense, for children with a variety of genes have a wider defense against disease. Just as with fingerprints, each of us has our own unique odor print, which is genetically programmed by a set of genes called the major histocompatibility complex—the same genes that also help command our immune system.

The pheromones ants use to communicate form a unique language, with each pheromone a letter in their "alphabet" that together forms words and silent sentences. If you've ever noticed how ants walk in lines, take note next time of their ingenious way of finding the shortest distance between two destinations. They make pheromone trails to guide their travels, so over time, the shorter distance trail will become more intense and stronger. While they may not have a brain that can do basic arithmetic or "know" what they are doing, the pheromones supply their memories.

Attack is not the only threat to a colony's survival. Ants can become infected with harmful microbes, especially parasitic fungal infections that can spread quickly and decimate a colony. Diseased ants know how to self-isolate as well. Infected ants will try to leave the nest and die on their own. Even a cocoon that's infected will start sending out signals—again with the help of pheromones—and other ants will show up to kill the cocoon. Ants are martyrs, models of what's called social immunity, which describes how individual behaviors can reduce disease for a whole community. These behaviors range from more common acts like the grooming of nestmates and removal of dead material from the main nest area to detecting and isolating an infectious or diseased brood.[37] Worker ants even take sick days. Nathalie Stroeymeyt, who was once a colleague of Erik Frank when they were at the University of Lausanne in Switzerland, has documented that after the threat of a foreign pathogen, the patterns of social interactions are significantly changed.[38] Stroeymeyt found that "not only did infected workers alter their behavior after exposure, but healthy workers altered their behavior toward their infected counterparts. They observed that both exposed and unexposed workers maintained their distance from indoor workers by active isolation—increasing their time outside away from the nest."[39] This should all sound familiar after our own experiences with the COVID-19 pandemic and quarantine.

Social colonies can thrive only when certain rules are set in place. For the ants, these rules have been encoded in their genome for millions of years. We're still learning how to overcome the curse of our higher-order thinking and emotional intelligence that leave us craving connection, touch, and individual autonomy. We're also trying to accept the fact that we tend to be bad at predicting the future. We like certainty and predictability—to know what's around the corner. Virtually every prediction I have heard made at the World Economic Forum from some of the most brilliant people has been off the mark, many times wildly so. That speaks volumes. As a society, we should focus less on models and fictional forecasts and more on simple preparedness. Work with the problems in front of you. Don't look back (yet); go forward and take it step-by-step. You think the ants have fancy digital models? They don't. But they respond better than we do when a crisis strikes.

A Brief Note about Termites

These wood-loving bugs may be the enemy of homeowners and a target of ants, but they too hold antiaging insights for us.* Just ask Judith Korb, an evolutionary biologist and ecologist at the University of Freiburg in Germany, who prefers to study termites (over ants and bees) to figure out how social factors and molecular processes influence aging. Bespectacled with delicate features and tufts of curly, tousled auburn hair, she has spent two decades in the trenches of tough fieldwork to unlock the wisdom of termites in their intricate mounds that are perfectly controlled temperature-wise year-round (these are meter-sized structures built by millimeter-sized insects). Like their fellow social insects that maintain exquisite civic hierarchies, termites (the "social cockroaches" of the planet†)[40] defy the logic of human capabilities in many ways, especially the queen—and her king. Indeed, there's a royal pair in this system and they are called the "reproductives."

In a termite colony, the king and queen are always together in their chamber. And interestingly, they each have eyes, whereas

*There are more than twenty-six hundred known termite species in the world. Africa is home to more than 660 species, and is by far the richest continent for termite diversity.

†Termites were recently bunched into the same taxonomic family as roaches. *Smithsonian Magazine* reported, "As far back as 1934 researchers noticed that the specialized microbes in the guts of termites are also present in the guts of some cockroaches." Decades later DNA analysis suggested that termites belonged to a branch of the cockroach family tree. That was confirmed in a 2007 paper that suggested termites should be lumped with the cockroaches near a group of roaches called *Cryptocercus*, which tunnel into wood. And in 2018, it was made official with another paper that defined termites as "eusocial cockroaches." In the paper, the researchers write, "Around 150 million years ago, eusocial termites evolved from within the cockroaches, 50 million years before eusocial Hymenoptera, such as bees and ants, appeared." Unlike the termites, however, cockroaches do not have colonies.

workers do not. In fact, on their "nuptial flight," Korb tells me, they see each other and go on a "tandem run," or mating flight. The queen controls the process: she'll emerge as a winged virgin from her colony, release pheromones to attract her future king, and then mate. But she'll first play hard to get and fly a dance of avoidance to ensure that she chooses the fastest and fittest male termite to be her partner for life. As soon as the young queen and future king meet, their wings immediately break off, and they scamper away together to find a new home—to found a new colony and start a family.

Some species of termite queen, such as the *Macrotermes bellicosus*, can remain fit and fertile until nearly the day the queen dies. The queen lays about twenty thousand eggs daily and reaches the age of twenty years, whereas workers, who have the same genome as the queen, are infertile and live for only a few months, aging gradually and experiencing senescence just as we do. The queen, however, can pump out eggs and proteins pretty much at full speed until the day she dies. Her secret? Korb found that in addition to being well protected from outside threats and being well-fed and catered to just like a queen ant, the termite queen also exhibits genetic signaling that is not the same as that of her workers whose genes begin to jump with age and then ultimately cause their demise and death.[41] But the queen termite can suppress these jumping genes like the queen ant can and activate pathways that destroy them before they move, thereby protecting her youth and longevity. It's these queens' hidden weapon against traditional aging.

We humans also harbor jumping genes (also called transposons), many of which have everything to do with our health and longevity. And they have been with us since our evolutionary beginning, some coming from ancient viruses and bacteria that inserted themselves into our DNA. Most jumping genes are not functional coding genes. Over the years, they were actually called "junk DNA." But now, new studies show that these DNA sequences help control other functional genes, so they certainly aren't junk and thus factor into our health, speed of aging, and risk for disease.[42] The more we study them, the more we may be better able to control ones that can ultimately de-age us or prevent premature decline. This may also involve some CRISPR technology. If we want to live long and die fast, perhaps the royal termite will be our model.

Korb amused me with her imagery of studying long-lived termite colonies in Africa. She feels horrible when she digs out a colony in search of the hard-to-get-to royal couple. The encounters with elephants and snakes pale in comparison to the encounters with the honeybees that cover her and her team as they conduct fieldwork. "They crawl into your clothes and shoes and sting you. After five stings they become really aggressive. It's annoying, but I love it."

Creature Cheat Sheet

If there's one thing the new coronavirus has taught us it's that some of us would do well to take more sick days and be more mindful of our behavior. Make no mistake: social animals, from bats and ants to humans, benefit mightily from their communities. They know the value of teamwork, shared labor, and helping a fellow in times of distress. They develop habits that foster individual and collective wellness and communicate effectively without uttering a single word. And, when necessary, each member knows how to "take one for the team."

This chapter covered a lot of ground on gene-editing technologies that are on the cusp of revolutionizing medicine. But most of us are not about to edit our genes today or age like the queen ant by virtue of a complex constellation of mysterious circumstances, some of which science is still trying to figure out. One of the greatest lessons from this chapter has everything to do with an ant's prophesy: its job. We know now that an ant's job determines its life span.

And so I ask you, Where do you work? What do you do for a living? Who and what surround you? How does your job factor into your health and health span? Many of us don't think about how our daily duties as workers, parents, and friends contribute to our well-being and longevity or how our work environments and settings participate in our health equation. But they directly and indirectly relate to encountering potential danger (or protection from threats), access to resources, finding and forging new and beneficial relationships, and developing risk factors for aging in general. Put simply, what you do for a living—and all that that encompasses, from people to places and exposures—matters. We all witnessed, for example, the risks that front-line and essential workers bore at the height of the pandemic versus those in jobs that shielded them from harm. Inequality in life spans no doubt has roots in socioeconomic disparities in health and mortality, but that inequality also hinges on the jobs we pursue and the workplace attributes that come with those occupations.

A few years ago, when researchers in health care analytics put a number on this phenomenon, they discovered that 10 to 38 percent of the differences in life expectancy across demographic groups can be explained by the different job conditions and experiences in those jobs.[43] That means our jobs do indeed take part in our longevity, and more so than we appreciate or imagine. Granted, not everyone can suddenly change careers or go back to earn an advanced degree and search for a job that comes with an inherently better, healthier life. But there are little things we each can be doing within our chosen professions to reduce those risks and maintain practices that help counter any dangers that are beyond our control.

An ant's fate is built into its title role. If the same could be said for your fate, how is your title role (or set of roles) influencing your behaviors and risks? And is there room for improvement? Can you start to build practices that limit or reduce those risks? See if you can come up with at least three good habits to focus on within your daily duties that can amount to your crowning achievement in tipping the scales of longevity in your favor. Or perhaps think about finding a new job.

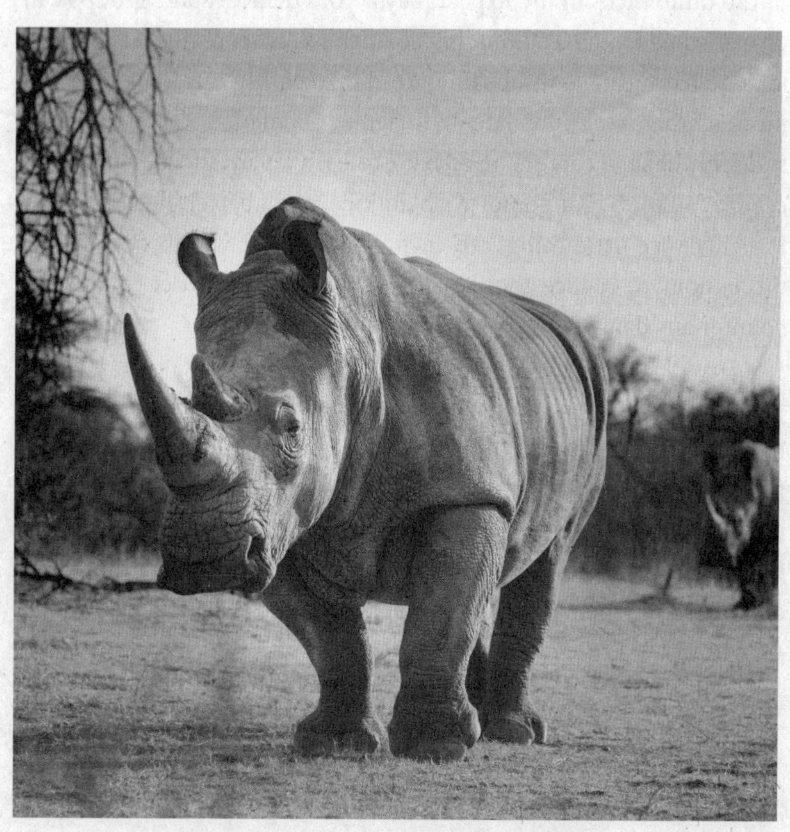

A white rhino in the South African veld.

8

Rhinos, Reproduction, and Running

Little Forces in Your Environment That Can Foment Big Changes in Your Fate

> *God is really only another artist. He invented the giraffe, the elephant, and the cat. He has no real style. He just keeps on trying other things.*
>
> —PABLO PICASSO

Pop quiz: What do rhinoceroses and horses have in common?

Answer: A long-lost relative from which the two species evolved that we think was the largest land mammal to have ever tramped the earth. Picture a rhino-like hornless creature forty feet in length (the length of a semitrailer), seventeen feet tall, and weighing about twenty tons (making it two and a half times as heavy as an elephant or a *Tyrannosaurus rex*). Some have described these animals as resembling big, hairless camels. No matter how we illustrate these fantastical characters in our minds, we can all agree that they are the terrestrial heavyweight champions of the mammalian world.

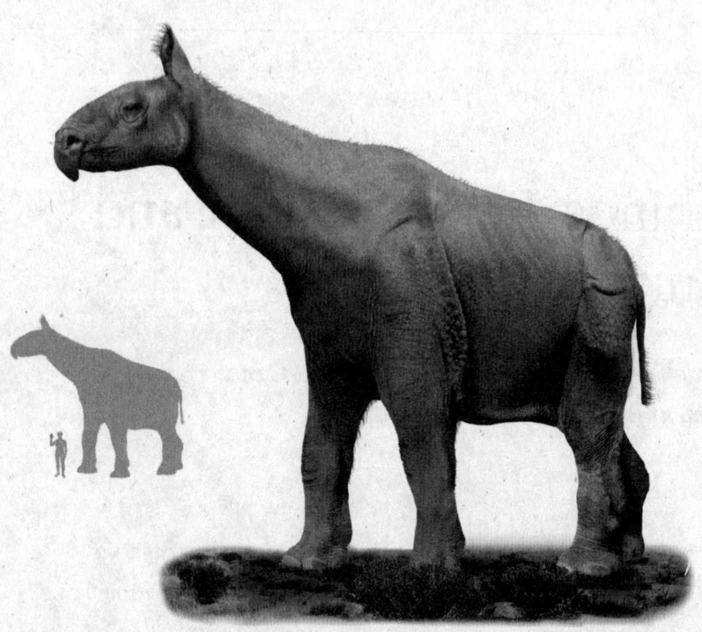

An artist's impression of an *Indricotherium* with a comparison (back left) to a human in size.

The Indricotherium ("Indric beast") lived during the late Oligocene, 34 to 23 million years ago. To put this into perspective, that's tens of millions of years after the last dinosaur died. The Oligocene period is the transition period between the Eocene, where Earth was populated with dinosaurs and the first iterations of mammals, and the modern world of the Miocene, where the mammal population grows and we see an ecosystem similar to ours today. In our oceans, the baleen and toothed whales emerged as their ancestors; population declined, partly because of the absence of echolocation, which they relied on for survival more and more as ocean temperature decreased, turning colder and murky. Without echolocation, a skill for locating objects using the reflection of sound, ancestral whales could not successfully navigate to find food or avoid deadly collisions.

Echolocation would evolve to help these animals "see" acoustically, an important survival tool.

The Indric beast's name is fitting: the word *Indric* (also transliterated as *Indrik*) is an altered version of the Russian word *edinorog*, which means unicorn. In Russian folklore, the mythological Indrik creature wears the crown as the king of all animals. It lives in seclusion on a mountain known as the Holy Mountain, where no other being can trespass. When the beast stirs, legend says, the earth trembles. This amazing and extremely large creature is thought to have legs similar to that of a deer and a head that resembles a horse's, and it is described having a horn on the front of its face. It looks vaguely similar to a rhinoceros, although the Indricotherium did not have horns.[1]

To think there was once a mammal that dwarfed the dinosaurs, which have hogged a lot of attention in our evolutionary story, is astounding. Where were the Indricotherium in my science books growing up? There's no explanation for why the obliterated reptiles have superseded most fossilized mammals as the objects of our prehistoric adoration. Perhaps they are popular simply because they've always enjoyed great marketing courtesy of movies, documentaries, children's books, museum exhibitions, and headline news that accompany each new discovery of a previously unknown dinosaur species. And unlike many dinosaurs, no complete set of bones of an Indricotherium has yet been found.

We owe more of our own history—and biology—to these original unicorns than to any of the Jurassic characters. Solitary animals that could live into their eighties, the *Indricotherium* invested in their progeny much like we do, with long gestational periods and close parenting after birth. Though we may never know for sure, it is thought that females carried their unborn young for two years. (Gestation periods of large mammals are generally proportional to their size.) After giving birth, the baby's mother sought isolation with her newborn, which she would then care for for another three years to protect the vulnerable youngster from meat-eating predators (like the now-extinct ferocious *Hyaenodon*) until it was large enough to be safe.

When these ancestral rhinos were roaming our planet, terrestrial Earth didn't look like it does today. The earth was dry, and scrub vegetation was interspersed with open areas.* The Indricotherium had a major advantage in this ecosystem: it could reach the tops of trees due to its size, which added sustenance, as most other animals at that time couldn't. Similar to today's rhinos, the Indricotherium also likely had a prehensile upper lip that made eating leaves from tall trees easy. (*Prehensile* means able to grasp and is a word classically used in the animal world for a limb or tail capable of grabbing.) We know nothing of their tails or much about their skin texture and coloring. Paleontologists' best guess is that their skin was thick, folded, gray, and hairless like that of modern rhinoceroses. Many creatures, including the elephant and the rhinoceros, have evolved to have little or no hair, as hair causes retention of body heat. The Indricotherium may have had large ears to help with the control of body heat, similar to the ears of the modern elephant.

Clearly the size of an Indricotherium meant they had very little threat from predators. So what led to their demise? These giants were taken out after 1 million years by their own Achilles' heel: leaf eaters wholly dependent on deciduous trees year-round did not fare well when the climate cooled as Earth went through a transition toward the end of the Oligocene period. For reasons still under study today, the weather changed and, with it, the scenery, flora, and fauna.

Fossils of several species of Indricotherium have been found in Mongolia, Kazakhstan, Pakistan, and China. We don't think they

*Indricotherium have had three different names since their discovery: *Paraceratherium*, *Indricotherium*, and *Baluchitherium*. In a *Guitar World* interview, Eddie Van Halen talked about the tenth track on his 1995 album, *Balance*, an instrumental titled, "Baluchitherium." Apparently, when his wife at the time, Valerie Bertinelli, heard the song for the first time, she said, "That sounds like a dinosaur song," and Eddie looked in a book to find the name of the biggest mammal that lived in the prehistoric age. Hence the name.

reached western Europe, but it's possible that one day, we'll find evidence to the contrary. We have globe-trotting adventure seeker Roy Chapman Andrews to thank for the discovery of the first *Indricotherium* fossil. Arguably the American Museum of Natural History's most prominent resident explorer, Andrews began his time at the museum as an assistant in the taxidermy department, doing odds and ends, and worked his way up to become director. Not only did he bring the world's first-known fossil dinosaur eggs to the museum in 1923, but the previous year, he also drove a fleet of Dodge cars westward from Peking through Mongolia, where his party found a skull and other fossilized body parts of Indricotherium. If Andrews brings to mind Indiana Jones, you wouldn't be alone. It has long been rumored that the iconic character was modeled after him.[2]

If Andrews were alive today, I'd introduce him to another legendary naturalist, Barbara Durrant, the director of reproductive physiology at San Diego Zoo Wildlife Alliance whose mission is to save white rhinos from extinction. Modern white rhinos, the largest rhinos in the world, not only give us a peek into the past that Andrews craved to reveal but may also inform our fertility needs. It sounds implausible

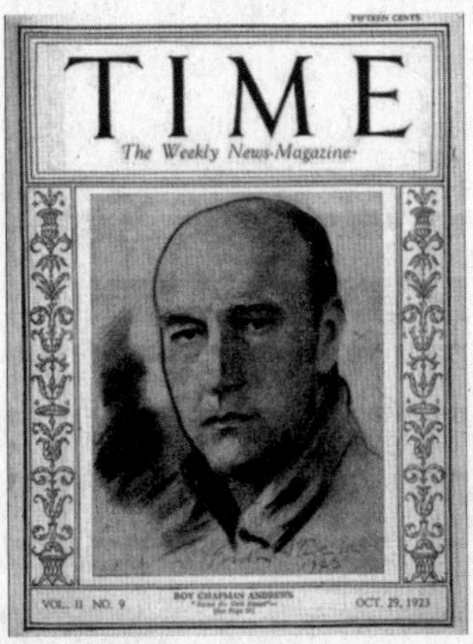

Cover of *Time* magazine on October 29, 1923, featuring Roy Chapman Andrews.

to say a rhino can teach us something about procreating, but Durrant may have discovered an unexpected source of infertility.

Problems with Procreation

An estimated 11 percent of women of reproductive age in the United States have experienced fertility problems, while among men, sperm counts in the United States and Europe appear to have declined by roughly half over the past fifty years.[3] Erectile dysfunction is increasing (and 26 percent of men who deal with it are under forty years old), and testosterone levels are declining by 1 percent each year.[4] There are many reasons, from physical conditions that disrupt healthy ovulation and sperm quality to delayed childbearing. But the costs of infertility are monumental and include both monetary and emotional sacrifices. Can the rhinos clue us in to at least some of this complicated story?

Barbara Durrant has an unusual job. Since receiving her PhD in 1979, she has worked at the San Diego Zoo, where she today uses some of the same reproductive science employed in human fertility research, in vitro fertilization, and embryo transfers to encourage pregnancies in species on the brink of extinction. The southern white rhinos are among her favorite subjects. On July 28, 2019, she became the proud godmother of Edward, the first southern white rhino born by artificial insemination in North America. Artificial insemination of southern white rhinos is rare, as the process is uniquely complicated, but young Edward has since been joined by a female calf named Future.

I learned a lot during my visit with Durrant on a warm October morning as she gave me a tour of the Nikita Kahn Rhino Rescue Center. Her sense of responsibility for these creatures is detectable in her warm demeanor; she's unmistakably devoted. When I was there, Edward's mother, Victoria, was still pregnant with him and being closely watched. Durrant had helped Victoria conceive through

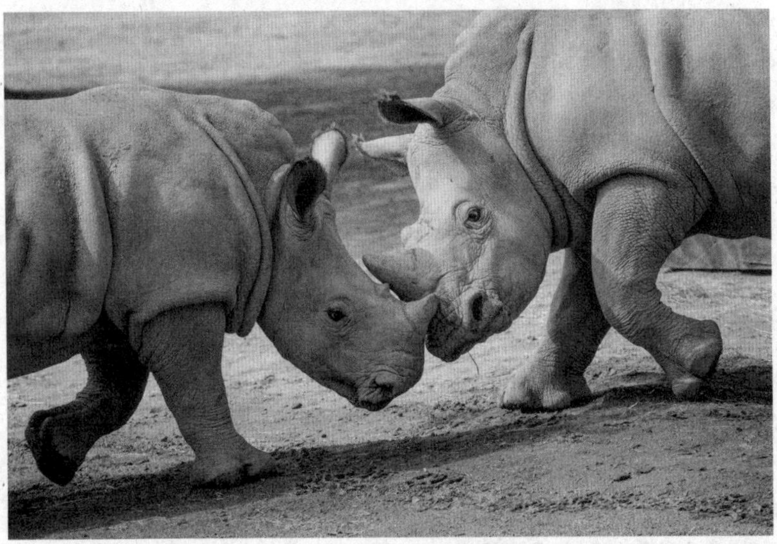

When Future (left) met Edward (right) at their home at the San Diego Zoo Safari Park, the two rhino calves became fast friends.

hormone-induced ovulation and artificial insemination with frozen semen from a southern white rhino.[5] DNA from both southern and northern white rhinos is banked at the institute in a facility called the Frozen Zoo, which houses samples from about ten thousand animals—a Noah's ark on ice. Edward was conceived the same month the last male northern white rhino died, leaving the remaining two females on the planet under protective guard from poachers at the Ol Pejeta Conservancy in Kenya. Unfortunately, these females are past breeding age.

A rhino's pregnancy lasts between sixteen and eighteen months. Victoria labored for only thirty minutes before her calf arrived weighing 148 pounds and standing up within twenty-five minutes. At six months, the calf topped 850 pounds. His birth caused much excitement, and enabled progress on one of the long-term goals of the zoo, which is to recover the northern white rhino. Northern and southern white rhinos differ in size, features, and feeding habits. The northern white rhino is smaller, with a flat skull and shorter front horn, while the larger southern white rhino sports a concave back and prominent shoulder hump. Durrant's plan is to use preserved skin cells from the northern white rhino to create stem cells that can then be programmed to develop into egg and sperm cells. It's riveting, edge-of-the-seat technology, as converting a skin cell into a stem cell is no easy task, a coup analogous to de-aging a cell back to its immature baby state, where it doesn't know what it will become (skin cell, nerve cell, muscle cell, gamete). Neither is reprogramming a stem cell to become a gamete (an egg or a sperm cell). But thanks to Nobel Prize–winning Japanese stem cell researcher Shinya Yamanaka, we know how to access the genes to perform this miraculous feat. The reset process involves four regulatory molecules now called the Yamanaka factors. Southern white rhinos like Future would then serve as surrogates, gestating the northern white rhino embryos through artificial insemination (inserting the sperm directly into the uterus), in vitro fertilization (joining the egg and sperm in a laboratory dish before inserting the mixture into the uterus), or an embryo transfer (transferring an already fertilized egg into the uterus). Durrant expects a northern white rhino calf to be birthed in this manner within ten to twenty years.

Contrary to what you might think, rhinos (Greek for "nose") are like big affectionate dogs—they know their names and come when you call for them. In their pen at the zoo, the rhinos sleep a lot during the day but become feistier in the late afternoon, and I was struck by the fact they don't suffer from joint issues despite their large body mass. They love to be touched; their skin is warm, tough, and supple all at once. In the wild, poachers kill them, and, like elephants, they lose their ability to eat well as their teeth deteriorate with age. But wild rhinos aren't known for having issues with fertility. It's the captive-born rhinos that develop infertility issues, which highlights some of the challenges of living in a zoo—challenges we face in our own "zoo" as we too find ourselves straying from nature. I was totally taken aback by what Durrant's work has uncovered as a likely source of her female rhinos' infertility: phytoestrogens—plant-based estrogens that naturally occur in many legumes. The rhinos were consuming phytoestrogens in their feed. It took her team eight years to identify the source of the fertility snags. But what was a difficult dilemma turned out to have an easy solution.

Let's Get Hormonal

Hormones are the body's biological messengers, produced in glands such as the pituitary and hypothalamus at the base of the brain, adrenals above the kidneys, ovaries in females, and testes in males. From there, they travel through the blood to other parts of the body, where they exert their effects. Hormones typically act at vanishingly small concentrations, docking at highly specific hormone receptors to transmit their messages to the target cells or tissues. The presence or absence of these receptors determines whether a particular cell will respond to the hormonal signal or ignore it. There are more than fifty hormones (and related molecules) that together control and coordinate nearly every bodily process—from your thinking brain to your growing hair.

The best-known hormones are the ones we deal with daily: Those that control appetite and digestion; sex-related hormones such as estrogen, progesterone, and testosterone; glucocorticoids such as cortisol, which regulate our response to stress; and thyroid hormone, which controls how many calories our bodies burn at rest. Insulin traffics how much glucose is in our blood; insufficient insulin or lack of response to insulin can lead to diabetes and a host of other health complications. Melatonin is required for our sleep/wake cycles. The brain's neurotransmitters such as dopamine, serotonin, and epinephrine affect our moods and decision-making. Growth hormone protects our tissues from breaking down and increases muscle mass and bone density when needed.

The dynamism of life is punctuated by hormones. Your age largely determines how and when many hormones get produced, especially those that affect reproduction. In women of childbearing age, the ovaries make the highest amount of estrogens, mostly in the form of estradiol, which induces monthly ovulation during an active menstrual cycle. During a normal twenty-eight-day cycle, estradiol levels peak around days eleven or twelve in the dominant follicle that hosts an egg cell. The estradiol change is identified by the hypothalamus, which signals the pituitary gland to release luteinizing hormone (LH) and follicle-stimulating hormone (FSH), which then trigger release of the egg (ovulation). The estradiol level change also stimulates the endometrium layer of the uterus to build up; the uterus lining is then shed when the estrogen level decreases (if there is no pregnancy), beginning menstruation. Young women produce large amounts of estradiol in their ovaries, and young men produce high levels of androgens, such as testosterone, in their testes; levels of both hormones decrease as we age. In men and postmenopausal women, estrogens do not come principally from the sex glands. Instead, fat and a variety of other types of cells produce estrogens, which mostly act where they are made rather than being secreted in large amounts into the blood.

The natural shifts in these sex hormone levels during the aging process are associated with other changes in the body, one of which is visibly obvious to us all: how our fat gets distributed. Older adults tend to have higher levels of body fat overall owing to factors like a slowing metabolism (our metabolism after age sixty declines by about 0.7 percent a year), gradual loss of muscle tissue, and a steady decline in physical activity as people lose motivation to exercise.[6] And the extra fat is more likely to be visceral—around our internal organs—than subcutaneous, or right under the skin, like baby fat.

Hormones and their effects are contextual; that is, the context in which they enter the bloodstream matters on how they affect an individual. This is important to understand because it relates directly to

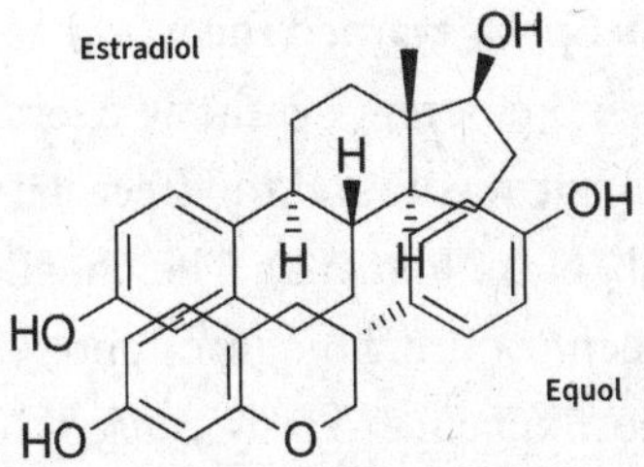

Comparison of estradiol structure (natural estrogen) and equol structure (isoflavone metabolite). Notice the striking similarity in the spatial arrangement of these two different molecules.

how dietary factors and chemical exposures can have various effects across the life span. By the same token, certain hormones can have nuanced effects across the life span too. A strong estrogen-like substance, for example, will have a different impact on a prepubescent girl than on a grown woman. And exposing a male fetus to unusually high levels of estrogen could have long-lasting effects on that fetus's fertility as an adult.

Endocrine-disrupting chemicals (EDCs) are increasingly talked about in scientific circles for how they potentially change a body's natural hormonal signaling patterns. Some of the most widely studied EDCs are chemicals that alter the balance of sex hormones in wildlife and contribute to adverse reproductive outcomes such as sex reversal or sterility in aquatic animals. Endocrine disruptors chiefly work by mimicking naturally occurring hormones in the body.

Natural estrogen (estradiol) and an estrogen-like compound from a soy-based isoflavone (equol) can look structurally nearly identical, confusing or blocking hormone receptors so that the natural hormone no longer works or even confuses the hormone-making tissue into making more or less of a particular hormone. One of the best-known EDCs that gained notoriety in the mid-twentieth century was DDT, the pesticide used widely to combat mosquitoes and the diseases they carry, such as malaria and typhus. By 1972, a decade after

Rachel Carson's *Silent Spring* warned the world about the dangers of rampant pesticide use, the potent synthetic chemical was banned in the United States after it was found to affect wild bird populations (and could potentially harm humans). The chemical was one of the reasons behind the decline during the 1950s and 1960s of our nation's mascot, the bald eagle. Exposure to DDT caused the majestic birds to lay eggs with brittle shells that cracked easily.

Industrial lubricants and plasticizers are chemicals that have been associated with declining reproductive health and increasing body mass index in humans. Some can also contribute to insulin resistance.[7] The biological mechanisms through which they exert their effects is complex, but we know they have the power to disrupt a body's normal metabolism and hormonal systems. These chemicals, most of them manufactured synthetics, are added to a wide variety of plastics to increase their flexibility, transparency, durability, and longevity. They are found in products as diverse as vinyl (PVC) wares (including baby bottles and food storage containers), paint, toys, air fresheners, and personal care and beauty goods. Although one category of these compounds, polychlorinated biphenyls (PCBs), once used as electrical insulators and flame retardants, was banned decades ago, they do not readily break down in the environment and so cycle through air, water, and soil—reaching us primarily through contaminated fish, meat, and dairy products.

More recently, long-term exposure to per- and polyfluoroalkyl substances (PFAS, pronounced "PEA-fass") has been implicated as potentially problematic too. PFAS have been linked to an increased risk of some cancers, immune system suppression (which can entail diminished responsiveness to vaccines), disrupted thyroid function, liver damage, problems with fetal development, and low birth weight. PFAS have been used commonly to coat and protect surfaces of various materials since the 1940s. And like PCBs, PFAS are "forever chemicals"—virtually indestructible compounds found everywhere: contaminated drinking water, electronics, furniture, nonstick cookware, waterproof clothes, food packaging (think pizza boxes, fast-food wrappers, and microwave popcorn bags), carpets and textiles, and even some cosmetics, dental floss, and athletic apparel (yes, your yoga pants). In 2022, the Environmental Protection Agency warned that these forever chemicals pose a greater danger to human health than previously thought, and the agency has begun to take aggressive action to better regulate the "contamination crisis."[8] In June 2022, the EPA drastically cut the safe level of PFAS down from what the agency had previously advised while also admitting there's no such thing as a safe level in our water systems, where most people are already unknowingly being exposed. The agency's goal is to have a zero tolerance policy.

It's impossible to avoid all exposures to these chemicals, especially the ones that persist in the environment, so we have to consider how these exposures could be contributing to preventable health challenges at special times in our lives, such as when—like the San Diego Zoo's rhinos—we're trying to get pregnant, sustain healthy pregnancies, and then nurse and nurture our children as they develop.

Developmental Origins of Disease

A lot can be mined from birth and death records if you're willing to look deeply and think critically. When David Barker, a professor of clinical epidemiology at the University of Southampton School of Medicine, pored over birth and death records in the United Kingdom, he noted a distinct relationship between low birth weight and a risk for dying from coronary heart disease as an adult. Wondering about the connection, Barker developed a hypothesis: that a baby born to a mother who was malnourished during pregnancy would be more susceptible later in life to chronic diseases such as diabetes, high blood pressure, heart disease, and obesity because the fetus had adapted to a nutritionally poor environment. His observations culminated in a paper published in the *Lancet* in 1989 in which he and his colleagues reported that among 5,654 men from Hertfordshire in southern England, those with the lowest birth weights and lowest weights at one year old had the greatest mortality from cardiovascular disease.[9]

Barker was not the first person to record the relationship between early life conditions and later disease. The Norwegian community doctor and researcher Anders Forsdahl had initially formulated the hypothesis in 1977, when he noted that a child's living conditions from the prenatal period through adolescence have an important impact on that child's risk of chronic disorders later in life, especially cardiovascular diseases after the age of forty.[10] His observations pointed to how programming of a body during vulnerable periods of development can ultimately affect health outcomes.

It should be duly noted that these relationships are just that—associations. They do not necessarily reflect direct cause and effect; early life exposures are not deterministic, though they may raise risk for certain ailments later. But that also gives us hope that by reducing early life exposures, we may be able to lessen the likelihood of disease later in life. In one of Barker's last public speeches, he stated, "The next generation does not have to suffer from heart disease or osteoporosis. These diseases are not mandated by the human genome. They barely existed one hundred years ago. They are unnecessary diseases. We could prevent them had we the will to do so."[11]

What are the diseases that can be affected by exposures during the fetal and developmental periods of childhood and adolescence? Most of the chronic ones we suffer from include: cardiovascular and pulmonary maladies; neurological ailments; immune-related conditions; disorders of reproduction and fertility; cancer; and metabolic disorders, including obesity and diabetes. Scientists who study this realm use a version of the following analogy: when a fifty-five-year-old man is diagnosed with Parkinson's, a thirty-five-year-old woman has breast cancer, a twenty-five-year-old man is infertile, a teenager is obese with metabolic syndrome and type 1 diabetes, a nine-year-old girl has asthma and food allergies, and a six-year-old boy has learning disabilities, the causes may not be found purely in their genetics.[12]

Although there is a genetic component to these conditions, variations in an individual's gene sequence likely account for only small and fluctuating risk. Instead, the common link among all these noncommunicable conditions is they likely had some environmental influence during early development—altered nutrition, stress, drugs, infections, or exposure to dangerous chemicals—that triggered epigenetic changes that stay with the body throughout life. When you hear about a typical Western diet—heavy in processed, refined flours, sugars, and bad fats—contributing to health conditions and even nuisances like acne, one of the mechanisms is through epigenetic signaling.[13]

Epigenetics literally means "on top of genetics" and refers to how your behaviors and environment can cause molecular changes in your DNA that affect the way your genes work. To be sure, your DNA's sequence is not changing, but epigenetic changes can influence how your body reads your DNA sequence and therefore which protein products get produced (or not). This can occur in a variety of ways.* The important thing to remember is that epigenetic changes affect which genes get turned on or off, thereby affecting your body's functionality. Epigenetic changes are the link between your lifestyle and genes.

Despite how complex living organisms are, with many opportunities for things to go wrong, development largely works well because there are built-in redundancies and backup plans for potential errors that could otherwise lead to serious malformations, defects, or problems. Cells have elaborate mechanisms to repair DNA as well

*Epigenetic changes can affect which genes are turned on by changing DNA methylation (adding a chemical group to DNA that can block the proteins in the body from being able to "read" the DNA), histone modification (these proteins bind tightly to DNA so that the genes encoded by the portion of the DNA cannot be turned on), or noncoding RNA (which regulates RNA and turns down the making of proteins).

as mechanisms to kill themselves in an orderly way if too many mutations are detected. Development is also exquisitely sensitive during certain stages in which small changes can have major outcomes. These are called "critical windows" of sensitivity.

There's no better way to illustrate this concept than with what I call the egg experiment. (I was originally told this by one of my early mentors at Johns Hopkins Hospital and one of the greatest cancer researchers of all time, Don Coffey.) If you take a fertilized egg and let it sit at room temperature for a few weeks, you get a rotten egg. But if you take that same egg and instead of letting it spoil on a counter for three weeks, you subject it to a cozy 99.5 degrees Fahrenheit and rotate it three times a day (it's best to choose an odd number to ensure the egg isn't in the same position two nights in a row), the outcome will be totally different: a chirping baby chick. Another entertaining example is in frog embryology: if you tilt a frog embryo at a critical time before the fertilized egg divides into two cells, you will get an embryo with two perfect heads; do the same thing thirty minutes later and the embryo will be completely normal. This simple experiment demonstrates the profound effect that environmental nuances can have as gravity and temperature turn chaos to order.

Perturbations that occur during critical windows in the course of a pregnancy can lead to dramatic birth defects—or no birth at all.[14] The effects of changes in hormones during the gestation of a fetus can be difficult to quantify and may not be manifest at birth, but the effects may clinically be present many years later. We learned that lesson the hard way from the story of diethylstilbestrol (DES), a synthetic estrogen that was administered to over 10 million women between 1938 and 1971. DES was initially thought to reduce the risk of miscarriage (which it turned out not to be effective at), and it was even recommended to many pregnant women as a routine preventive medicine.[15] So even women with no history of miscarriage were prescribed it. The chemical wound up in many products, including lotions, shampoo, and growth enhancers for chicken and cattle. Many years later it was learned that children born to DES-treated mothers would have reproductive issues or certain characteristic cancer conditions later in their lives. Adverse effects were first detected in 1971, decades after DES use had become commonplace. But that made sense, as the cancer (cancer of the cervix and vagina called clear cell adenocarcinoma) was seen in the daughters of the women who took DES, not in the mothers who were originally prescribed the hormone.[16]

One last example of critical windows of sensitivity that many women can recall is the use of thalidomide decades ago to control nausea from morning sickness during pregnancy. Fully 80 percent of babies whose mothers were prescribed the drug were born with severe limb defects if the mother took the drug between twenty and thirty-six days after fertilization (that is, in the first month or so of pregnancy). But if thalidomide was taken by the pregnant mother outside this critical window, the children did not have these defects. Again, this goes to show how *what*, *how much*, and *when* are important. Today, thalidomide is used to treat a skin condition as well as multiple myeloma, a rare blood cancer. It's also under study as a potential treatment for a wide array of conditions, which again goes to show that how a drug is used—under what circumstances, when, and at what dose—means everything. The exact mechanism of how thalidomide caused the teratogenic deformities in children is still unknown.

Developmental disruption can also lead to more subtle alterations that cause adverse health outcomes and increased risk for disease that may not manifest until many years later. Reduced fetal growth, often one of the results of exposure to nicotine in utero, is strongly associated with chronic conditions later in life, such as heart disease, diabetes, and obesity. Physicians recommend certain guidelines to pregnant women for many good reasons: avoid drug X, take prenatal vitamins containing folate (to help prevent some major birth defects of a baby's brain and spine), don't smoke or drink alcohol, avoid exposure to noxious chemicals and infectious agents, and so on. Insults to fetuses can have devastating and permanent repercussions.

Among the first studies to provide early, undeniable clues to a cause-and-effect relationship between the prenatal experience and lifelong consequences was the now-famous Dutch Famine Birth Cohort Study.[17] Known as the Hongerwinter ("Hunger Winter") in Dutch, the Dutch famine took place near the end of World War II during the winter of 1944–1945 in the Nazi-occupied part of the Netherlands, especially in Amsterdam and the densely populated western provinces. A Nazi blockade cut off food and fuel shipments from farm areas, leaving millions starving. Rations were as low as four hundred to eight hundred calories a day—less than a quarter of what an adult should consume. More than twenty thousand people died of starvation. Those who survived, some 4.5 million people, relied on soup kitchens until the Allies arrived in May 1945 and liberation of the area alleviated the famine. Carl Zimmer of the *New York Times* explained that because the Hunger Winter "started and ended so abruptly, it has served as an unplanned experiment in human health. Pregnant women, it turns out, were uniquely vulnerable, and the children they gave birth to have been influenced by the famine throughout their lives. When they became adults, they ended up a few pounds heavier than average. In middle age, they had higher levels of triglycerides and LDL cholesterol. They also experienced higher rates of such conditions as obesity, diabetes, and schizophrenia."[18] The Dutch Famine Birth Cohort Study (which David Barker was part of) showed that the famine experienced by the mothers caused epigenetic changes in their children that were manifested later in life as a predisposition to disease; some of these effects were passed to the next generation.[19] And when that generation had their own children, those offspring were also shorter than average and had increased fat and poorer health later in life. This alarming observation was among the first to show the power of epigenetic changes, which can be passed on through multiple generations.

Scientists are still figuring out how this happens at the molecular level. "How on earth can your body remember the environment it was exposed to in the womb—and remember that decades later?"[20] asked Bas Heijmans, a geneticist at Leiden University Medical Center in the Netherlands, in a *New York Times* article. He and his colleagues at Columbia University published a potential answer: that certain genes had been turned off by the paucity of calories (through changing of the epigenome and not the DNA sequence) and that these gene expression changes remained affected as the child grew up.[21] Plenty of competing ideas about how exactly these epigenetic changes took root are under study, for much mystery still remains. But the overall finding prevails: the type and availability of nutrients during pregnancy and infancy may have profound impacts on an individual's life. We also know that developmental programming does not stop at birth but continues throughout early life, probably at least until adolescence.

The Rhinos Reclaim Their Fertility

The rhinos in the San Diego Zoo weren't starving. That was what was so perplexing: they seemed to be living in an optimized environment. So what was the problem that took eight years to figure out? (I've already hinted at the answer.)

One of the most striking differences between the lives of wild animals versus the lives of their peers in captivity is often diet. Although the scientists and zookeepers who care for captive animals do their best to serve nutritious foods typical of an animal's natural diet, there can be unintended mistakes. When Barbara Durrant and her team were faced with infertile southern white rhino females, they realized they ought to look into the role phytoestrogens could be playing.

While roaming wild, white rhinos graze on grasses or whatever else is edible on the grounds they walk.[22] They can gobble up these short grasses faster than you and I could mow them; it takes about 120 pounds of grasses a day to keep up with a rhino's metabolic needs. In captivity, where the animals are not grazing all day, they're fed store-bought pellets, which are mainly made of dried soy and alfalfa, cheap and readily available natural sources of protein. But these pellets also naturally contain a lot of phytoestrogens, which have been implicated in fertility challenges in other species.

Phytoestrogens are estrogen-like (estrogenic) compounds derived from plants and are ubiquitous in human and animal diets. The phytoestrogens do not have as much estrogen activity as the hormone estradiol, but they still bind to the estrogen receptor and signal the cells like estrogen. Research conducted by Dr. Christopher Tubbs of the San Diego Zoo demonstrated that phytoestrogens "consumed in the diet and absorbed into the bloodstream can interact with an animal's estrogen receptors," which gives them "the potential to disrupt developmental and reproductive processes regulated by estrogens."[23]

The most common sources of phytoestrogen exposure to humans are soy products—but not the obvious ones (edamame, miso, tofu, tempeh). Soybean-derived foods creep into our diets in many ways, whether intentionally or not, from soy-based products like soy cheese, milk, burgers, ice cream, bacon bits, and even infant formulas to textured soy flour and soy protein isolate used in a dizzying array of processed and packaged foods. Soy is found in 60 percent or more of processed foods, in everything from sports drinks to granola bars and even doughnuts.[24] To see for yourself, look for variations of "textured vegetable/soy protein" on an ingredients label. Soy is a popular food and additive because it is an inexpensive, cholesterol-free, vegetarian protein that has plenty of fiber and no lactose. It also helps with binding ingredients and keeping a food moist.

We often hear about the good effects soy phytoestrogens have on human health, as they have been promoted as healthy alternatives to synthetic estrogens. Women going through menopause say soy phytoestrogens help them endure symptoms like hot flashes and night sweats because the soy phytoestrogens act like real estrogen. Postmenopausal women hear that soy can prevent bone loss and osteoporosis for the same reason—the phytoestrogens mimic estrogen in the body. Soy is a central ingredient to a traditional Asian diet, and because Asian populations have historically enjoyed lower rates of cardiovascular disease, menopausal symptoms, breast and prostate cancer, diabetes, and obesity than those in the West, such an observation has led to the belief that eating more soy products may reduce the risk of these diseases.[25]

Food claims have to be approved by the FDA, and in 1999 the FDA allowed the claim that eating soy daily reduces the risk of heart disease. Afterward, the number of foods that included soy as an ingredient went up dramatically.[26] But well-designed studies don't definitively prove any of these claims. Determining if phytoestrogens increase or reduce the risk of developing breast cancer has proven to be one of the most challenging human health impacts to address. It is well established that estrogens promote breast tumorigenesis, and that parameters which increase lifetime estrogen exposure (such as early menarche, short-duration breastfeeding, and low parity) are associated with elevated breast cancer risk. But the effect of phytoestrogens on breast cancer risk has still not been determined definitively. It would be very difficult to do prospective studies as there are so many variables to consider, including the race and age of the patients, the dose of phytoestrogen, the context of the phytoestrogen (what are you eating with them), the duration of the exposure, as well as the other hormones of the patient, among many.[27]

Can dietary phytoestrogens be toxic to our systems and, in particular, our fertility? Can we get too much of a good thing? Observational studies over the decades have raised concerns. An observation made in 1946 started concern over this issue. It was reported, at the time, that sheep grazing on red clover, which is high in phytoestrogens, were infertile. Two decades later, the effect of red clover on fertility was also seen in cows. Then in the 1980s, zoo-based cheetahs eating soy had fertility issues. In each of these animal situations, fertility returned when the phytoestrogen was reduced or eliminated from the diet. Some studies in women have also shown reproductive health issues with high levels of phytoestrogen ingestion.[28]

When Durrant and her team significantly reduced phytoestrogens from the white rhino feed in 2014, a fourteen-year-old female who'd never given birth before soon showed rising levels of progesterone, indicative of pregnancy. This female had been breeding since 2007, but she had never conceived until her diet changed. This was a big step forward, but her progesterone level began to drop two months before her due date and the calf was delivered stillborn. Durrant did not lose hope. Other successful pregnancies followed in her white rhinos that had never reproduced previously. Durrant's discovery culminated in a 2019 paper for the American Society for Microbiology.[29] What does microbiology have to do with fertility? This is where the story gets even more interesting.

Within each of us lives a community of microbes housed largely in our gut that interacts with our own biology and commands much of our metabolism, neurochemistry, immunity, and perhaps even fertility. It's called the microbiome and has been one of medicine's most talked about subjects in recent years. The health of an animal depends on the microbial composition of its microbiome. And this is true whether we're talking about a human or a rhino. Durrant has written on this topic and made the observation that the southern white rhino metabolized and absorbed the soy phytoestrogens in a manner that reduced her ability to carry a child. When Durrant and colleagues looked at another rhino species, the greater one-horned rhino, who can eat soy pellets and still deliver baby rhinos, she showed that different bacteria in the gut (a different microbiome) appeared to be responsible for the difference. The bacteria in the GI tract of the southern white rhino are different from those in the one-horned rhino. Think of it as with a different soil, a different seed will grow. Each species of rhino has different soil in its GI tract. The one-horned rhino can eat phytoestrogens and have no issue with its fertility, while this clearly isn't the case for the southern white rhino. Durrant's work to elucidate this was critical in understanding the role of the gut, the microbiome, and hormone metabolism and absorption.[30]

The microbes in our guts help metabolize what we consume. And in the process of breaking down dietary compounds, they create active metabolites that can then go on to affect virtually every system in the body, including those related to hormones. Scientists are increasingly astonished by how much our microbial comrades in our guts regulate our own physiology, a phenomenon we'll explore more in chapter 9. But all of this raises another intriguing question: How much does our own microbiome contribute to our fertility? And how can changes to our microbiome alter fertility for better or worse?

Before I answer these, I'll put some of the debate to rest by saying that soy phytoestrogens are perfectly safe for humans when consumed in moderation—preferably from natural, less processed sources (more edamame, less soy protein isolate, and no supplements). Soy earns neither the health halo nor health hazard label. And we should remember that any ingredient can be problematic when devoured to extreme (water included). Eating more than 100 mg of soy isoflavones (which is a lot—equivalent to about 6 ounces of tempeh or 16 cups of soy milk) daily has been linked to a change in ovarian function, but moderate soy consumption has not been demonstrated to be an issue as of yet in adults.[31] It may actually indirectly confer benefits at the right amount by reducing your consumption of saturated fats in red meat and increasing your fiber intake—a double bonus.

When it comes to soy-based formula for babies, however, we need more data to answer questions about soy's effects at this critical-window age. In 2018, Children's Hospital of Philadelphia published a scientific study demonstrating that "infants who consumed soy-based formula as newborns had differences in some reproductive-system cells and tissues, compared to those who used cow-milk formula or were breastfed."[32] The differences were noted among the girls, who showed signs of responses to estrogen exposure in their vaginal and uterine cells. The authors of the NIH-funded study were quick to point out, however, that the differences between the breast-fed babies and those fed soy milk were small and did not seem to be an issue in their reproductive development.[33] For babies who cannot, for whatever reason, receive breast milk or properly digest milk, soy-based formulas may be warranted. But you may be surprised to learn that soy formula accounts for up to 25 percent of formula sales in the United States—something that deserves further thought and study.[34]

In what I hope is the not-too-distant future, we'll learn how to manage soy consumption for ideal health and even potentially manipulate our microbiomes to reap soy's rewards without any downsides. Which brings me to answer the question about the microbiome's impact on fertility: yes, the strength and function of your microbiome serve an important part in the story of your health from matters of fertility to matters of your heart, brain, nervous system, immunity, and overall metabolism.

The southern white rhinos teach us not only that diet can have profound effects on our biology, but also that those effects can result from subtle, seemingly superficial changes. The idea that small changes can have big effects dovetails with the butterfly effect I raised in an earlier chapter. Think of the individual who commits to walking thirty minutes a day and loses twenty pounds over a year or, conversely, the person who decides to reduce consumption of sugar by switching to sugar substitutes in the forms of aspartame, sucralose, and saccharin. You might assume that's a healthy swap to save calories and avoid the downstream effects of too much sugar. But substances in these artificial sweeteners can change the composition of your microbiome to the extent they may ultimately lead to increased insulin resistance, diabetes, and obesity. Again, small changes can have monumental consequences. We are indeed "robust but fragile," a phrase used to describe how, for example, complex systems can be paradoxically resilient and vulnerable at the same time.

For anyone who suffers from fertility issues, it may not necessarily be something offensive in the diet but rather something else small and simple that adds up. Things like chronic poor sleep, lack of physical activity, and too much psychological stress may seem innocuous but can have enormous effects. For many people seeking healthier, longer lives, starting with the basics—better nutrition and more movement—is most doable and motivates one to make other improvements in behavior and habits.

Remember that one of the tenets of a healthful diet is to try to eat as close to nature as possible and as much like your ancestors as you can. Depending on where you are from in the world, your body evolved over many centuries—hundreds of generations—for certain foods, and we need to respect this. Earlier I covered how we evolved to eat and digest meat along with our chimp ancestors, but for some populations, meat-centric diets are not healthful. In fact, so-called vegetarian genes have recently been discovered. Genetic variations have evolved in populations that have historically favored plant-based diets, such as in India, Africa, and parts of East Asia, that allow these people to process omega-3 and omega-6 fatty acids more efficiently, converting them into compounds necessary for early brain development and controlling inflammation.[35] (People who eat meat and fish can get plenty of their omegas directly from those foods.) Similarly, genetic variations have been found among the Inuit in Greenland, who mainly eat seafood and are uniquely adapted to a marine-based diet. We don't know when these adaptations occurred in evolution, but one thing we can conclude is that we can use this genomic information to try to tailor our diets so they match our genome. This personalized nutrition is a burgeoning area of research and study. We may soon be able to tell, through simple genetic analyses, who should stick with a wholly plant-based diet.

We are complex systems. Yet within that complexity, there is also simplicity—rhymes and reasons, as well as a certain level of adaptability. Our internal programming may be somewhat fixed from our early life experiences, but it's not all static and immutable. In San Diego, Edward and Future hold the keys to keeping Earth's unicorns alive and thriving. And you and I can do what we're able to prevent what may lie in wait for us. We may not be able to change our past environments, but we can shape the ones we enter going forward. To this end, I'll share one more little-known secret that rhinos tell us: how to exercise.

The Run-Stop-Run Recipe

Earlier I said that rhinos are remarkably free of joint pain despite their massiveness (and lounging habits). But I also learned that they are the fastest of all the land mammals that weigh over two thousand pounds (white rhinos can clock in at five thousand pounds, making them the world's second-largest land mammal behind elephants). They can charge when they need to, reaching speeds over thirty miles an hour and sustaining that for about a mile. By comparison, the fastest humans reach speeds of only twenty-eight miles per hour in a short hundred-meter sprint.*

Wild animals don't spend a full hour on a treadmill, but they aren't sedentary for most of the day. They move about routinely and engage in brief periods of high-intensity movements when necessary (or when playing). There's something to learn from that strategy to

*The current record holder for being the fastest human runner is retired Jamaican sprinter Usain Bolt, who ran the hundred-meter dash in 9.58 seconds, which translates to about 27.5 miles per hour when he hit full stride in the race. Studies suggest that human speed on land is limited not by the strength of our bones and tendons but rather by our bipedal stride that leaves us hanging in the air—and during the brief moments that our feet are hitting the ground, we have to exert a lot of force. Put simply, we're limited by how quickly we can reposition our legs and have time to propel ourselves off the ground. Four-legged creatures have the leg up on this one.

stay fit because we're more likely to either commit to one-hour exercise routines or do nothing at all (and those one-hour commitments are often surrounded by hours of sitting in front of our computers).

Over and over again, the science tells us that regular movement is key to health, and it doesn't take all that much. A mere two minutes of activity an hour extends life considerably, and even three seconds a day of resistance training—contracting your arm muscles as hard as possible—can increase your biceps' strength by as much as 12 percent after a month![36] We've gotten used to thinking we need to engage in rigorous exercise for long periods of time to reap the rewards. Not so. There's a lot we can do from our desks at work or in our homes or at a local park without any equipment whatsoever. Simply getting off our butts at least twice an hour for those two minutes to jump up and down or take a quick stroll will confer benefits. But there is something to be said for short bursts of activity during which you push yourself hard and then back off to recover, then repeat. It's nature's best exercise. It's how most animals stay fit naturally in their environments as they hunt, play, run from predators, and survive.

Whether it's interval training or a game of tennis, which happens to be one of the sports most linked to longevity, all of us can find something to participate in that's physically demanding and gets us active without the need to become endurance athletes. In fact, all the evidence to date points to more benefits from moderate amounts of moderately strenuous exercise—not the extremes of too gentle or too rigorous. It's nature's happy middle ground. There's nothing natural about counting down the minutes spent on a gym machine.

So why do sports like tennis win over solitary engagements such as cycling, swimming, and running? Not only do most partnered or team sports involve the run-stop-run recipe, but with other people at play, you gain a social component. It's one thing to boost your heart rate, but it's wholly another thing to do that while sharing the experience. Being social helps reduce stress and makes us feel connected, which directly affects our health. And if you need more proof, consider this: in a beautifully done study spanning twenty-five years that looked at the impact of different types of sports and physical activities on longevity, the results spoke for themselves—people who played tennis gained nearly a decade more of life (compared to their couch potato counterparts), while the gym rats (who participated in "health club activities") earned a paltry 1.5 years extra.[37] I'll take the extra ten years. And I do love tennis.

Putting the Long in Longevity

The environmental forces we've covered—including exposures, nutrition, and exercise—mean that our longevity is largely up to us. Your genes account for much less than you'd think when it comes to your life spans. New calculations based on analyses of large ancestry databases have genes accounting for under 7 percent of how long people live, a profound change from previous estimates that had genes accounting for as much as 20 to 30 percent.[38] Put simply, our longevity is based mostly on our lifestyle choices: what we eat and drink, how much we move, what kind of stress wears on us, and even other factors like the quality of our relationships, whom we marry, the strength of our social networks, and our access to health care and education. Even personality traits like conscientiousness, friendliness, and positive attitude can factor into longevity. To me, this fact is tremendously empowering, and optimistic. Our genes are not our fate. As humans, we can use our intelligence and higher processing to make the decisions to enable us to avoid disease.

One study in particular—a collaboration between Google's life-extension spin-off Calico and the genetics company Ancestry—involved more than fifty-four million family trees (amounting to four hundred million people who were born from the nineteenth century to the mid-twentieth century).[39] The researchers looked at the life spans of married couples, finding that they shared similar life spans—more so than brothers and sisters. The study went on to show an amazing life-span correlation with longevity of the nongenetic in-laws! Can you imagine that I can tell you how long you'll live more accurately based on how long your mother-in-law lived than by sequencing your entire genome?!

Such an outcome obviously suggests a strong influence of nongenetic forces because spouses or in-laws do not typically have genetic variants in common. Other factors they probably do have in common, however, include things like eating and exercise habits, having access to clean water, being literate, living far from disease outbreaks, respecting and complying with doctors' recommendations, and not smoking. This makes sense: people tend to marry others who enjoy the same lifestyles. You don't generally see the lounge lizard coupled with a marathoner or the teetotaler married to the party animal. Again, to me, this finding is incredibly powerful and exciting; more than 90 percent of our longevity is in our own hands. We are each in charge of our future.

Creature Cheat Sheet

Your environment matters from the moment you're a ball of living cells in a womb to a screaming baby, hormonal teenager, and thoughtful adult hoping to raise good humans (and yourself along the way). We often don't think about the small and subtle changes we can make in daily life that translate to big outcomes in our health and longevity. But as exemplified by rhinos, those delicate small edits affect not only how our genes behave but also how our internal microbial partners show up to help or hinder us. DNA may be static, but how it behaves through epigenetic forces can change everything. We want to protect not only our inherited DNA but how it acts in the environment, and even how we choose to exercise can play into our longevity. We have more control of our fate than we realize.

While you're not going to change the exposures and events that epigenetically shaped who you are today, you can certainly have an impact going forward and reshape your biology and DNA's behavior through your daily habits. You also can help support the ideal environment for the people around you, including children who are not yet mature and attuned to serve themselves best.

To that end, here are some chief takeaways: Be mindful of exposures, especially during vulnerable periods in life, such as when you're pregnant and raising your children. Chemical exposures can be stealthy in today's world, be they synthetic ones in our air, water, consumables, and household goods or natural ingredients like soy in foods and formulas that have unknown effects in different people at various ages. In the next decade or so, each one of us may benefit from personalized nutrition that can tell us what we should be consuming to respect our unique biology and the indelible relationship between our gut bugs and human cells. Two minutes of physical activity an hour minimum is necessary to meet the body's demand for movement. Short bursts of activity throughout the day are ideal, and when you carve out time for longer stretches of exercise, go for interval training or engage in team sports that have the dual effect of striking the sweet spot: achieving those short bursts of activity and socializing. Any racket sport—from tennis to pickleball—will hit the spot. Remember that moderate amounts of moderately strenuous exercise are nature's happy middle ground.

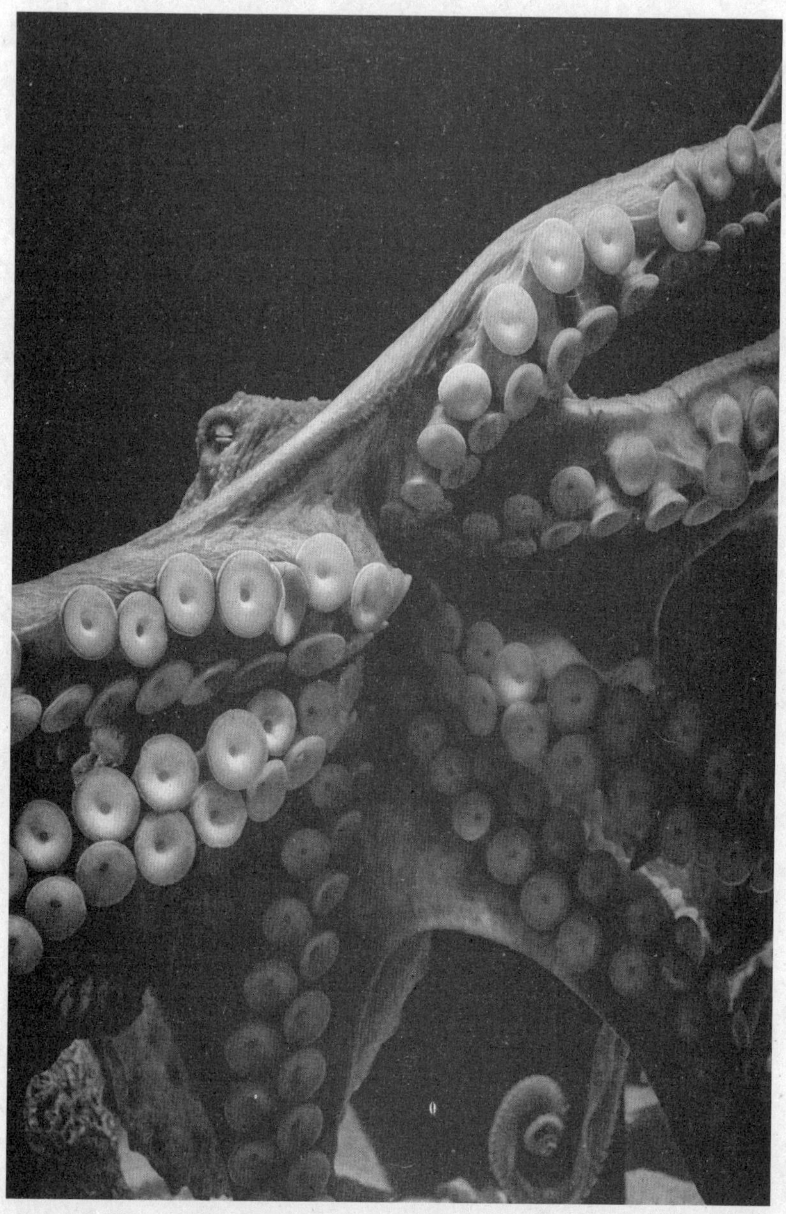

The nine-brained octopus.

9

Smart Suckers and Demented Dolphins

On Intelligence and Thinking Straight Forever

> *The measure of intelligence is the ability to change.*
>
> *Everything should be made as simple as possible, but no simpler.*
>
> —ALBERT EINSTEIN

Have you ever wondered what it means to be intelligent? Is it being able to solve advanced math equations? To invent something that revolutionizes an industry? The ability to learn (quickly), adapt (swiftly), and make difficult decisions in an instant? Or how about the opposite—to unlearn and relearn as new data come in to invalidate what you previously believed? When plants grow toward the sun, is that intelligence? Is a dog who reliably sniffs out cancer or low blood sugar on par with master sommeliers who can detect the vintage of a century-old Château Latour? Raccoons are renowned for their lock-picking skills, squirrels are masters at evading elaborate tricks to prevent them from getting into bird feeders for a savory snack, and pigs can understand emotions and recognize themselves in mirrors at a younger age (relative to their life span) than humans can. So again, what defines intelligence?

Most scientists cringe to define such slippery terms as *conscience*, *mind*, *sentience*, and *intelligence*. Even the word *intelligence* has interesting origins: from the Latin *inter* ("between") and *legere* ("choose"), as if being able to choose wisely between things were all it took. Intelligence is notoriously difficult to measure. We may lean on IQ tests and SAT scores, but even these are terribly narrow-minded metrics (and constantly under attack). The three capabilities scientists often study to analyze intelligence are self-control, self-awareness, and memory, but even these focal points can be unimaginative and limiting. In one of my favorite books, *The Lives of a Cell*, Lewis Thomas writes about another aspect to intelligence rarely acknowledged by us humans: group effort in thought and execution of an idea. As he notes:

> A solitary ant, afield, cannot be considered to have much of anything on his mind; indeed, with only a few neurons strung together by fibers, he can't be imagined to have a mind at all, much less a thought. He is more like a ganglion on legs. Four ants together, or ten, encircling a dead moth on a path, begin to look more like an idea. They fumble and shove, gradually moving the food toward the Hill, but as though by blind chance. It is only when you watch the dense mass of thousands of ants, crowded together around the Hill, blackening the ground, that you begin to see the whole beast, and now you observe it thinking, planning, calculating. It is an intelligence, a kind of live computer, with crawling bits for its wits.[1]

As Carl Zimmer of the *New York Times* pointed out, "Intelligent animals don't rely on fixed responses to survive"; instinct and reflexes may be smart adaptations in and of themselves, but true intelligence requires the ability to invent new behaviors, adapt on the fly, and make contextual decisions.[2] The study of animal intelligence, or cognition, is a nascent field that is increasingly cluing us in to the meaning of "smart." We may think we sit on top of the animal kingdom, but when it comes to intelligence, that viewpoint is grossly oversimplified.

Other questions to ponder: What do you *need* to be intelligent? An education? Good genes? A sixth sense? The ability to take risks? A bunch of neurons that make up a nimble brain? Or how about a bunch of suckers dotting eight long, meandering arms? Octopuses* are highly intelligent creatures with nine brains, but they don't live long and most don't like to socialize. So how did these loners get to be so ingenious? Why do they grow smart, live fast, and die young?

The Outsmarting Octopus

In the 2016 Academy Award–winning sci-fi thriller *Arrival*, based on the 1998 novella *Story of Your Life* by Ted Chiang, Amy Adams plays a linguistics professor, Dr. Louise Banks, who is sent to try and communicate with extraterrestrials when spaceships land on our planet. They don't know if the aliens are hostile or friendly. As fearful nations teeter on the verge of war in the confusion, Banks and her crew must race against time to find a way to communicate with the extraterrestrials, who speak in a cryptic language using palindrome phrases written with circular symbols.

Without getting into the details of the story, consider the following: Somebody, inspired by Ted Chiang's descriptions, had to come up with how to represent these intelligent beings on screen. They are called "heptapods" for their seven limbs, and though they are beastly in size compared to humans, they don't look too dissimilar from earthly cephalopods. This is hardly coincidence. Cephalopods are the most intelligent, most mobile, and largest of all mollusks and include

*Note that the plural form is preferably octopuses rather than octopi. The word comes from Greek, not Latin.

squids, octopuses, cuttlefish, and chambered nautiluses. (Mollusks are one of the largest and most diverse class of animals on Earth, including over fifty thousand species like snails, clams, scallops, and oysters.) Cephalopods can tell us a lot about what it means to be intelligent, especially the octopuses that present a paradox that evolutionary biologists are still trying to figure out: Why do they possess such large brains if they don't live that long?

Their "brain," mind you, is much more than a doughnut-shaped organ in their physical head. They are said to have nine brains, eight of which reside along their eight arms where two-thirds of an octopus's half a billion neurons zip around messages, allowing the blobby sea creature to touch, smell, and taste. Each arm works like its own minibrain, able to act independently. It was finally shown in 2011 that the central brain of the octopus processes the creature's sight and also is charged with some control over its arms.[3]

The brain requires a lot of energy to function, so the scientific argument goes that the larger the brain (which requires more energy), the more intelligence it has, or otherwise evolution wouldn't let it take up so much energy.[4] Humans invest a lot, as the human brain is larger than expected for our bodies (compared to other primates and to mammals in general) and consumes an outstanding 20 percent of our total energy budget despite representing only 2 percent of our body mass.[5] The encephalization quotient (EQ) offers a more precise measure, estimating intelligence by comparing an animal's brain to that of a typical creature of the same size. It isn't a perfect measure, but it is pretty good. The concluding fact is that the octopus's brain-to-body ratio is the largest of any invertebrate. It's also larger than that of many vertebrates, although not mammals.

Now here's the absurdity: all that brainpower doesn't help them live long lives. Although a giant Pacific octopus can live up to the age of a human kindergartner (five years), some species of octopuses eke out only a six-month existence. That's not a good return on investment. Peter Godfrey-Smith of the University of Sydney, who studies animal life and the birth of the mind, says it's a bit like spending a vast amount of money to earn an advanced degree and then having only two years to make use of it.[6] Such a contradiction gives scientists plenty to study. Godfrey-Smith and others who observe octopuses think they're watching the closest thing we'll get to meeting an intelligent alien. What I love about these animals is that they not only share a history with us on this planet, but also show us that evolution constructed minds twice over. And it did so with different blueprints, building blocks, and even zip codes.

Philosophers may enjoy speculating about the whole mind-body problem and how our consciousness arose, but nothing poses quite such a challenge or offers such intriguing clues as these soft bodies with many minds. Our last common ancestor existed six hundred million years ago and was thought to resemble a flattened worm, perhaps only millimeters long. Yet somewhere along the evolutionary line, octopuses and their cephalopod siblings developed high-resolution, camera-like eyes that focus an image on a retina. And so did we, totally independently—an example of convergent evolution. Two vastly different species arrived at exactly the same eyesight technology, which gives pause for thought about the process of evolution. The same goes for our brains.

Brains are the crowning case of convergent evolution—the process by which unrelated or distantly related species evolve similar traits independently to adapt to similar physical necessities and navigate the same kind of world. The tendency of complex nervous systems to evolve in certain ways is probably universal—not just on Earth, but also in other worlds. Evolution tends to arrive at the same solutions over and over again because they are the ones that work. Anatomically our brain is certainly very different from the brain of the octopus, but both brains perform many of the same functions, such as long- and short-term memory, sleep, image recognition, and play.[7] Researchers have even shown that octopuses can distinguish between two humans dressed identically.[8]

If you haven't kept up with stories of octopuses making headlines for their extraordinary talents, let me say that their celebrity status goes back decades. (For a visual tour of their delightful and entertaining feats, see "Octopuses 101" by *National Geographic*'s WILD video library online.) A 1959 paper was among the first to detail an attempt to teach octopuses to perform a task.[9] The study occurred at the Naples Zoological Station in Italy under the leadership of Peter Dews, a doctor and researcher who spent most of his professional career at Harvard Medical School. In his experiments with the Italian octopuses, Dews tried to train three of them to pull and release a lever in exchange for food. Two of them, Albert and Bertram, succeeded in a "reasonably consistent" manner, but the one named Charles was not so compliant. Charles resisted the experiment; he not only warded off Dews and his team by squirting water at anyone who approached the tank, but also grabbed and dragged the light suspended above the water into the tank and applied so much force to the lever that it broke—"forcing the early termination of the experiment," Dews wrote. Disappointed, Dews thought his experiment had mostly failed, but since then, true tales of octopuses' cleverness have become legend.

They've been seen plotting great escapes from aquariums, navigating mazes, solving puzzles, squirting jets of water to deter predators, camouflaging themselves into invisibility like masters of disguise, opening screw-top jars to reach concealed food (and getting their whole bodies in and out of those jars), using tools in the wild like stacking rocks to protect the entrances to their dens, and using coconut shells as armor. Octopus behavior is legendary, and so is their biology. Octopus arms grow back if you slice them off, they have a complicated genome (2.7 billions of letters compared with our 3 billion letters), and have similar complexity in proteins found in their blood to what we have. In an amazing *National Geographic* video clip placed online in 2007, a 600-pound octopus can fit through a hole the size of a quarter, because they have no bones in them.[10] And as Dews discovered, they can be quite unruly and uncooperative, beguiling scientists who try to study them.

Although we have to be careful about anthropomorphizing animals—a fundamental precept of animal psychology called Morgan's canon says higher mental faculties should only be considered as explanations if lower faculties with simpler processing could not explain a behavior—the octopus leaves much for us to ponder in our definition of intelligence. Morgan's canon is named after the nineteenth-century British zoologist and psychologist C. Lloyd Morgan, who was particularly interested in "mental evolution," a term he used to describe the borderline between intelligence and instinct.[11] For example, Morgan had a terrier named Tony who could open the garden's gate. If you were in Morgan's yard and saw the gate being opened, you would conclude that Tony was brilliant by this "final behavior." Morgan, though, had watched Tony gradually learn the behavior through much trial and error and concluded there was no "insight" that led to the final event of opening the gate. The dog had been trained to open the gate; he wasn't employing some clever problem-solving. This distinction was critically important in the growth of the idea of behaviorism, the theory that much of human and animal behavior is explained in terms of conditioning, without needing thoughts or feelings. Such an idea can actually help us humans understand why people (ourselves included) behave the way they do. Often it could be based more on prior conditioning than on thoughtful, in-the-moment reasoning. To some degree, we all base decisions on a combination of reflexes from previous experience combined with intelligent input on the spot. Acknowledging this can assist us in making better, more thoughtful decisions that lead to healthy changes in our behavior—changes that help us live longer than the smart octopus.

"Grow Smart and Die Young"

Piero Amodio is a Cambridge University–trained biologist and psychologist who studies animal behavior and cognition. Spirited and youthful, he seems like your cool tenth-grade science teacher who never tires of talking about the oddest features of the sea's surrealist characters. He's had a love for cephalopods since his boyhood growing up in Naples, not too far from the zoological station where Dews conducted his experiments and where Amodio is a research fellow today at the Stazione Zoologica Anton Dohrn. The Mediterranean has been his lifelong playground.

"For as long as I've had a memory, I've taken to the sea," he tells me. "I spent hours on snorkeling expeditions and free diving down two, three meters to find and catch octopuses." It was his version of a video game, playing against a cunning opponent with artful hiding skills. And when he did happen to momentarily snag one, he often found himself soon holding an empty bag in a cloud of ink spurted out of the cephalopod as if to say, "See ya later!"

He never took the octopuses home if he happened to catch any. He merely wanted to try to interact with them. "The fun part was to see if I was good enough to find them, as they can hide so well," he says. "They can turn invisible by cloaking their appearance into their background or try to pretend not to be there by showing specific shapes to visually throw you off. You can hold your breath for a minute or two and move your fingers in front of them. Or you can remove the rock they wrap themselves around."

Amodio defines intelligence as a collection of complex abilities: problem-solving, physical cognition (acquiring and using information from the physical world), and social cognition (understanding other creatures). Social cognition is sometimes referred to as "theory of mind," or being able to infer someone else's thinking and adjust your behavior accordingly. Amodio offers an example from the avian world to help explain: if you're a bird that notices another bird around that can see where you're hiding food, you'll move the food when the other bird goes away.

One of the reasons Amodio studies animals other than those in our direct lineage is that apes are the most studied model for intelligence. But they aren't the only one. "There are different evolutionary paths leading to intelligence," he notes, leading creatures to have different cognitive experiences. The way octopuses perceive emotion is probably different from the way we do, although Amodio is quick to point out that there's no way to measure things like emotion in an octopus. So although there are certain evolutionary benefits to feeling scared, for instance, we cannot show an octopus to be "scared." Our ability to experience a wide array of emotions, some of them quite complex, is probably another layer to our intelligence that sets us apart from other animals. Appreciating our capacity to bring emotions into our thinking can improve our problem-solving and decision-making. It is critically important that we realize when emotions are having a role in our decisions, for better or worse.

In 2018, Amodio published a paper with five other scientists that received international media coverage.[12] That paper, "Grow Smart and Die Young," reviews two common theories about the development of intelligence. According to the *ecological intelligence hypothesis*, intelligence evolves as an adaptation for finding food. Smarter animals can find food more reliably and quickly. They can learn to remember which trees bear fruit, for example, use tools to obtain the food and store it, and know the right season to go back for more. The *social intelligence hypothesis* says that wiser animals cooperate and learn from other members of the same species. Maintaining interpersonal relationships, while mutually useful to individuals and a society, is not necessarily easy. It demands a certain level of mental faculties and cooperation that includes using powers of reasoning, or bringing in our sensibilities when we make and sustain friendships. Both forces may have given rise to various forms of intelligence, though here again, octopuses surprise us because they tend to be loners, which is rare for intelligent creatures. They don't use their wits to engage in elaborate social relationships and underwater mingling. There is no octopus "culture," another feature that sets them apart from us. And therein lies a potential takeaway: sometimes it may be valuable to think outside the influence of others or the dominant culture, to be our own creatures, and to essentially get out of our own heads.*

The fact that our brains are centralized does have its limitations. What if, like the octopus, we could have limbs that could act and carry out instructions on their own or in coordination with one another?[13] Granted, that may never literally happen. But by studying the octopus's brainy multitasking, robotics engineers are beginning to find applications for new technology in bots. This way of thinking is even having influence in military settings, which are mimicking it for troop and command structures.

There's another reason Amodio's team thinks octopuses could have gotten so clever. Zimmer described this reason in his 2018 *New York Times* piece: 500 million years ago, he wrote, the snail-like ancestors of the octopus evolved to use their covering as a flotation device. The shells would be filled with varying amounts of gas as a means of moving deeper in the ocean or moving toward the surface. About 275 million years ago, the ancestor of the cephalopods lost the external shell as part of their evolution. The actual reason for this isn't clear, but it led to their ability to move more easily around the ocean floor and enter places that weren't possible with a shell. But the lack of a shell did open the cephalopods to be easier for certain predators to attack. The threat of being eaten may have led them to evolve bigger and more functioning brains to be able to hide, escape, and enable survival. Though the evolution of the octopus optimized

*In addition to his work in his native Italy, Amodio serves as a National Geographic Explorer, leading the first scientific expedition to study the elusive larger Pacific striped octopus in the wild. Unlike its siblings, this species of octopus happens to be highly social. Perhaps he'll find a new revelation to incorporate into our understanding of the mystery of octopus intelligence.

their ability to move and camouflage, those characteristics don't completely protect the octopus from harm. Soft-bodied octopuses couldn't expect to survive as long in the wild as those with shells, and so their new big brains evolved at the expense of a shorter life.[14]

Although humans have both ecological and social intelligence, octopuses teach us to embrace other forms of intelligence too. Not everyone can excel at math, paint a masterpiece, perform brain surgery, or fly a spaceship. We each bring our unique ways of thinking, reasoning, and problem-solving to the world, and we should appreciate those differences. Whether we're a human or an octopus, one truth remains the same: a good life is about being able to adapt to our environment, learn from experience, and overcome obstacles. Whatever wits you have to achieve those goals make up intelligence. And perhaps one day we'll be able to incorporate the octopus's multi-brained, multitasking prowess into bioengineering advances to our benefit—without splintering our centralized brain across our fingers and toes. Another critically important lesson from the octopus is the value of short-term versus long-term gain. Many medical or other interventions can make us feel better or stronger today, but the implications for tomorrow can be significant. Taking growth hormone, for example, might make you "look better" today but may significantly shorten your life.

If you're wondering how octopuses die, this is where the story gets even more interesting. And tragically gruesome. After mating, octopuses pretty much self-destruct on cue, entering a death spiral that can include self-mutilation as if they've gone crazy. The females in particular steal the grisly show. The female octopus will lay the eggs, and then she stops eating and begins to slowly die. When the eggs hatch, she is likely already dead. In captivity, females will actually go a step further and try to harm themselves.[15] Males also deteriorate and perish soon after performing their mating duties, but again it's the females who enter a most bizarre course of events. This wild orchestra that ends in a quick death has vexed scientists for a long time, but we finally now think that it owes its origins to the machinations of the octopus's optic glands, which are functionally similar to our pituitary gland, which pumps out many essential hormones. When scientists remove the optic glands, located between the eyes, the death march is halted and an octopus's fate is totally changed: the creature will return to feeding, growing, and can live a longer life. We don't fully understand all the signaling that goes on during this incredibly unique death process, but clues are starting to come in and reveal a surprising culprit: cholesterol.

Although cholesterol tends to be couched in negative terms, healthy levels are required by the body where cholesterol serves important functions, acting as a building block for tissues, cell membranes, and vital substances such as many hormones. Vitamin D, for instance, is made in your skin cells on exposure to UV light using cholesterol (in those skin cells) as a precursor molecule. Nobody realized, however, that this same molecule, cholesterol, that helps support life can also act as a self-destruct hormone. And yes, to be sure, cholesterol is itself a steroid hormone. When scientists dug a little deeper into the chemical composition of the female octopus's optic glands' output after breeding, they found a breathtaking connection between the animal's hormone biology and inevitable death.

Once spawning has occurred, the optic glands in a female octopus undergo dramatic changes and begin producing large amounts of steroid hormones, and among them is 7-dehydrocholesterol (7-DHC), a precursor to our cholesterol molecule. An inherited genetic disorder in humans, Smith-Lemli-Opitz syndrome (SLOS), enables 7-DHC to build up in the blood, as the enzyme that converts it to cholesterol is dysfunctional.[16] Hallmarks of the disorder in children include severe developmental and behavioral issues and the same repetitive self-injury observed in the octopus's end-of-life demise. When the scientists published these findings in 2022, they noted that such a discovery shows the power of hormonal disruption—in this case, the effects that cholesterol signaling can have on an animal's fate.[17] The death process of the octopus is more complex than just involving one molecule, but it is interesting to see that the optics glands participate in a function other than reproduction, and the correlation to the human disease SLOS.[18]

Scientists continue to debate why the octopus can be so smart but miss out on a long life. Population control remains a prevailing theory. But then how do we explain the magic of one of their undersea opposites: an improbable creature with no brain whatsoever that might just be able to live forever? Hail to the immortal jellyfish.

Immortal Jellyfish?

I should clear up some confusion people have about octopuses versus jellyfish, for although these two species are both invertebrates with tentacles, they are not closely related. Jellyfish, which are not "fish" because they don't have a backbone, are not very smart; they have very simple sensory organs and no brain to process any information. One characteristic, however, worth noting about a particular species of jellyfish, the *Turritopsis dohrnii* (the "immortal jellyfish"), is that they are able to revert back to a juvenile form after becoming sexually mature. This ability is an extraordinary survival skill that comes in handy when there's a serious threat or harm incurred from physical damage, age, or even starvation. If surviving suddenly seems at stake, sometimes starting all over again and going back in time, so to speak, can help. Second chances. Smaller than the size of your pinky fingernail, it's the only known animal to leap back in its development process to reboot itself and be "born again."[19]

The regeneration process, called cellular transdifferentiation, is a lot more complex than an animal magically aging in reverse like Benjamin Button in the movie *The Curious Case of Benjamin Button* (2008). Dying adult cells are transformed into new healthy cells that bud off and re-create a whole new but genetically identical jellyfish that has skipped the earliest phase of life. It's a style of cloning all its own. These immortals cheat death repeatedly—and after reproducing sexually they roll back their biological clocks.

To understand how this happens, picture a jellyfish in your mind with its roundish parachute top (what's called the bell) and flowing trailing tentacles below. That's called a medusa, or an adult jellyfish. But jellyfish don't start out that way. They begin in a larval state after a jellyfish egg has been fertilized. In this stage, they are shaped like small cigars that spiral through the water in search of a rock or other hard surface on which to attach. Then the larva continues to change, eventually taking the form of a small sea anemone, which is named a polyp.[20] Eventually, when conditions are right, the polyp buds to release many swimming medusas that then spawn and die. (Scientists who describe this life cycle compare it to a butterfly's, with a caterpillar the equivalent of a polyp.) But here's where the immortal jellyfish exhibits eternal life: When a medusa dies, it falls to the bottom of the ocean and its cells start to change their order and architecture into a polyp, from which arises a new jellyfish. These regenerated medusas have begun anew, skipping the larval stage altogether.[21] They rise from their own ashes, and they can do this over and over again, like magic or an evolutionary trick.

Humans might never be able to achieve such a feat, but in 2022 a team of scientists in Spain published a mapping of this jellyfish species' genome in a bid to find clues relevant to human aging and efforts to improve our health span.[22] The researchers compared the *T. dohrnii* genome to that of a closely related species that does not have the ability to rebirth itself after reproduction. One of the key discoveries they write about in their paper is that it's not a single molecular pathway that gives *T. dohrnii* their immortality—it's a combination of many pathways that somehow synergize.[23] Such a finding relates to us: Extending health span won't focus on any single pathway or a simple drug. It's the combination of pathways—and the alchemy of those pathways—that will equate with a longer, healthier life. This new research also suggests that the *T. dohrnii* is probably better at repairing and replicating its DNA and maintaining its stem cells. And the spotlight on stem cells is an important clue.

The *T. dohrnii*'s "undying" talent has parallels and likely even applications in our use of stem cells, which is also a process by which one type of cell is converted into another. The phenomenon may offer us new knowledge that could yield ways to develop very specialized neurons from stem cells to treat conditions such as Parkinson's disease by enabling doctors to place the new functioning neurons, derived in a test tube, into the brain of patients where the original neurons are no longer functioning. These immortal jellyfish are hard to study, but the handful of scientists around the world who do try to study them like to say these creatures are among those that lie at the root of the tree of life. If they do hold the secret to life, however, it's not a result of the kind of intelligence we think of. In the next chapter, we'll explore the importance of stem cells, which are a special class of cells that are as close to being immortal as humanly possible. They may hold the key to our own regeneration in our quest for skirting premature death—without our returning to an infantile state and reliving childhood and adolescence.

Demented Dolphins

What if we don't crave immortality? What if we simply wish to hold on to our mental faculties for as long as we have on this planet? Could dolphins hold the key to our understanding of—and prevention of—neurodegeneration?

Scientists have long wondered about the consequences of living decades past our fertile years. Most animals tend to die shortly after their fertility window closes, but dolphins also live long after they are capable of having children. European researchers began to develop the idea that living long after the end of fertility might be linked to Alzheimer's disease in humans and animals alike when they studied dead dolphins washed ashore on the Spanish coast between 2003 and 2006.[24] The dolphins had become stranded for reasons we don't know, though theories abound—from poor water quality to confusion created by changes in the earth's magnetic field. In any case, the stranded dolphins afforded the researchers an opportunity to study their brains, which showed the infamous beta-amyloid plaques and tau protein tangles characteristic of dementia that gum up neuronal connections, inflame the brain, and render it dysfunctional.

Thanks in part to this discovery, researchers in a seminal 2017 study, led by a team at the University of Oxford, were able to conclude that Alzheimer's is a disease not of old age but of a long post-fertility life span, resulting from changes in our physiology after we can no longer procreate.[25] The consequences of living to see our children and grandchildren grow up? Higher risk for dementia and diabetes. The connection? Altered insulin signaling.

The connection between insulin signaling and brain health may not seem so obvious. After all, when we think about insulin, it's diabetes that comes to mind. But here's the thing: insulin regulates levels of sugar (or glucose) in the blood, and in doing so, it has a lot of downstream effects that can reach the brain. In fact, talk about Alzheimer's today often brings diabetes into the conversation. In 2005, a year after chronic inflammation landed on the cover of *Time* magazine in an article that linked virtually all chronic and degenerative diseases to it, studies describing Alzheimer's as a third type of diabetes began to make a quiet appearance in the scientific literature.[26] To help you grasp this phenomenon, I'll present a quick primer on glucose metabolism.

Glucose is the body's chief source of energy. It's the main sugar found in your blood and comes mostly from the carbohydrates you consume. Because it's so vital to life, the body can make glucose from other molecules, including fats and proteins. Glucose has to get to

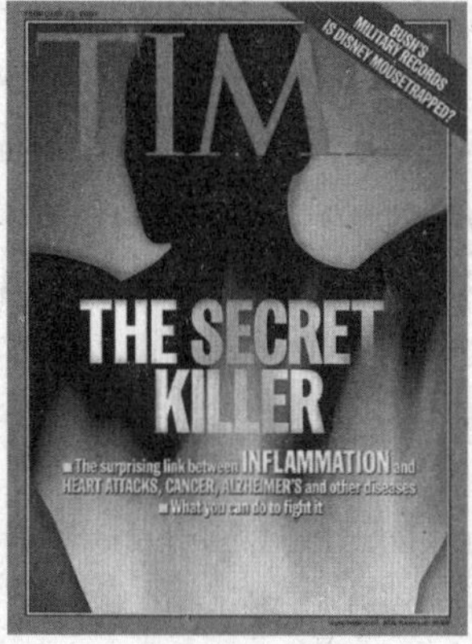

the right cells in the body that need it, and insulin enables that to happen. Insulin is secreted by the pancreas in response to sensors in the pancreas noting elevated sugar in the blood, mainly from eating food, and it facilitates the glucose's entry to our cells and either its use or its trapping in the cells (to be stored for later use). A feedback loop is present, so when insulin is elevated for long periods of time the receptors (the sensors) on the cells are downregulated and the cells become less responsive to insulin. This is what insulin resistance is. When someone with insulin resistance eats, the blood sugar goes up, but the cells don't respond efficiently to the insulin and the blood sugar stays elevated. More insulin is then required to get the same effect, and this can end as type 2 diabetes. As an aside, snacking during the day keeps insulin elevated and over time leads to resistance (manifest as the elevated hemoglobin A1C level [HbgA1C] at your doctor's visit, the ninety-day average of your blood sugar). If someone is less responsive to insulin, and sugar in the blood is elevated, this can lead to some serious issues over time, including heart disease, nerve function problems, a poor immune system, and even a higher risk of Alzheimer's disease.

By definition, people with uncontrolled diabetes have high blood sugar because their body cannot transport glucose efficiently into cells, where it can be safely stored for energy. And this sugar in the blood can inflict a lot of damage, leading to blindness, nerve damage, susceptibility to infections, heart disease, and Alzheimer's. Throughout this chain of events, inflammation runs rampant in the body. Type 2 diabetes incidence is rising dramatically around the globe, especially in areas where obesity and sedentary behavior are becoming more the norm.[27] (Type 1 diabetes is an autoimmune disease with a different etiology and is documented to have been around for much longer.)

The biology I just described happens in the brain too: neurons become unable to respond to the insulin these cells need to perform essential tasks, including memory and learning. We think that insulin resistance may spark the formation of those infamous plaques present in Alzheimer's disease, and some researchers believe that insulin resistance is central to the cognitive decline in people with Alzheimer's disease too. Research has shown that insulin resistance predicts the development of Alzheimer's disease and that people with prediabetes or diabetes have an increased risk of predementia and mild cognitive impairment, which often progress to full-blown Alzheimer's disease. By some measures, being diabetic more than doubles your risk for Alzheimer's. And once signs of disease set in, it's generally considered impossible to reverse course.

Our insulin signaling system with its feedback loops is a critically important part of our evolution and that of the dolphins. It allows us to take in calories from food for use by our cells and, importantly, store them for use later, and it has the positive effect of prolonging life span beyond the fertile years. But this system has potential faults, and long-term risk of diabetes and, potentially, Alzheimer's are chief among them. The system needs to be maintained and optimized because, as without attention, these maladies can become manifest. If you're still struggling to grasp the connection between insulin and longevity, consider the following: Insulin is among the body's most vital hormones in coordinating so much of our daily physiology directly and indirectly. The insulin pathway not only is intimately involved with our growth and development (and fertility) when we are young but also has a big hand in metabolism, stress and stress resistance, survival of brain cells, and preservation of memory throughout our lives—all of which ultimately influence life span and, more important, our health span.

The study of drugs to reverse Alzheimer's disease is littered with failures, partly because there aren't great model systems in which to study the drugs before starting the human clinical trials. While a mouse can be engineered to have the Alzheimer's associated plaques, they don't appear to manifest the disease with symptoms. We aren't going to try to develop drugs in dolphins, but we can certainly learn more from their behaviors about this horrible disease.

We can also learn from bottlenose dolphins, which have an exceptional feature to their insulin system: they can switch insulin resistance on and off.[28] During the day, these dolphins snack continuously and stay in an insulin-resistant mode to make sure there's enough blood sugar to feed their hungry brains. It's advantageous for them to be insulin resistant because they eat a high-protein, low-carb (low sugar) diet, so the condition ensures enough blood sugar to sustain their brain's demands. But at night, when they are in a fasting state, these dolphins switch off their insulin resistance. Scientists have already found a "fasting gene" that is abnormally turned on in people with diabetes; such a finding could be evidence that there's a way to control diabetes in humans. This offers potential for a breakthrough, as something has to tell the fasting gene to turn off in the dolphins. If we can figure this out, a new treatment for type 2 diabetes may be on the horizon.[29]

Not everyone with Alzheimer's also has problems with insulin control, as the disease is complicated, with no single explanation. Other hormones are likely at play too, as Alzheimer's disproportionately affects women; recent studies are looking into how estrogen signaling can affect risk for the disease.* But upward of 80 percent of patients—men and women—with Alzheimer's have a dysfunctional insulin signaling system, so gaining the upper hand on insulin is key—and not only for preventing cognitive decline. Insulin signaling is central to our metabolism, which has a role in a lot of our biology, from our waistlines to our brains.

Interestingly, dogs are another potential model for Alzheimer's disease. They get something called canine cognitive dysfunction, and studies have demonstrated it can affect from 14 to 35 percent of dogs who live to an older age. An ongoing study at the University of Washington, the Dog Aging Project, is studying illness in over 15,000 dogs enrolled by their owners. The work is being done by a huge consortium of scientists across many institutions around the world (Elinor Karlsson is among them). In 2022, one of their studies from this data set identified a top risk factor for dementia in dogs that mirrors a big risk factor for humans: lack of exercise.[30] The study found pretty drastic increases in canine cognitive dysfunction in sedentary dogs. This again could be linked to the insulin pathway, as exercise is one of the key modulators of this pathway. Although the finding is observational, it's a key to take seriously. And I'll add that exercise is one of the ways we help support that insulin signaling pathway and control our blood sugar. This latest study by the Dog Aging Project did not look at a dog's insulin signaling, but future research will likely find more correlations for us to learn from (and help our pets improve their health and life spans too).

For many people, the dread of developing dementia eclipses fears of cancer or even death itself. Someone in the world develops

*If loss of estrogen in postmenopausal women increases risk for Alzheimer's disease, we also know that giving women estrogen in this phase in life can up the risk for certain hormone-sensitive cancers like breast cancer. We may in the future be able to prevent both diseases through nifty tricks that stimulate estrogen receptors in the brain but block estrogen activity in other parts of the body (e.g., the breast). Such targeted therapy innovations are not far away.

dementia every three seconds; the numbers are reaching epidemic levels as the general population ages. But we can push back against these statistics by controlling what we can today. Dementia typically develops silently decades before symptoms show up. The misfires in the brain that manifest in disease later in life do not happen overnight—they accumulate over many years or decades. So, whether you're twenty-three, thirty-two, fifty-five, or eighty-five, start today.

Creature Cheat Sheet

Intelligence comes in many different forms and can be defined in a multitude of ways. Some of the smartest species on the planet, such as octopuses, predate us by a long shot and evolved their "intelligence" on an entirely separate branch on the tree of life. They teach us to appreciate different characteristics of intelligence aside from test scores and gregariousness. Brainpower alone will not help you live longer. But preserving your mental faculties will go a long way to help you stay cognitively intact, and one way you can do that is by maintaining healthy blood sugar balance in the body *and brain*. Keep your insulin-signaling system normal and fit. This will also have the effect of lowering inflammation. We often think of the ills of diabetes on our metabolism and weight, but blood sugar imbalances factor mightily into our brain function, levels of inflammation, and ability to think straight for as long as we're alive.

Regulating insulin levels is achievable with attention first and foremost to dietary habits. The following tips build on ideas we've covered in previous chapters:

- Follow a low-glycemic index diet that minimizes excess sugar intake (a Mediterranean-style diet gets my vote) and includes natural prebiotics found in foods like apples, onions, asparagus, and bananas (see the next chapter).
- Maintain a regular meal schedule. Eat your meals at the same time daily to support the body's natural homeostasis, or your body's preferred, balanced state of being. Erratic, inconsistent eating schedules are stressful on the body and promote adverse biological events such as surges in stress hormones.
- No snacking. It can disrupt your body's natural rhythms and hormonal signaling.

Watch your body mass index (BMI), a key indicator of the line between normal weight and overweight and a general measure of risk for disease.

When your BMI ticks up, it can mean your body is shifting out of balance. With age, especially when you're over forty, making blood sugar balance can be more challenging to control for a variety of reasons. This can lead to the weight gain detected by BMI, especially extra fat around your waistline (belly fat) indicative of an imbalance. Belly fat is usually the unhealthy visceral kind that wraps itself around vital organs and secretes hormones that further contribute to the imbalance. The good news is that with vigilance, you can bring it back into healthy balance.

Finally, I encourage you to work on your emotional and social intelligence in the spirit of supporting optimal brain function. While it's okay to act like an octopus and be a loner on occasion, we're not antisocial creatures. We need one another in a multitude of ways and our sociality factors mightily into our cognition. Connection protects against cognitive decline, a fact proven over and over again and one that we'll explore in more detail in the last chapter. For now, think about how you can improve your connections in your everyday relationships. Be bold like the octopus and look for an escape from the confines of your "aquarium" and reach out to other people. Be a befriender. (And if you haven't seen the remarkable film *My Octopus Teacher*, watch how one man befriends an octopus and has a life-changing experience.)

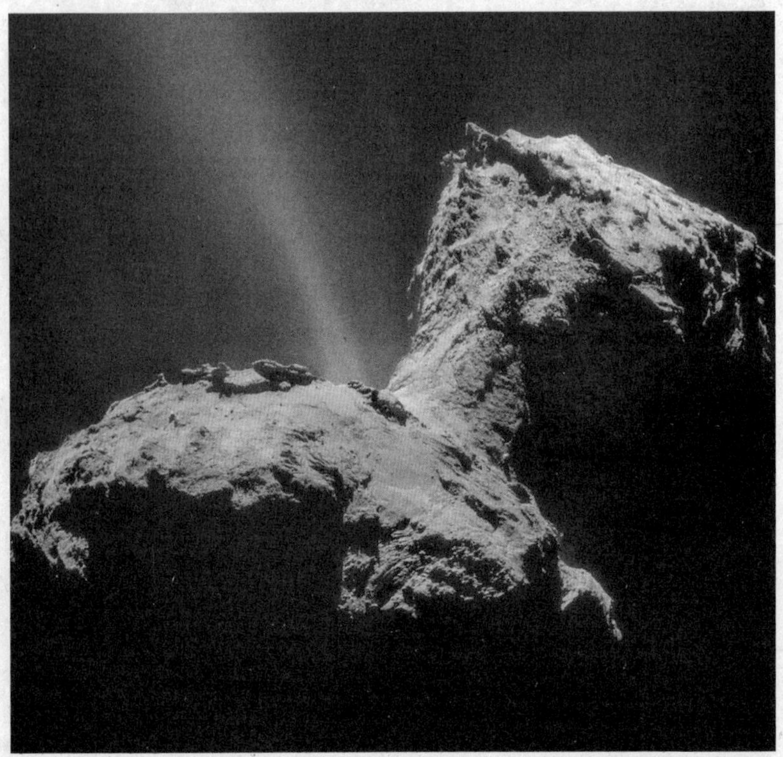

A stunning photo taken of Comet 67P/Churyumov-Gerasimenko on January 31, 2015. The comet was discovered on October 22, 1969, by scientists at the Alma-Ata Observatory in Russia. It's the first comet to be orbited and landed upon by robots from Earth. Churyumov-Gerasimenko loops around the sun in an orbit that crosses those of Jupiter and Mars, approaching but not reaching Earth's orbit. What you see here are jets of organic molecules and molecular oxygen emerging from the comet. "67P" indicates that this was the sixty-seventh periodic comet discovered. Churyumov and Gerasimenko are the names of the discoverers.

10

The Hitchhikers

Microbes, Biomes, and Immortal Stem Cells

> *The nitrogen in our DNA, the calcium in our teeth, the iron in our blood, the carbon in our apple pies were made in the interiors of collapsing stars. We are made of starstuff.*
>
> —CARL SAGAN

The idea that intelligence has evolved more than once in different species and through alternative routes raises a lot of intriguing questions, the most pressing ones being: Where did all this life come from? If our last common ancestor with the octopuses was a wormlike creature 600 million years ago, what happened after that?

More than half a billion years ago, something big happened. Pretty much everything we see today in our natural world leaped, crawled, squirmed, flew, slithered, walked, swayed, blew, danced, and ran out of what's called the Cambrian explosion, the period (approximately 53 million years) where there was a tremendous amount of evolution and change in the organisms residing on Earth. ("Cambria" is the Roman name for Wales, where Adam Sedgwick, a renowned English geologist and Anglican priest, studied rock strata dating from this period and named the period. Charles Darwin is known to have attended his lectures.) Earth went from hosting mostly aquatic muck and simple single-celled prokaryotic organisms in the sea to welcoming multicellular eukaryotic organisms that would eventually make it onto land.

Our planet looked very different during the Cambrian period, the earliest geological time period of the Paleozoic era (the "time of ancient life"). *LiveScience* described it this way: "In the early Cambrian, *Earth* was generally cold but was gradually warming as the glaciers of the late Proterozoic Eon receded. Tectonic evidence suggests that the single supercontinent Rodinia broke apart and by the early to mid-Cambrian there were two continents. Gondwana, near the South Pole, was a supercontinent that later formed much of the land area of modern Africa, Australia, South America, Antarctica and parts of Asia. Laurentia, nearer the equator, was composed of landmasses that currently make up much of North America and part of Europe. Increased coastal area and flooding due to glacial retreat created more shallow sea environments."[1]

In the beginning of the Cambrian period, the ocean floor was a thick layer of mud covered by microbial life. It was the oxygenation of the oceans during the Cambrian explosion that likely helped support the blast, bloom, and diversification of life. The proverbial tree of life took root, but the resulting bursts of new life did not happen linearly with a gradual increase in oxygen levels. New studies point to fluctuating rises and falls in oxygen ("pulses") over tens of millions of years as the chemistry of the oceans and, in turn, their inhabitants changed. As new life-forms emerged and sets of predators and prey became established, a coevolutionary arms race of sorts began that further accelerated the diversification.

The trilobites, a now-extinct marine invertebrate (they somewhat resembled cockroaches), ruled as one of the most common animals of the Cambrian period and became one of evolution's greatest success stories, surviving 300 million years.[2]

Scientists debate ad nauseam what triggered this Cambrian explosion, from tectonic events whose geologic force had physical, chemical, and biological effects, to those pendulum swings in oxygen levels that ultimately supported new life. Whatever sparked the explosion, it split the earth's 4.6-billion-year history into two distinct, uneven historical "sides": before complex life-forms and after their birth and evolution. Earth continued to look very different during this period. North of the tropics was predominantly open ocean, and the landmass was a supercontinent in the south called Gondwanaland. Five major extinction events would occur throughout the rest of our geologic history, including the one that terminated *T. rex* and other dinosaurs.* But the Cambrian period marks a pivotal dividing line—a ground zero of sorts for life as we know it. Fossils are a way of looking back at the simple record of what animals walked the earth years ago. The Cambrian period is the turning point between few fossils to many all across the world. The animals emerged during this period, just tens of millions of years ago,[3] which is short in the geology world![†] We humans are more recent arrivals. If Earth's timeline were represented by a twenty-four-hour day, we knocked on the door a fraction of a second before midnight.

We've been here for less than 1 percent of the earth's history. Another way to conceptualize this is to hold out your arm and clip a sliver of a fingernail; that's less than the duration that we've existed on the earth. Compare that with a horseshoe crab, which happens to be one of the best examples of a "living fossil"; they have existed virtually unchanged for the past 445 million years. Not only do these

*About 75 percent of all species, including the dinosaurs, went extinct sixty-six million years ago when an asteroid, dubbed Chicxulub, at least six miles wide, landed in what is now known as the Yucatán Peninsula. Almost every living organism on Earth perished as the impact's effects reverberated around the planet. The buildup of soot in the atmosphere blocked the vast majority of sunlight from reaching the planet, prohibiting photosynthesis, which led to massive die-offs. Within a few years, life bounced back, starting with bacteria.

†If you want to see physical evidence of the boundary between the Precambrian era and the Cambrian period, a small handful of rock sections filled with fossils can be found in Asia (Siberia) and North America (on the southern shores of eastern Canada).

TIMELINE of 4.6-BILLION-YEAR-OLD EARTH

	Age	Percent of age of the earth
Prokaryotes (simple cells)	3.5–3.8 billion years	76–82%
Eukaryotes (complex cells)	2.0 billion years	57%
Multicellular life	1.0 billion years	22%
Simple animals	600 million years	13%
Fish and Cambrian explosion	500 million years	11%
Mammals	200 million years	4%
Birds	150 million years	3%
Appearance of Homo on Earth	2.5 million years	0.05%
Modern humans	200,000 years	0.004%

helmet-shaped hardy mortals date back to the Cambrian period (predating the dinosaurs), but they also outlasted six mass extinctions and today provide lifelines to us all. Their milky-blue blood, which owes its hue to the same copper seen in octopuses' blood, provides the only known natural source of a substance (limulus amebocyte lysate) that can detect toxins produced by bacteria. Pharmaceutical companies around the world rely on these crabs to produce safe, toxin-free injectable medicines, including vaccines, as well as other sterile medical products that can come into contact with blood, such as artificial knees and hips.*

Theories of how and why the Cambrian explosion happened abounded. Even Darwin got into the game to try and explain the sudden presence of the complex animals.[4] The oxygen theory is but one of many hypotheses. But if all of this really boils down to a focus on

*In 1977, the FDA approved the horseshoe crab's toxin-detecting ingredient for use in testing drugs and vaccines, as the crab's blood will clot immediately if bacterial toxins are present. The reaction allows drug companies to ensure their products are not contaminated; it's a litmus test of sorts. Although they are bled and returned to the sea, conservationists worry that their population could be in jeopardy, as many end up dying afterward. In 2016, a synthetic alternative to crab lysate, recombinant factor C (rFC), was approved as an alternative in Europe. It was officially approved by the FDA in 2020.

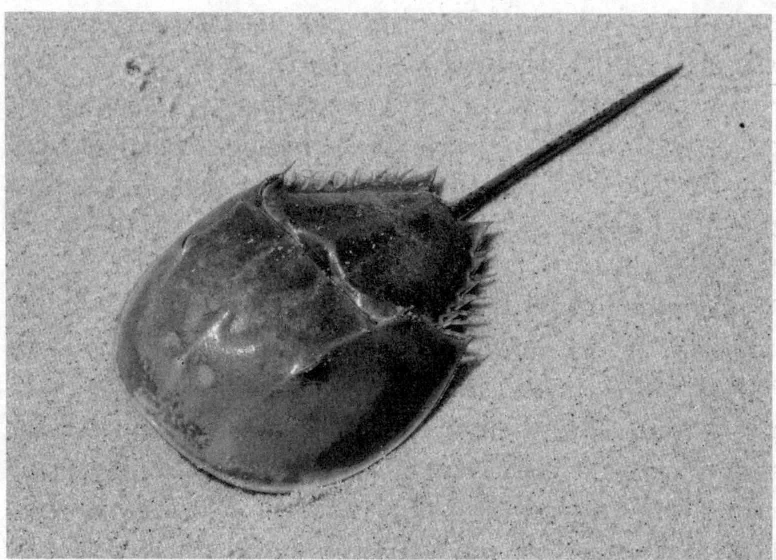

Atlantic horseshoe crab (*Limulus polyphemus*). Also called the American horseshoe crab—it's the only species of horseshoe crab found in North America.

oxygen, why did certain organisms live probably more than a billion years with oxygen without changing prior to the Cambrian period? They clearly needed oxygen, but maybe getting more wasn't always good? Of all the theories, the cancer one really pushes the envelope and deserves attention. Could it be that we owe the origins of complex life to cancer's smart machinery?[5]

The Cancer Theory

We all know that we need oxygen to live, but it may not have always been that way. Through its combustion via metabolism, Emma Hammarlund of the University of Southern Denmark has noted, "oxygen may provide an unparalleled way for animals to produce energy."[6] (Isn't it funny to think that our metabolism is a slow form of combustion, using oxygen to turn food into energy through a series of reactions?) But the transition to this fuel type wasn't straightforward.

Some 2.4 billion years ago, the advent of photosynthesis in the plant kingdom led to the accumulation of oxygen to levels that were likely toxic to many microorganisms; they lacked enzymes to protect themselves from reactive forms of oxygen, which are unstable molecules that can do damage, disrupting structures of key compounds. Over time, selective pressure favored the organisms that could use oxygen for energy and protect against damage from oxidative stress.[7]

But what if oxygen wasn't the primary cause for the Cambrian explosion? In 2018, geobiologist Hammarlund offered a radical new idea, proposing that the changes on Earth during the Cambrian explosion might have started within animals' own biology.[8] She bases this provocative proposition on evidence from proteins found in tumors. Contrary to the oxygen theory, which revolves around changes in the environment that triggered massive evolution, this cancer theory points to origins from within. Here's how this could be possible.

First, consider two important facts. The first is that stem cells are the key to the survival of multicellular organisms and have to constantly repopulate their tissues. They are said to be pluripotent for their ability to differentiate and give rise to all other cell types that make up our tissues. The trillions of cells in our body must be replenished continually to keep us going, some more often than others. Stem cells that quietly reside in our tissues make this possible. But the second fact to keep in mind is that stem cells do not like lots of oxygen because it robs them of the ability to make new cells; they differentiate to mature cells in its presence. But there are still things not clear, as stem cells are present in other environments, including those that have plenty of oxygen like the skin and retina, as well as in cancers. As we study cancer cells in the laboratory, we are getting a glimpse into how we preserve our stem cells in tissues drenched in oxygen.[9]

Cancerous cells are evolutionary marvels—nature's evil geniuses. What starts as a single rogue cell makes the leap to a multicellular entity by copying itself over and over again. (Sound familiar? It's what our animal ancestors did.) All cancers have stem cells, and they help keep the tumor thriving whether there is a lot of oxygen present or not. And just like stem cells hanging out in healthy tissues, cancer stem cells are immortal. They are a subpopulation of cells within a tumor that can self-renew by dividing and give rise to the many cell types that constitute the tumor.[10] They employ a specific biologic mechanism, however, to deal with oxygen: a protein, called HIF-2-alpha (HIF stands for hypoxia-inducible factor).

The HIF-2-alpha (α) protein is part of the HIF complex that is integral to our body's function. Think of it as a sensor and communicating molecule for telling the body we need more oxygen or nutrients in a certain area. For example, HIF-2α stimulates new blood vessel formation (to enable more oxygen delivery to tissues) and can tell the kidney to produce more of the hormone erythropoietin, which then signals the bone marrow to make more oxygen-carrying red blood cells. When you ascend a tall mountain and reach a high altitude where the lower air pressure means oxygen is not so easily pushed into your lungs, these proteins are working in overdrive.

HIF-2α proteins are unique to vertebrate animals. And here's the important part of the story: these proteins existed before animals had red blood cells. As Hammarlund's study noted, this supports the idea that animals had to find a way to control and maintain the properties of stem cells before they could soak their tissues in oxygen with blood.[11] This further deemphasizes the role of oxygen in the external environment to fuel life's evolution. Her study also brings to light questions about the potential benefits of low oxygen (hypoxia). Might it be good for our bodies sometimes? One instance that Hammarlund mentions is the process of procreating; early on in pregnancy, when the embryo is rapidly dividing, hypoxia acts as a signal to drive normal placental development before the fetus is fully attached to the mother's blood supply.[12]

The adaptation to leverage oxygen's powers doesn't come without its drawbacks. Yes, we could finally evolve complex organs and big brains, but now we rely on oxygen to survive, and those large brains suck up a lot of energy. Permanent damage sets in after four minutes deprived of oxygen, and death soon follows. The other pitfall is that when the HIF proteins work in an uncontrolled way, cancer looms as those proteins promote the growth and progression of the disease by altering the structure and function of tissues. This suggests that cancer could very well be an inevitable side effect of being able to take advantage of oxygen's energy-releasing abilities.[13]

Studies in stem cell technology are accelerating as part of antiaging research, but there remains a lot to learn. Popular science likes to say these cells could be a cure for many diseases, allow us to regrow injured tissue, and even be the secret to immortality. But human stem cells are generally immortal only in cultures and in embryonic states. In other words, there's a difference between embryonic stem cells and adult stem cells—the cells you carry around after you're past the embryonic phase in utero. Adult stem cells are critically important (they are different from embryonic stem cells). The adult stem cells are normally specific to a particular organ or location and are limited in what they can differentiate into. The stem cells in your bone marrow, for example, can differentiate into different blood cells, but you can't expect them to suddenly replace brain or pancreatic cells. Shinya Yamanaka, previously highlighted in chapter 8, was awarded the Nobel Prize in Physiology or Medicine (with John Gurdon) in 2012 for the discovery that mature adult cells can be converted to pluripotent stem cells with the addition of a bunch of four key growth regulatory proteins (now called "Yamanaka factors," mentioned briefly also in chapter 8), and this opened up the potential of making these cells for an individual person for a personalized stem cell treatment. In a big step forward, Yamanaka and colleagues at Kyoto University in Japan announced in early 2022 that the placement of transplanted corneal tissues derived from induced pluripotent stem cells improved vision in three of the four almost-blind subjects without any negative effects.[14]

The future of these cells to treat disease is certainly exciting, but also just as exciting is to understand how stem cells work to better understand and treat disease. At a lengthy dinner with Yamanaka in Kyoto, we discussed the role of stem cells in wound healing. If you fall and skin your elbow, for example, stem cells are activated and enable wound healing to begin. In fact, the wound healing (the scab) grows larger than the original skin section, stops growing, and involutes to fit in the skin section that was missing. The original wound-healing process almost looks like a cancer—crazy growth—but the stopping and involution are an elegant reminder of the difference between stem cells and cancer. If we understood this better, there may be a cancer treatment idea hiding here.

Put simply, stem cells are unsung heroes of our evolutionary past and may very well become the lauded heroes of our future longevity.

The Space Theory

Perhaps the most tantalizing, even far-fetched idea, about the origins of life also came in 2018 when an impressive array of thirty-three authors from well-respected global institutions wrote a paper arguing for panspermia: the seeding of life on Earth from outer space. They hypothesized:

> Life may have been seeded here on Earth by life-bearing comets as soon as conditions on Earth allowed it to flourish (about or just before 4.1 billion years ago); and living organisms such as space-resistant and space-hardy bacteria, viruses, more complex eukaryotic cells, fertilized ova, and seeds have been continuously delivered ever since to Earth so being one important driver of further terrestrial evolution which has resulted in considerable genetic diversity and which has led to the emergence of mankind.[15]

To explain the abrupt appearance of animals during the Cambrian explosion, the authors suggest that "cryopreserved Squid and/or Octopus eggs, arrived in icy bolides several hundred million years ago" and that this helps explain "the Octopus' sudden emergence on Earth ca. 270 million years ago."[16] You read that right: they put alien octopuses and squids from the stars on the table. To bolster their argument, they state that a "miracle" would have been needed for the origins of life to have occurred on its own on Earth. And the origin of new genetic information? According to this new theory, genetic material arrived on Earth in the form of space-born viruses, which they call "among the most information-rich natural systems in the known Universe." They write, "The most crucial genes relevant to evolution of hominids, as indeed all species of plants and animals, seems likely in many instances to be of external origin, being transferred across the galaxy largely as information rich virions."[17]

Alien origins of life is not a novel concept; scientists have exchanged views on this possibility for as long as the origin of life has been one of the great unsolved mysteries of science (which is to say, forever). These conversations don't include how God fits in; that's another chapter in this unfinished story. Even the origins of water remain unknown and debated, with new evidence suggesting that too may have come from outer space. In 2020, a team of scientists from Washington University and France's University of Lorraine showed that most of Earth's water could have formed from hydrogen delivered by certain meteorites.[18] Although it's great fodder for many sci-fi narratives, the notion of cross-pollination across the universe is not fiction. And it's not a one-way street, so to speak. It's possible that we ourselves on Earth have already seeded otherworldly places. When Earth took a hit sixty-six million years ago as an enormous asteroid struck the planet and eviscerated most life, including the dinosaurs, the impact had its own enormous power to spew debris that escaped our gravitational pull and found its way billions of miles away. We know from computer modeling done by scientists at Los Alamos

National Laboratory in New Mexico that some of the "earth-vomit" from the Chicxulub asteroid would have been launched into orbit around the sun, and over time, remnants of Earth end up on other planets and moons in our solar system.[19]

If you need more evidence, consider that pieces of Mars found on Earth come from the same sequence of events: an asteroid hits the planet, debris from impact spurts into the galaxy, and ejecta eventually lands on other planets and moons. A 2013 study in the journal *Astrobiology* estimated that over 1 to 2 billion years ago, tens of thousands of pounds of impact rubble from Chicxulub, potentially carrying life, may have landed on our distant planets and moons.[20] All three moons are believed to have promising habitats for life. What's more, computer modeling also indicates that at least some of the drifting debris ejected from Earth still harbored living microbes. As thriller author Douglas Preston states in the *New Yorker*, "The asteroid may have sown life throughout the solar system, even as it ravaged life on Earth."[21]

The Hitchhikers and Us

Carl Sagan was a prescient scientist who startled people with his extraordinary, provocative knowledge of the universe and ways of explaining complex astrophysics to everyday people on our "pale blue dot," as he called our planet. He remains one of the greatest science communicators in history. When he said we're all made of stars, I can only imagine how many people scratched their heads and wanted to call his bluff. But he was right. We may never know whether microbes and viruses came from another galaxy; the fact is we're all ultimately built of star stuff, and as disturbing as that may seem for some people, we must appreciate this wisdom. After all, it's who we are.

As I previously noted, we are more viral than human, with more viral genetic material inside our genome than our own genes. Those ancient viral particles have helped us to survive and to become who we are and informed how we function. I've also already described how we harbor trillions of microbes in general, especially bacteria, though we still haven't been able to quantify the precise ratio between microbial cells that comprise our "microbiome" and our own. The 10:1 ratio you might have heard about may not be accurate, but even if it's about 3:1 or 1:1 between our "pure" selves and microbial hitchhikers, the fact is that we're dependent on microbial life.[22] There are about five hundred to one thousand bacterial species in each of our intestinal tracts, alongside a large and yet-to-be-determined number of viruses, fungi, and other microbes.

Our microbiome probably has as much to say about our metabolism and digestion (remember the rhinos and their fertility challenges rooted in changes in their gut health) as it does about our intelligence and risk for cognitive decline. In fact, scientists are now mapping the brain's microbiome to learn what bacteria the brain can harbor and how to decipher friendly colonies from ones that might incite brain decline and dysfunction, from depression to dementias. So not only does the gut's microbiome communicate with and influence the brain, but also the brain likely harbors its own resident microbes that have an impact on its function and risk for disease. Research in this area is finally taking place using new technologies that make it easier to study brain tissue in living people. The results might shatter old dogma that once said the brain is a sterile environment. And I should underscore that the microbiome in general—the sum of all microbes that live in and on us in a mostly symbiotic relationship—has a profound role in the health and functioning of our brains, as well as our immunity and general levels of inflammation. Collectively, our microbiome serves many functions that we haven't begun to crack.

Your gut's microbiome takes center stage in speaking with your brain and nervous system through what's called the gut-brain axis—a unique and complex two-way highway. You probably don't think of your gut and brain being connected the way you see your limbs linked up to your brain. But you've no doubt experienced this hidden connection through nerve-racking experiences that leave you, for example, with butterflies in your stomach. The main "highway" between gut and brain is the vagus nerve (derived from the Latin word for "wandering" because this cranial nerve has the longest course). The vagus nerve serves as the primary channel of information between the hundreds of millions of nerve cells in your central nervous system and your intestinal nervous system. We have an intestinal (enteric) nervous system, which is reliant on similar neurons and neurotransmitters found in the brain and spinal cord, the reason the intestinal nervous system is termed the "second brain."[23] Incredibly, both the central and enteric nervous systems are created from the same embryonic tissue during early-stage fetal development, and they share a lifelong bond via that vagus nerve. There's also an axis to your skin, the gut-brain-skin axis, to complete the loop. Hence, when you experience strong emotions, such as fear or embarrassment, your stomach may hurt and your skin may turn you as white as a ghost or flush red. The bacteria in your gut also make use of this highway through the body, sending out chemicals that communicate with your brain.

Suffice to say that our bodies are complex ecosystems, with many interactions that scientists can't even begin to describe because we don't have the tools or the language to do this yet. New studies show that more than 99 percent of our internal microbes are unknown to science in any detail.[24] And it has been estimated (but is also debatable) that Earth could contain nearly one trillion species, with only one-thousandth of 1 percent now identified—which is to say that 99.999 percent of all species remain undiscovered (and likely hiding in plain sight until we develop technologies to identify them).[25] Deep under the sea, from which we were all born, with or without a brain, less than a fifth of life is identifiable.[26]

Even how our cells generate energy is dependent on bacteria. Our mitochondria—the tiny organelles in our cells that produce the chemical energy our cells need (in the form of adenosine triphosphate, or ATP)—are also ancient hitchhikers. It's thought that mitochondria, which have their own DNA containing thirty-seven genes, originated in bacteria more than a billion years ago. One evolutionary biologist once defined it in this way: "Mitochondria originated by permanent enslavement of purple non-sulfur bacteria."[27] In other words, some ancient, primitive bacteria long ago evolved into mitochondria that were swallowed up by a primitive eukaryotic host cell and they started working together in ways that made them inseparable. When our forebears left Africa some 200,000 years ago, they descended from a common ancestor affectionately termed mitochondrial Eve—the maternal ancestor of all human beings. (As each person's mitochondrial genome is inherited from their biological mother.[28])

Mitochondria are involved in many bodily processes, from helping decide which cells should be destroyed to storing calcium and generating heat. When something goes awry with mitochondria or their DNA becomes damaged, trouble looms. Many conditions—from organ dysfunction to degenerative diseases and accelerated aging—can be linked to mitochondrial problems. I should add that most mitochondrial diseases are due to mutations in nuclear DNA—not the mitochondrial DNA.[29] And your DNA's mutations affect products that then reach the mitochondria. If the mitochondria cannot function properly, a range of medical problems can ensue depending on which cells are affected (and where). Mitochondria research is another exploding field that requires multidisciplinary studies across many areas of medicine. The complexity of these diseases, and whether they are inherited or develop over time, demands a translational approach.

Mitochondria are like ancient microbial partners in life. But of course there are other microbes we'd best avoid that try to partner with us. To that end, we briefly return to one of our star scientists whose work on one comma-shaped bacterium, an ancient companion to our evolution, shows us the essence of natural selection, or our evolution in motion.

Evolutionary Pressures on Our Genome

Not all microbes are friendly. In the discussion of Elinor Karlsson's work on dogs in chapter 2, I mentioned that her work has taken her outside the doghouses, so to speak. One fascinating piece to the story of microbes that she's also studying is susceptibility to cholera, one of the most dreaded diseases in human history. Which genes protect people from cholera? This area of her work does not involve dogs, but it's worth mentioning within the context of genomics. Cholera is not a disease we in the Western world worry about because it's well controlled and there are effective treatments for it when it rarely emerges.

Cholera is an infectious and often fatal disease caused by a bacterium (*Vibrio cholerae*) that wreaks havoc in the small intestine, causing torrential diarrhea and vomiting that can kill in a matter of hours. It's often contracted from infected food and water supplies and kills tens of thousands of people a year in many parts of the world. But some people have a genetic advantage against this disease that has evolved relatively quickly and recently. The genomes of people who live in Bangladesh, where cholera is endemic and still ravages over 100,000 people a year, have developed ways to fight the disease.

We are observing human evolution unfolding before us. The first cholera pandemic raged through India beginning in 1817. The disease itself has the power to change an entire gene pool because of how many children it can kill. This led Karlsson and her colleagues "to suspect that it was exerting evolutionary pressure on the people in the region, as malaria has been shown to do in Africa."[30] (People who carry the genetic mutation for sickle cell anemia have an advantage when infected with malaria, which is caused by a parasitic infection. This was selected for in sub-Saharan Africa, where malaria is endemic and one of the major causes of death. It's human evolution in fast-forward in response to a serious challenge to survival. We've long known that the sickle mutation is highly common in populations from areas of the world where malaria is very frequent, with sometimes 10 to 40 percent of the population carrying this mutation. Now we know why: the mutation helps those populations who have it survive in their environment.[31]) Microbes and the infectious diseases they inflict have been driving human evolution for millennia, and especially since we started living in closer quarters with the advent of agriculture and building communities.

By the time children in Bangladesh are fifteen years old, half of them have been infected with the cholera bacterium. Many of these individuals suffer mild symptoms or don't get sick at all, which could mean they have advantageous adaptations to counter the infection.[32] Karlsson sought to find out why this is so. She and her colleagues from the International Centre for Diarrhoeal Disease Research in Bangladesh used a novel statistical method that pinpoints sections of the genome that are under the influence of natural selection.[33] These are areas in the human genome that scientists have determined are likely to reflect relatively new evolutionary changes brought on by pressures in a unique environment.

The group demonstrated that over three hundred regions of DNA in these families had been affected by the cholera evolutionary pressure over the course of many generations. More and more we are going to see individual genes or sets of genes that define who will be susceptible to a particular pathogen and who will tolerate exposure to the pathogen. Over time, this will enable individualized preventive and treatment strategies rather than the current treat-everyone-the-same paradigm.[34]

What's going on behind the scenes of this evolution in action? Karlsson's team dug deep into the mechanism, discovering that one set of genes changing in response to cholera encodes an ion channel for potassium that will cause a chloride influx into the intestines. This is not surprising because the toxin produced by the cholera germ activates these channels to release large amounts of chloride that then trigger the severe diarrhea characteristic of the illness—another of the genes-modulated inflammation hindering the body's immune response. And yet a third set of genes plays a role in detecting pathogens and firing up the antipathogen inflammatory process. Identifying disease processes like these that change under the influence of formidable forces such as lethal germs in the environment is nothing short of extraordinary. Karlsson's recent findings might not lead to new cholera treatments immediately, but they establish a fundamental foundation for new fields of study. If we can understand how we've evolved under the pressures of potentially fatal germs, perhaps we can design more powerful vaccines to better protect ourselves against not just cholera but also other infectious ailments as well. Again, all of this goes to show the power of microbes in our systems to help—or hurt—us.

Creature Cheat Sheet

We are more than an ecosystem. We are a metaorganism—a living collective of microbes in and around us that has been with us since long before humankind. These microorganisms hitched a ride with our primate ancestors to help them thrive and make us whole. What I take from this knowledge is that life is complex and evolution has been slow, so we shouldn't try to force major changes to human biology unless we're treating an illness because unnecessary interventions (which could simply be through an extreme diet or supplement regimen) will disrupt this complex system in ways we cannot predict, and the chances that they will be beneficial are extremely low, if at all. But we can look at our evolution as a way to gain clues to tweak our system without going to extremes.

Now that we're beginning to know the power of our microbiome, we can nurture it as best we can through healthy habits—an optimized diet, sound sleep, sufficient movement, and so on. All the strategies we think of when it comes to living a healthy life apply to nurturing our microbiomes. An added tip is to choose to eat more prebiotic foods. A prebiotic is a type of fiber that we cannot digest but serves as food for the bacteria, yeast, and other organisms in our bodies, helping to support good bacteria in the gut. Prebiotics come from garlic, onions, leeks, asparagus, bananas, oats, apples, dandelion greens, flaxseeds, and even cocoa (chocolate!). However, I wouldn't focus too much on consuming probiotics or eating foods with good bacteria in them because the secret to a healthy microbiome is to have a diverse one with lots of species. All the studies of late show that diversity, not necessarily a specific microbiome profile, is the key. If you eat foods with one or two different species in them (say, lots of yogurt with *Lactobacillus* and *Streptococcus*), they can overwhelm the bacteria that are supposed to be there, so any probiotic food in excess is probably not good. Prebiotics nevertheless will feed your gut bugs, support their proliferation, and contribute to that diverse flora.

Animals in nature generally eat the same things daily. Hence, their microbiomes and their diversity are usually stable. Our diet prides itself on diversity: trying new things all the time, and even eating many things that aren't real food. One of the unique things about people who live in blue zones (regions of the world with a higher-than-usual number of people who live much longer than average) is that they have relatively consistent diets, akin to wild animals. That doesn't go to say their diets are not diverse in nature and don't include a wide variety of foods, but their diets are reliably stable and exclude exotic processed grub not ideal for human consumption.

Whether or not our earthly intelligence came from outer space will probably be bandied about for centuries to come. We are just scratching the surface now with DNA sequencing efforts of various species, and as databases grow and newer ways to analyze the other "omics" of organisms arise, we will learn more. New sequencing technologies offer new ways of identifying hidden species in and around us. And no matter where we came from in the universe, the hitchhikers of our evolutionary past, from stem cells to microbial allies, are part of our complexity that makes us human.

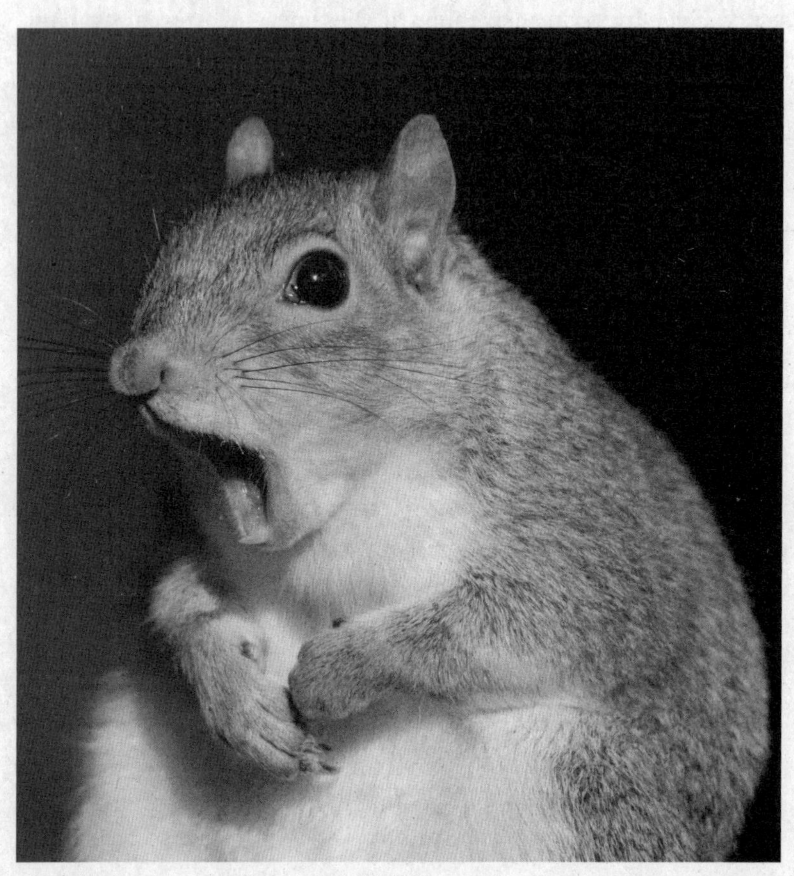

A gray squirrel yawning.

11

Positivity, Personality, and Pain

When Does a Bad Mood Kill? What Pigs, Squirrels, and Albatrosses Teach Us

> *We mortals with immortal minds are only born for sufferings and joys, and one could almost say that the most excellent receive joy through sufferings.*
>
> —LUDWIG VAN BEETHOVEN

What happens when an animal in the wild endures a traumatic injury, picks up a nasty infection, or develops cancer that settles in the bones and kindles excruciating pain? Animals don't go to the pharmacy or emergency room. They have to suffer through pain, sometimes prolonged pain. Or do they?

Sadie, our family dog for twelve years, died during the pandemic in fall 2021. She was half Bernese mountain dog and half Great Pyrenees, an amazing and loving protector of our family weighing in at more than 120 pounds, with bearish features. She was quite unaware of her size. Over the course of her life, she had surgery (at least once) on each of her knees. Toward the end of her life, she hobbled around the house and clearly had difficulty walking, but she almost never showed us she was in pain. She would let out a yelp if something hurt her for a fleeting moment, but she never acted as if she was in constant agony and she never complained. She was always happy and wanted to be part of our family fun, and still greeted me daily expressing her joy and love with a bounty of excited moans and kisses. And in her eyes, I saw love and happiness—never pain.

The word *pain* comes from the Latin word *poena*, which translates to penalty or punishment. In Greek mythology, Poena is the personified spirit of punishment or vengeance and the attendant to Nemesis, the goddess of divine retribution (the word *subpoena* is derived from these same roots). Pain has been with us since long before the modern human tribe separated from our apelike ancestors and took to walking upright. We are the only mammal adapted exclusively to stand upright on two legs and stride (hence, we're bipedal). Most other mammalian bipeds hop or waddle. To walk, we simply tilt forward slightly and then keep up with our displaced center of mass, which is located within the pelvis. Our bipedalism empowers us in many ways; it also makes us more vulnerable to painful injuries in our knees, back, and hips.

It's unfortunate that the word *pain* implies revenge, as if it's our fault or that we somehow deserve it. Well, sometimes it *is* our fault, like when we touch a hot stove, get a tattoo, or run a red light and sustain an injury in an otherwise avoidable accident. And sometimes it's paradoxically pleasurable, such as when you exert yourself physically and wake up to sore muscles the next day, or you sit through several more minutes of an unbearably hot sauna, or you order an eye-wateringly hot dish filled with chilies. I'll briefly touch on this last example, which so many people can relate to, as it has great relevance for studying pain.

Zaria Gorvett wrote for the BBC that "pain [is] a uniquely human indulgence." We eat food that causes pain, such as chilies, for sport. The active ingredient in chilies responsible for the burn is capsaicin, and while this chemical won't cause a problem, you feel its heat because it happens to bind to TrpV1, part of a family of temperature-sensitive receptors in our tongue. These receptors alert the body to potentially damaging heat or cold. When TrpV1 is turned on, a message shoots up to the brain as if the tongue was touching something very hot (even though it's not).[1] Capsaicin is used routinely in labs that aim to learn more about pain and its processes, especially in experiments employing humans. It's impossible to get rats to eat chile-laced foods; they cannot overcome their instinctive aversion to the spicy hot sensation. Capsaicin is also paradoxically used to treat pain topically. When applied to the skin, it causes the quick release of the pain molecule substance P and leads to an accompanying pain sensation, but capsaicin ends up depleting substance P from presynaptic neurons, eventually raising the body's temporary pain threshold.

Ask a roomful of people to describe pain, and you will get a roomful of different answers depending on each person's experience of it, though I think we can all concede that pain is a necessary evil in our existence. The poet Lord Byron once said that "the great object of life is sensation—to feel that we exist, even though in pain." After all, we pinch ourselves to feel the pain indicative of being alive or not dreaming.

What amazes me about pain in my patients is that its level isn't predictable. I have patients with cancer all over their body yet don't complain about much pain, whereas others have tremendous pain despite a very small cancer. It isn't that some people are tougher than others; it is the location of the cancer, how fast the cancer is growing, and how our individual brains are wired—the neuronal circuitry and influence of certain brain chemicals—that determine the experience of pain. When cancer grows very slowly, the body can adapt and accommodate more easily than it does to a fast-growing tumor; thus, there is more pain if the cancer grows quickly. This is not too unlike the experience of sitting in a warm bath in which the temperature slowly increases. You can tolerate the hotter temperatures as they rise, whereas jumping into a hot tub might feel immediately unpleasant and even intolerable.

Pain is simply a brain perception of something going on. The dream of all doctors is to have pain as a warning, and then once the doctor and patient are aware, they can work toward turning the pain off and dealing with the root cause. The continued pain offers little benefit, although it does tell me if cancer therapy is working. I can almost 100 percent predict the result of a scan if I follow the pain of the patient. We have medicines that help turn off pain, but they affect all nerves in the body, which is why pain management is so difficult, with so many side effects.

Despite centuries of study, pain is sorely misunderstood and stigmatized. We still don't know a lot about how it works or how we can manage it without powerful drugs that can be addictive. We've witnessed the harrowing opioid crisis that has affected millions of Americans. But pain does serve a purpose: self-preservation. It's the ultimate teacher, telling us what to keep away from, what to tend to, where to pay attention, and when to rest and heal. Pain may be one of our greatest forces for behavioral change, especially in the short term when it's acute and prevents us from everyday activities. But what happens when pain persists and becomes a disease all on its own? What purpose does that serve, if any? And how do we explain never-ending pain that has no obvious source? Some people can pinpoint the original source of their pain, but over time, pain can evolve and manifest in disparate diseases and diagnoses that can be challenging to define and manage, let alone cure.

According to the International Association for the Study of Pain, chronic pain is defined as "pain that lasts or recurs for more than three months" and disrupts everyday activities and quality of life; it's one of the most common reasons people seek medical care. Chronic pain is a global problem that has reached epidemic proportions, affecting at least 20 to 30 percent of the general population worldwide and individuals of all ages, races, and genders.[2] But no two sufferers of chronic pain are alike. And your definition of the numbers on that classic 1 to 10 pain scale is different from anyone else's, with your past experiences of pain factoring into how you perceive pain when it strikes. If you've broken bones, developed arthritis or migraines, passed a kidney stone, injured your back, sustained a third-degree burn, or given birth, for example, your definition of pain is relative to those most painful experiences, and it can change over time.

Some can even experience physical pain after emotional stress or trauma, as can be seen in military personnel home from war and dealing with posttraumatic stress disorder (PTSD). Some of the most elusive pain of all can come from body parts no longer there, as in the case of phantom limb syndrome, when a person feels pain from an arm or leg that has been amputated or lost in an accident. Despite the absence of the body part, the nerve endings at the site of the lost appendage send pain signals to the brain as if the limb were there; a mix-up in nervous system signals can leave someone in agony.

Stat News wrote about long COVID pain and made the interesting argument that one reason that persistent pain can go undiagnosed for so long is that health care workers are not educated how to diagnose, describe, or treat it. And while research into understanding chronic pain has improved, our country's investment pales in relation to many other less common conditions.[3] At last count, the United States spent more than ten times the amount on research for cancer and brain diseases funded by the National Institutes of Health than for chronic pain.[4] Yet chronic pain affects far more people than cancer, diabetes, or even heart disease: one in six of us lives with pain daily. Disabling pain affects almost 20 million Americans today and may limit them from working and doing many of the daily activities we take for granted.[5] It also can affect their self-image, their social lives, and their ability to connect with others.

What makes pain such a mysterious condition is how it's tied to our emotions and even our memories, which is why chronic pain can play into our eating patterns and affect our moods, confidence, and sleeping habits, and trigger other problems like anxiety, depression, and chronic fatigue. Pain and emotion circuits overlap in the brain. New research shows that the circuitry in the brain responsible for pleasure and motivation is changed by the experience of pain, particularly when it's ongoing; pain can even trigger disordered eating habits that lead to weight gain and obesity.[6] Somehow the chronic pain messes with satiety signals—feelings of fullness—in the brain and spurs cravings for foods high in fat and carbohydrates. What's more, the disrupted eating behavior is also accompanied by structural changes in the nucleus accumbens, a primitive part of the brain that happens to be responsible for decision-making. These new findings are shifting how doctors not only view underlying causes of obesity but also understand pain's far-reaching impacts on the body, brain, and human behavior.

Interestingly, although there are accounts of chronic pain (and attempts to prevent or treat it) in pets and farm animals, we don't have much data on chronic pain in wild animals. Does this signal a gap in our knowledge or a reality in the natural world? Some scientists have hypothesized that if wild animals don't experience chronic pain, then it exists in humans and domesticated animals to elicit help.[7] It's the pain paradox: solicit help from others for the sake of survival when you're hurting (rather than retreating alone to die like a wounded animal in the woods), but at the cost of suffering more and prolonging pain. It's a beautiful, albeit counterintuitive, idea: our ancestors who were motivated to ask for help survived in greater numbers than did the staunchly stoic and thick-skinned. This has been dubbed the "pain of altruism."

One case in point is to consider childbirth. We are the only species that recruits help in giving birth; expectant mothers do not try to isolate themselves when the cervical dilation heralds the beginning of the birth process and imminent (painful) contractions. We humans also have the distinct ability to communicate distress through emotional tears, a phenomenon not observed in other primates. Put those two things together, and we arrive at a definition—and experience—of pain that is truly unique to us in our survival and propagation on the planet.

The so-called pain of altruism also works in reverse: studies show that acting altruistically can relieve not only acute induced physical pain but also chronic pain among cancer patients.[8] Science has long documented that random acts of kindness can trigger the release of feel-good neurochemicals like dopamine and oxytocin, but only recently has it shown that performing altruistic actions can also confer an analgesic type of pain relief, which may further help explain why someone would go out of their way to help others despite personal costs incurred.

In one such series of experiments in China and published in the *Proceedings of the National Academy of Sciences,* researchers asked volunteers to donate money to help orphans.[9] The volunteers were also asked how much they thought their donations helped the kids. Each of the participants then underwent a functional MRI scan, which looks at brain activity involving pain while experiencing electrical shocks. The researchers documented that those who had donated showed less brain response to the shock than did those who refused to donate. They also found that the more a volunteer felt their donation had helped the orphans, the less that volunteer's brain responded to the shock, and the participants reported feeling less pain too.[10]

In another experiment, researchers compared cancer patients experiencing pain who cooked and cleaned for others with similar patients who did so only for themselves. And once again, they found that those helping others reported less pain overall.[11] Altruism needn't be financial; it can simply be a kind act of donating time. If, by helping others, we can help buffer our own unpleasant conditions, that's a relatively easy effort for a potentially huge payoff.

The Biology of Pain

Rumors long maintained that animals other than humans don't experience pain, but that is patently false. All mammals have a similar nervous system to sense pain and respond to it. Bears, for instance, have impressive neurological functions; their uncanny ability to taste, smell, and hear enables them to thrive, and a minor touch on their fur can elicit a reaction. All evidence supports that they feel pain in a manner similar to humans.[12] No scientific evidence suggests that bears feel less pain than other mammals, including humans. And chronic induction of pain, as happens when bears are captured in traps for conservation, research, or management, has been shown to have adverse effects on their bodies—lowering their overall condition and accelerating their aging process. Indeed, chronic pain can age us all. I sometimes wonder how much Sadie's hidden pain toward the end of her life hastened her physical decline that eventually forced us to put her to sleep once her quality of life was gone.

But the rumor that the brain has no pain center—that the brain has no sensory receptors, which would send signals to the spinal cord and brain, to alter to painful stimuli—is true.[13] The brain can't experience pain itself, yet it's what tells you that you're in pain, be it from a deep laceration, arthritis, a stomachache, or sciatica. The brain is so insensitive to painful stimuli that neurosurgeons do not apply anesthesia to the brain tissue they operate on, allowing patients to be completely responsive for the whole procedure. Yet the brain "feels" all our pain; it is the organ through which we interpret, evaluate, and experience all the sensory signals from the body. This enigma is made even more mysterious by the fact no one can "see" pain.[14] Even experiments that employ brain scans cannot tell how exactly the brain constructs the experience of pain. But we're starting to understand more.

Other structures in our head and neck have pain receptors. Headaches, for example, are usually caused by problems with one of these structures relaying the pain to the brain but not originating there.[15] Migraines remain somewhat of a conundrum; the activation of sensory pain receptors potentially in the meninges, the lining of the brain, but again not in the brain itself, could be to blame, but we don't know what activates these receptors. Other culprits could include changes in brain chemicals such as the very neurotransmitters—glutamate, serotonin, and dopamine—that play a role in the pain of a migraine; shifting levels and abnormal activity of these chemicals could contribute to the onset and trajectory of an attack. People who experience dizziness, double vision, and lack of coordination during the onset of a migraine (what's called an aura) might owe their pain to changes in the lower part of the brain, the brain stem—the physical structure that connects the brain to the spinal cord and serves many roles, including the regulation of the cardiac and respiratory systems, as well as the control of consciousness and the process of sleeping.

The brain stem's interactions with one nerve in particular—the trigeminal (three-part) nerve—could also be a culprit. This nerve is how you feel your face and it helps you chew and swallow. It's also responsible for a rare condition that's considered one of the most painful things anyone can experience: trigeminal neuralgia, or tic douloureux, a painful tic or wince. On the pain scale of 1 to 10, sufferers give a number greater than 10 and describe the exquisitely electric, episodic stabbing pain that shoots across the face as enough to motivate one to consider suicide.

Most experiences of pain begin in those sensory receptors, the nociceptors (receptors for *noci*, which is the Latin word for "harm"), specialized nerve endings throughout the body and in most of the organs. These sentries respond to basic kinds of painful, threatening triggers: temperature (extreme heat or cold), pressure, some chemicals (such as capsaicin), and damage. Nociceptors then convey the hurt on to the brain via the spinal cord. Once received by the brain, neurons in the brain's cortex convert this input into the feeling of pain. Most nociceptive pain results from an injury or an invasive disease affecting one of the body's physical structures.

But how pain signals are ultimately translated into painful sensations can be influenced by a person's emotional state because the parts of the brain that are associated with sensory perception share real estate with the parts of the brain that are involved in the processing of emotions. This is why doctors are clear to separate pure nociception pain signals and the more complex form of pain joined with unpleasant emotional and cognitive experience that results when our nociceptors are turned on. It's no wonder that multiple regions are activated in response to painful stimuli, including networks that are also involved in emotion, cognition, memory, and decision-making. This helps explain why people with depression report that they experience more pain in their daily life, and inducing a low mood in otherwise normal people increases pain ratings and lowers tolerance to pain.

A *National Geographic* article on the science of pain explained it this way: "The same stimulus doesn't produce the same activation pattern every time, indicating that a person's experience of pain can vary even when the injuries are similar. This flexibility serves us well, raising our pain tolerance in situations that demand it—for instance, when carrying a scorching bowl of soup from the microwave to the kitchen counter. The mind knows that dropping the bowl midway would result in greater misery than the brief anguish caused by holding the bowl, so it tolerates the momentary suffering."[16] Irene Tracey, a neuroscientist at the University of Oxford, is among those who have pioneered this kind of research into pain's mysterious nuances.[17] She's performed a lot of experiments on human volunteers using pinpricks to their skin, pulses of heat, and that beloved ingredient capsaicin from hot peppers to trigger harmless momentary pain—and record the volunteers' tolerance.[18]

The idea that our pain can be tolerated differently brings us to the concept of a set point—and to a fascinating new piece of information that's changing how we write about pain science and perhaps how people with low tolerance for pain who suffer with chronic pain for which there's no obvious source might be able to handle it.

Glia, which literally means "glue" in Greek, were discovered in the mid-1800s when scientists were searching for the brain's connective tissue, but for more than a century after that, they were cast as a passive support staff for the more glamorous and electrically excitable neurons until new science forced scientists to rethink this glue's role. Glia feed neurons by transporting nutrients, help neurons communicate by releasing neurotransmitters and other signaling molecules, and even assist neurons with taking out their trash and cleaning up their dead. This neuronal pruning, or clipping away of extra branches on neurons to help fine-tune their developing connections—getting rid of little-used connections to allow the neurons to focus on strengthening more frequently used ones—makes glia the cellular gardeners of our nervous system. There are several different types of glia, each with its own special function. Microglia, for example, scavenge and eliminate dead cells and other materials, as well as protect the brain from invading microbes; oligodendrocytes generate the myelin sheaths around the axons in the brain and spinal cord; and radial glia serve as guides for developing neurons as they migrate to their end destinations.[19]

Overall, the neuron-glia networks ensure the development, maintenance, and function of the brain. The size and density of this network, by the way, may explain why we have superior cognitive abilities compared to larger-brained animals like elephants. A more

Brain Size and Neuron Count

	Capybara (largest rodent, non-primate)	*Rhesus Macaque (primate)*	*Western Gorilla (primate)*	*Human (primate)*	*African Bush Elephant (non-primate*
Brain weight	48.2 grams	69.8 grams	377 grams	1,232 grams	2,848 grams
# of cerebral cortex neurons	0.3 billion neurons	1.71 billion neurons	9.1 billion neurons	16.3 billion neurons	5.59 billion neurons
Total # of brain neurons	1.6 billion neurons	6.38 billion neurons	33 billion neurons	86 billion neurons	257 billion neurons

When it comes to intelligence, overall brain size isn't everything. The human brain is much smaller than that of an elephant or whale. But there are far more neurons in the human cerebral cortex than that of the elephant or whale.[20]

intricate network means more highways and roadside assistance, if you will, for the neuronal connections that make us clever beings. Location counts. The African elephant brain, for instance, is about three times larger than the human brain and contains three times more neurons than the average human brain. But more than 97 percent of the neurons in the elephant brain are found in the cerebellum at the back of the brain, which coordinates voluntary movements like walking, whereas we house the majority of neurons (and their glial glue) in our cerebral cortex, which grants us more cognition and higher orders of thinking.[21]

Now the glia are increasingly being scrutinized for directing pain signals that fuel chronic pain.

The Glue of Chronic Pain

Some types of glia look like starfish-shaped neurons, while others resemble oddball Lego parts or nondescript blobs, but all glia are there to nourish and protect the neurons around them. Glial cells are far more numerous than neurons—perhaps ten times greater in number. They are scattered through the nervous system and occupy almost half its space. And while they don't transmit nerve impulses, they are serious multitaskers with their own language using waves of calcium and chemical messengers. Glial cells are part of the neurological conversation that takes place as we learn and form new memories, and they have the power to regulate pain signals by, say, increasing or decreasing their intensity or duration along pain pathways from the periphery to the central nervous system and brain. A growing library of papers shows how this works in rodent models, with more focus on human models underway.[22]

It is the mismanagement of this glial sculpting of sensory neurons that we now think leads chronic pain to develop: overactive glia accelerate the pain system into a vicious inflammatory cycle that provokes the nerves into generating a perpetual pain alarm. If this is true, then targeting the glia with therapeutics to change their behavior may seem like a logical solution to treating chronic pain, but glia happen to be incredibly versatile and chameleonlike; they can quickly evade a dead end in a pain pathway to transmit a pain signal using another path. Unfortunately, we can't just shut the glia down entirely because they are too important (and painkillers don't help because those drugs target neurons that transmit nerve impulses, not glia that communicate in their own language). My hope is that future research will untangle the glia's complicated behaviors so we can find new approaches to treating chronic pain.

There are also new hints that glial cells assist with controlling animal behavior in general. Have you ever wondered how you know to stop performing a task because continuing to try is a waste of precious energy? When a behavior doesn't yield the desired outcome, after several tries, animals stop the behavior, which can be calculated (and energy saving, though my hunch is that stubborn humans spend more time trying).[23] How does the brain identify behavioral failures and raise the "it's okay to quit now" flag? Research into the glial system has uncovered that it may be the real messenger here as it integrates information from certain neurons to force the quit.[24] For example, when zebra fish give up on performing an impossible and overwhelming task (that involves their sight and motor skills), their glia integrate information from certain neurons to pull out the "stop" sign.

Although the glia are gaining the spotlight in pain research, they are certainly among a long list of players in the story of Poena. Other research shows that our immune cells and our mitochondria—the powerhouses of our cells, which originated in bacteria more than a billion years ago—deserve greater attention. Between the glia and other pain-related forces, there's a lot to unlock in the kingdom of pain. Once we can shine a brighter light on their secrets, maybe we can tweak our individual set point for pain.

Set-Point Theory of Pain

Set-point theory is frequently talked about in weight-loss circles. It goes like this: Each one of us has an intrinsic set point for ideal weight, meaning there is a biological control method that actively regulates weight toward a predetermined number for each person. The body prefers to stay within a certain range of weight, and it will do whatever it can to remain in that range, but there are limits. If that set point becomes dysregulated because of prolonged (and often extreme) overeating or undereating, the results are evident, and sometimes dramatic, in weight gain or loss. This can potentially create a new set point. Similarly, we each carry a baseline tolerance for pain. Within a certain range, we can deal with pain. The body can cope with daily fluctuations too as long as the pain stays within the range. By "cope," I mean we can tolerate some pain without it interfering with our lives. The range varies immensely among individuals based on a variety of factors, from inherent biology and underlying genetics to previous bouts with pain and ingrained perceptions colored by emotions and mental states. (As another aside, a significant percentage of our capacity to experience happiness is genetic: we are born with it. This could imply that we each have an approximate default level of happiness, which we tend to return to over time, barring significant events that can change things dramatically. Happiness set points have to be combined with pain set points in the calculation of our overall pain experience.)[25]

We all know people who have a high tolerance for pain, some of whom seek out adversity and painful experiences like participating in endurance events, consuming ridiculously spicy foods, or even gravitating toward painful sexual activities. Experiments dating back to the early 1980s show that our penchant for riding the pain-pleasure line is about thrill seeking; we enjoy taking constrained risks so long as they don't cause lasting damage and intolerable pain. Perhaps it's part of our survival tools. But what happens when those constrained risks lose their constraint? What happens when our set point for pain gets reconfigured for the worst? Can you change your set point for pain so it's back in the more tolerable range? When it comes to treating chronic pain, no single technique is guaranteed to produce complete relief, but there are solutions.

Apart from using medicine for pain—or surgery, or alternative mind-body treatments like acupuncture and biofeedback, or novel therapies like deep-brain stimulation—I have a radical approach to suggest adding to any pain management repertoire: work on your personality, and that includes working on your environment and sociality. I prescribe this rather strange idea after taking cues from happy domestic pigs and ground squirrels, plus a few stressed-out albatrosses filing (or flying) for divorce. We've already covered the importance of your environment within the context of growth, development, and fertility, but another angle here will show just how key environmental forces can be to the experience of pain—through the lens of personality.

Positive Pigs, Bold Squirrels, and Cheating Albatrosses

On July 12, 1998, France defeated Brazil in the finals of the World Cup of soccer, claiming its first World Cup victory. The event, which twenty-six million avid French sports fans—40 percent of the country's population—watched, afforded French scientists the opportunity to raise the question: Does an exceptional positive sporting event lead to a decrease in deaths from heart attacks? You'd think the emotional stress that triggers high blood pressure, plus the alcohol consumption around such an occasion, would increase the incidence of fatal heart attacks. But how about the diametrically opposed effects caused by the zeal, hope, and collective euphoria brought on by the win? The circumstances motivated researchers to have a look at the death counts and do some math. They counted the number of deaths from all causes for June and July in 1997 and 1998 and reported their surprising findings in the May 2003 issue of *Heart*.[26]

They found that the number of deaths in general (from all causes) remained the same for the five days before and after the World Cup final among both men and women. But when the researchers looked at the number of heart attack deaths, they spotted a significant discrepancy. An average of thirty-three heart attack deaths were reported among men on each of the five days preceding and following the World Cup soccer final but only twenty-three heart attack deaths occurred on the day of the final when France beat Brazil. A similar trend was documented among women: before and after the final, twenty-eight women died of heart attacks, but on the day itself, only eighteen suffered fatal attacks. Moreover, the number of fatal heart attacks also fell to twenty-three among men two days later on Bastille Day, a national holiday in France. No such differences were documented in the previous year. The authors of the study suggested that the combination of less physical activity and the satisfaction of the national victory had a calming effect that ultimately reduced risk for heart troubles (an effect that then carried over to the day off from work). They also noted that a previous study showed that British emergency rooms were less busy when England hosted the 1996 European soccer championship, and there were fewer emergency psychiatric admissions in Scotland during the World Cup finals. A summary of this amazing finding detailed on WebMD concluded, "Music may soothe the savage breast (a famous line in William Congreve's 1697 play *The Mourning Bride*), but it takes a major victory to soothe the heart of the average sports fan."[27]

If optimism can protect against adverse health outcomes, then does pessimism prompt bad outcomes? The first noteworthy study to tease apart the optimism-pessimism puzzle over a long period of time began in the 1960s when a team of Mayo Clinic doctors evaluated 723 subjects over thirty years.[28] After conducting medical evaluations and classifying each individual as optimistic, pessimistic, or mixed based on a psychological test, they marked their calendars and checked in on their participants thirty years later. Who was more likely to have died? The pessimists. For every ten-point increase in pessimism on their optimism–pessimism test, the death rate rose a whopping 19 percent. Another way to interpret this is to say the optimists lived on average 19 percent longer than the pessimists, which for the people who made it into their eighties was an additional sixteen years of life.[29]

Interestingly, the majority of the people were classified as mixed in terms of their optimism/pessimism profile, which probably reflects the general population. But more interesting still was the fact that fewer people were labeled as purely optimistic compared to pessimists (124 were classified as optimistic, 518 as mixed, and 197 as pessimistic). So maybe those of us who are a mixed bag also tend to lean toward pessimism. Urban legend certainly says we have more negative than positive thoughts a day, but that's not so easy to prove.

In another study that also began in the mid-1960s, researchers looked at 6,959 students who took a comprehensive personality test when they entered the University of North Carolina. During the next forty years, 476 of the people died from a variety of causes, with cancer being the most common. All in all, pessimism took a substantial toll; the most pessimistic individuals had a 42 percent higher rate of death than the most optimistic.[30] The mechanisms through which optimism boosts longevity are multifaceted, from the biological effects of reduced stress to the fact that a good outlook on life motivates people to engage in health-promoting activities and have more social interactions (people enjoy being around them more).

Over the past several decades, there have been many other supporting studies of the health-promoting effects of an optimistic personality. Much research has been done on the connection between a high level of optimism and good health, described well in Goodin and Bull's research paper, appropriately titled "Optimism and the

Experience of Pain: Benefits of Seeing the Glass as Half Full." The authors state that optimism "is linked to both enhanced physiological recovery and psychosocial adjustment to coronary artery bypass surgery, bone marrow transplant, postpartum depression, traumatic brain injury, Alzheimer's disease, lung cancer, breast cancer, and failed *in vitro* fertilization."[31] Newer research demonstrates that high levels of hope have been found to be related to lower levels of pain, psychological distress, and functional disability in patients with chronic illnesses.[32]

I notice these associations daily when I see patients, and so my clinical style is to be an optimist. I don't want to give false hope, but I think a major role of a physician is to educate patients about the possibilities for treating their diseases, both those that are available now and those that may be available in the near future. I know it is demoralizing as a patient to feel out of control, but by ensuring patients understand what is going on, I hope I can at least reduce some stress—and perhaps even enable them to have a better outcome through their new optimism.

It's important to note that acceptance of pain is not about giving up but rather reframing and contextualizing pain as a part of life and—this is the critical element—learning how to live more effectively in spite of it. A 2011 study in the *Journal of Pain* noted that this entails "accepting what cannot be changed, reducing unsuccessful attempts at eliminating pain, and engaging in valued activities despite pain. Studies have shown that individuals with high levels of pain acceptance report significantly lower levels of pain and pain-related disability."[33] The hard part, of course, is the learning process. How do you learn to be more optimistic if you do not naturally see the glass as half full? Programs are being developed by clinicians and researchers to train for optimism, to shift expectation from negative to positive. These programs often include thinking techniques that require envisioning an imaginary future in which everything has turned out in the most optimal way.

You can do this easily on your own, without registering for a training class, by taking time to imagine things turning out well for you and writing down (journaling) your wishes and what it's like to achieve them. Be realistic but playful, detailed but open-minded to anything. If challenges or anxious thoughts intrude, write down how you can solve or overcome them. You can also incorporate this type of mental processing in meditation or a guided visualization exercise, or by simply taking a few minutes for some deep breathing and letting only positive thoughts enter your mind. And if negative thoughts trespass, try to look at them from a distance as if you're detached from them and they are merely passing by. One of the worst offenders to optimism is catastrophizing—thinking the worst will happen and amplifying the severity of a situation, which leads to irrational thoughts and a distortion of actual reality. Not only does catastrophizing make pain worse; it also makes pain persist longer. And people who tend to catastrophize by habit are a lot more prone to chronic pain.

This is not to say there's no value in grief and feeling glum. Forced optimism can backfire when too much inauthentic positivity leads to denialism and hiding dark emotions that demand we process them. I'm not asking you to fake a smile despite real pain, but there are things you can do to cultivate a genuine smile despite pain. And it's perfectly fine to be optimistic but occasionally cranky or irritable. Your mood and general outlook on life are not mutually exclusive. But the two do interact to help determine your overall personality and approach to life in response to positive or negative events.

The domestic pig (*Sus scrofa domesticus*) is an interesting animal to study and compare with humans. Pigs are among a growing list of research subjects in the relatively young scientific field of animal personality. Pigs share a number of cognitive capacities with humans, such as self-awareness, experiencing emotions, and playfulness.[34] Studies on the domestic pig tell us that mood and personality interact to influence thinking, how our biases come into play within our environment, and decision-making. And therein lies a key word:

environment. It turns out that our environments can make or break our moods (and those of pigs).

In pigs, personality is frequently measured by watching how the animals cope under different circumstances. Pigs that are deemed proactive, characterized by more active and consistent behavior, are not the same as reactive pigs that behave more passively and erratically. In studies on humans, proactivity and reactivity have been linked to extraversion and neuroticism, respectively, with extroverts more optimistic and those with neurotic tendencies more pessimistic. In one particularly illuminating 2016 study done by a group of researchers in the United Kingdom who specialize in animal behavior and welfare, a litter of pigs that included both proactive and reactive swine was placed in one of two environments known to influence their moods.[35] One environment, designed to be more feel-goody, was more comfortable, playful, and roomy than the other. It had a couple of more square feet per pig and the addition of straw, which pigs love to play with and use as their bedding. Research has long shown that the addition of straw to a pigpen can enhance pigs' welfare.

To conduct the experiment, the pigs were trained to associate two separate feeding bowls with different outcomes. One bowl contained sugary treats, which represented a positive outcome, and the other, filled with coffee beans, promoted the negative outcome.

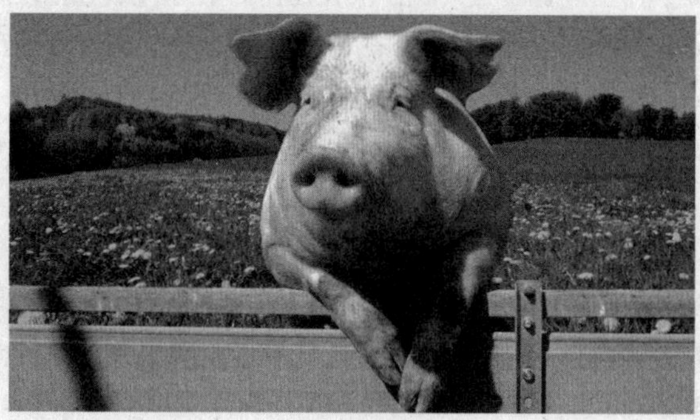

One happy pig.

Then the researchers introduced a third bowl that would act as the litmus test for identifying how optimistic or pessimistic each pig was. The researchers watched to see whether the pigs approached this bowl expecting more sweets (and thus another positive outcome) and were optimists. As it turned out, the proactive pigs were more likely to respond optimistically regardless, but the optimism of the reactive pigs hinged on their moods. Reactive pigs living in the roomier feel-good environment were much more likely to be optimistic about the feeding bowl with an unknown inside. The pigs living in a smaller, more barren environment acted pessimistically. The experiment also revealed what the researchers assumed was true from the start: humans are not unique in combining longer-term personality traits, such as a penchant to have a gloomy or conversely sunny outlook, with shorter-term mood biases when making judgments. Our personalities color our decisions, and our moods can be influenced heavily by our environments, which means we do have some control in protecting our preferred moods.[36]

If you want to tip the scales in favor of being hopeful and reap the health rewards, you need to be mindful of your living quarters, what (and most definitely, whom) you surround yourself with, and where you spend your leisure time (watching TV alone in your living room or taking a walk with a friend). This advice may sound obvious or trite, but not until recently has science really drilled down on the significance of the personality-mood-outlook-outcome phenomenon.

Other scientists have recorded findings in squirrels that point out once again that personality matters. A three-year study published in 2021 that was done by a team of researchers from the University of California, Davis and the Rocky Mountain Biological Laboratory in Colorado is the first to document personality in golden-mantled ground squirrels, which are common across the western United States and parts of Canada.[37] The researchers recorded four main traits: boldness, aggressiveness, activity level, and sociability.[38] They noted that bolder, more social squirrels earn an advantage over their shyer counterparts; the gregarious ones move more quickly, command the use of more space and places to perch themselves, and gain more access to resources. These effects ultimately favor the social squirrels' survival. It pays to be convivial, and maybe a little brash.

Although pain and pain management within the context of personality was not part of this study, we can draw some conclusions nevertheless. There is a lot that each of us has control over, and many things, such as health, where we have only partial control, so we have to use the power we have to tip the scales in our favor. This means taking a good look at our lifestyles, because work on the things that we can affect—our moods, our environments, whom we associate with, where we choose to spend our time—and the other aspects like pain and how we feel will improve. Maybe it will not alleviate all of our symptoms, but it will have a major influence.

New research into people with personality disorders, such as narcissism and borderline personality disorder, finds they report higher levels of pain and may even be at a higher risk for cognitive decline (and dementias, including Alzheimer's).[39] This newer research too highlights the power of personality. In particular, the research shows that people who are organized, responsible, goal directed, and gregarious and have high levels of self-discipline ("conscientiousness") may be less likely to develop cognitive decline and impairments than those who are moody or emotionally unstable ("neurotic"). My hunch is the research on pain and personality and cognition and personality will increasingly overlap. Our patterns of thinking and behaving—our personality traits—all go hand in hand with how we perceive pain and how our brains function overall.

In addition to working on your personality through your surroundings, it also helps to be mindful of your thoughts. This goes back to what I mentioned about catastrophizing. Cycles of negativity will pronounce and prolong pain. See if you can pause and take note of your thoughts when they turn sour and start to reframe them by saying, for example, "Okay, well, I know I have pain. But even with the pain I could still walk a mile and listen to a great podcast," or "Even though I have pain today, I'm starting to learn new ways to move that are going to help with my pain." Start small. Subtle reductions in negativity will go a long way to not only help you manage pain but also diminish the fear and anxiety that often accompany and aggravate pain.

I'll add one more idea that's not for everyone but should be noted: when pain strikes, try swearing. Scientists have studied the power of uttering an unbecoming curse word to induce a stress-related analgesia.[40] Some have called it the fastest-acting pain reliever of all of them. How this works is still unknown but theories abound, from how swearing provokes our emotions and in doing so may trigger a calming response from the autonomic nervous system, to the fact that swearing distracts us because it's funny. The F-word is rated in the top 1 percent of funniest words. In one study, scientists from the Keele University and the University of Oxford in the United Kingdom invented fake obscenities—"twizpipe" and "fouch"—and compared them to classics. There was no change in pain threshold or in any of the biological correlates to pain with the manufactured words, but the F-word increased pain threshold and pain tolerance, each by over 30 percent.[41]

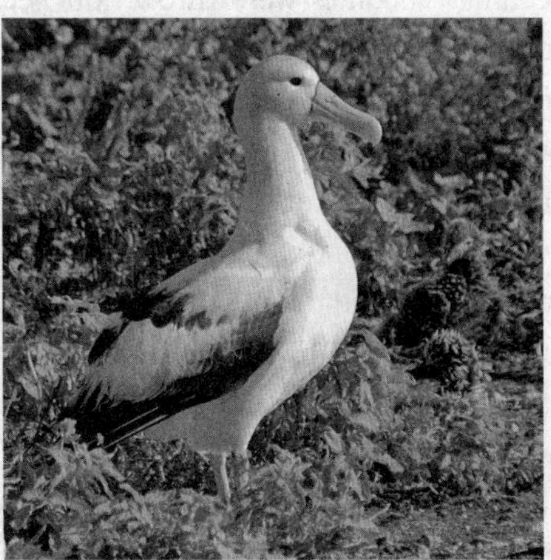

A short-tailed albatross on Midway Atoll's Eastern Island.

Now for those albatrosses. These large seafaring aviators share something in common with us that most people don't think about: they are socially monogamous animals by nature along with more than 90 percent of other birds. Albatrosses choose a partner to mate with and are with them generally for life, but divorce is not beneath them when life gets rough. In a study published in 2021, which culminated after analyzing data on more than fifteen thousand black-browed albatross breeding pairs over fifteen years in the Falkland Islands, conservation biologists in Portugal chronicled something peculiar: during stressful periods, notably years when the weather was unusually warmer, divorce rates went up.[42] Although albatrosses are known to uncouple or separate from their partners in search of better ones when they fail to reproduce, this study found that bad mates weren't the only reason to divorce. Albatross divorce rates were the highest in the years the sea temperature was highest, *even when the couples bred successfully that year*.

Albatross separation rate is usually 1 to 3 percent a year but has increased recently to approximately 8 percent a year, potentially due to the increased temperature of the oceans. As sea surface temperatures rose and adversely affected sources of food for these foraging birds, their breeding schedules were thrown off because the albatrosses had to travel farther to find food before returning to their customary breeding grounds. And breeding schedules out of sync with what's normal and expected are stressful on partnerships.

This is yet another example of how environment affects our decisions, even our ability to maintain our fidelities. The authors of the study proposed a provocative theory, the "partner-blaming hypothesis." As Francesco Ventura, University of Lisbon coauthor, said to the *Guardian*, "We propose this partner-blaming hypothesis—with which a stressed female might feel this physiological stress, and attribute these higher stress levels to a poor performance of the male," and then ditch him.[43] She conflates the stress caused by environmental conditions with some fault of her partner's. (Female albatrosses file for divorce first, declaring their singledom by showing up the following year for breeding season with different males. The exes don't squabble.)

We can learn much from studying these feathered friends, for when things get stressful, our tendency as humans is to blame: our spouses, our workplaces, our government. Take a step back and look at the whole situation with your uniquely human powers of reasoning, and many times you will see things in a different way. I have a personal strategy I try to follow (although am not always successful) to never respond the same day to a stressor. I let it go overnight, and think about the bigger picture. My next day's response is many times different than my immediate, reflexive response would have been.

Albatrosses are among the longest-lived birds. The world's oldest known wild bird is a Laysan albatross named Wisdom, who still lays eggs with a partner she's had since at least 2012 (if not far longer). She's seventy years old and has flown millions of miles, but returns to her same nest every year on Midway Atoll, the world's largest colony of albatrosses, located about fifteen hundred miles northwest of the Hawaiian Islands.[44] She must know a thing or two about how to make a partnership last. If I could communicate with Wisdom, a name so fitting, I'd ask about the secrets to courtship, bonding, and long-lived relationships. But we have another species to turn to for those nuggets of wisdom. And though they may be an animal you've never heard of, you'll soon fall in love with voles just like they fall in love with each other.

Creature Cheat Sheet

Pain is a game of chutes and ladders—you have good days and bad days but stay within a range (hopefully). To change your set point, employ the power of altruism, positive thinking/optimism, bold sociality, and a feel-good environment. Work on your attitude and personality. Seek help and employ a professional therapist when necessary to find solutions to your emotional, psychological pain that could be influencing your physical pain. A good practice is to keep a pain journal and write about your experiences and pain-free hopes for the future. Picturing a future where everything has turned out as best as possible, for instance, has been shown to increase optimism in terms of expecting favorable outcomes. Even better, this increase in optimism has been found to be independent of changes in positive mood. In other words, you can still be moody one day but sustain a healthy level of optimism. And when you need something to hit you with no pain, try music. In the words of Bob Marley: "One good thing about music, when it hits you, you feel no pain."

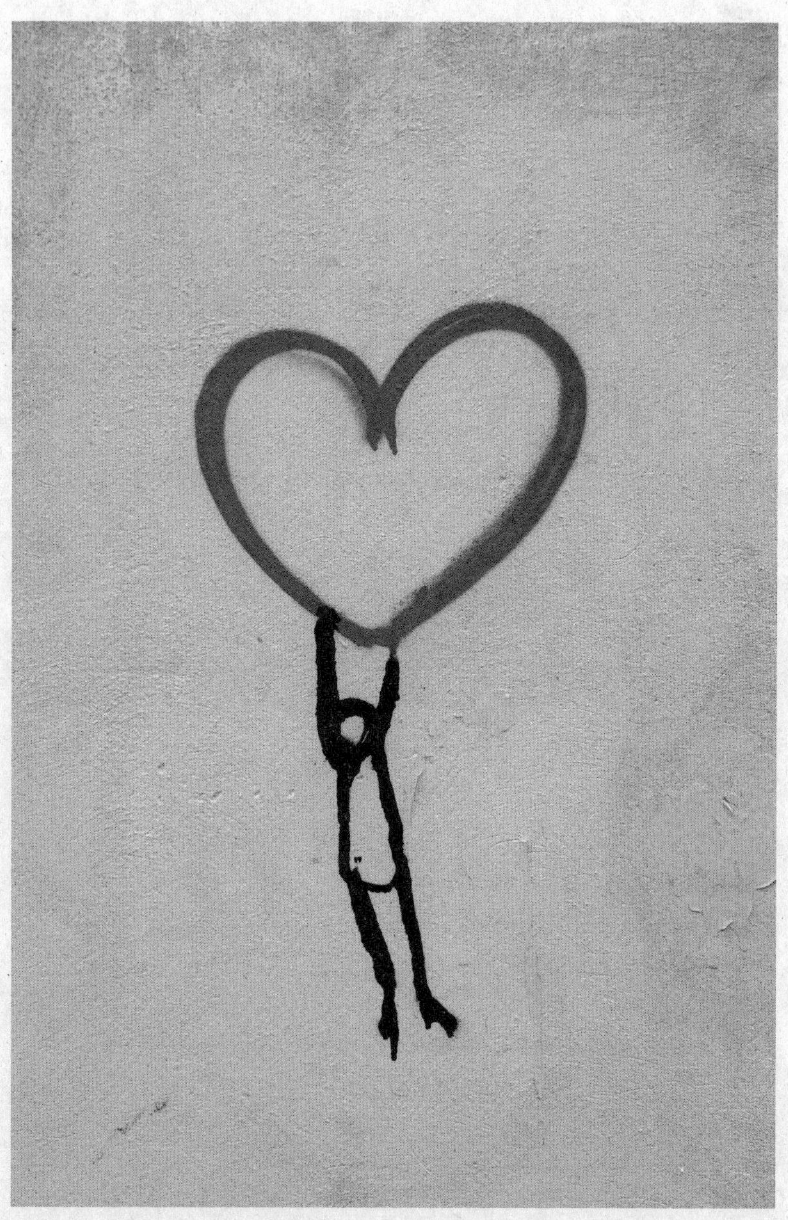

Street art (graffiti) in Florence, Italy.

12

Bonding, Sex, and the Law of Love

Why We Need One Another—and Mother Nature—Now and Forever

> *One word frees us of all the weight and pain of life: that word is love.*
>
> —SOPHOCLES

Eight hugs a day. Eight. That's roughly one hug per working hour. If you can commit to that, maybe you'll live longer and love better.

Talk to strangers.

Be nice, openhearted, and of service to others.

Embrace the weirdness of everyone around you (you included).

And immerse yourself in nature whenever and wherever you can.

There. That's it. The sine qua non of life and longevity. I just gave away some of the main lessons of this final chapter, which covers what we humans crave the most: connection; strong, enriching bonds with others; and love.

"I cry every day," Paul J. Zak tells me. He adds that it doesn't take much to bring him to tears—a rom-com movie, an emotive commercial, a heartfelt moment with a loved one. He's not someone who looks like a casual crier. Zak is a towering square-jawed man with patrician good looks, an enviable amount of hair for being in his seventh decade, and an air of authority; his alert blue eyes and open, curious face atop broad shoulders exude the kind of stoicism seen in a choice few people. Zak could easily play a senator in some epic movie about ancient Rome (and he does claim some Hollywood fame: he has created and voiced some of the science scenes for movies, including the blockbuster *The Amazing Spider-Man*). But once he starts talking, you quickly sense that Zak indeed has a soft side, one that he admits grows mushier the older he gets. "I'm a hugger," he says. "And I've trained myself to be much warmer than I was in my youth" (he also worries less about crying in public). The media have dubbed him Dr. Love.[1]

Zak is the founding director of the Center for Neuroeconomics Studies and a professor of economics, psychology, and management at Claremont Graduate University in Southern California. He is one of the pioneers in the emerging field of neuroeconomics, which studies the neurological and molecular roots of how humans make decisions regarding their economic behavior. He has spent the past two decades researching the neuroscience behind our connectivity, happiness, and effective teamwork in business settings. His research, which has taken him from the Pentagon to Fortune 500 boardrooms to the rain forests of Papua New Guinea, uncovers how stories shape our brains, tie strangers together, and move us to be more empathic and generous. And his target—his obsession, if you will—is a molecule we all produce: oxytocin. In his seminal 2012 book, *The Moral Molecule: The Source of Love and Prosperity*, Zak recounts his unlikely discovery of oxytocin as the key driver of trust, love, and morality—in other words, the things that distinguish us as humans. It's the "cuddle hormone," the brain chemical that oozes when we feel nurtured as babies; are unconditionally loved and cared for as children by our parents; make good friends; grow up and turn into warmhearted, productive adults; lust after our romantic partners and meet our mates; and eventually parent our own progeny.[2]

The molecule lies at the heart of momentous, life-affirming activities such as birth, lactation, social bonding, and sexual pleasure (including arousal and orgasm). And while it has traditionally (and stereotypically) been attributed mostly to a woman's biology, especially as it relates to childbirth, breastfeeding, and postpartum attachment to her children, it serves a vital role in every human's experience.[3] Women have 30 percent more oxytocin than men, but men definitely have the hormone, and through a series of experiments, Zak and his colleagues have helped establish the key role of oxytocin in a myriad of human behaviors, including generosity, empathy, and trust. He's not alone in these revelations, for a small coterie of scientists around the world have increasingly been linking oxytocin to a panoply of human behaviors, as well as to behaviors in other mammals.

The hormone was identified in 1909 when Sir Henry H. Dale found that an extract from the human pituitary caused the uterus of a pregnant cat to contract. Dale named the substance oxytocin, borrowing from the Greek words for "swift birth." It has been recorded as early as 1911 that doctors began using the pituitary gland extract to stimulate uterine contractions, and modern synthetic oxytocin (Pitocin) continues to be used worldwide to stimulate uterine contractions and promote labor.[4] Pitocin, for example, can be delivered intravenously to help trigger labor in a pregnancy two weeks past the due date or speed it up if a woman's water breaks without labor following. Dale subsequently found that oxytocin also enables the release of breast milk in a lactating mother.* The hormone oxytocin contracts the smooth-muscle cells surrounding the milk ducts of the female breast to move milk into the nipple for the infant to drink.

*Dale also went down in history for helping to discover the chemical transmission of nerve impulses through the actions of acetylcholine. In 1936 he shared the Nobel Prize in Physiology or Medicine with German pharmacologist Otto Loewi for their findings.

Zak points out that when we believe that someone trusts us, we instinctively trust that person back, and this alters our behavior because trust allows heightened positive interactions with others. Ultimately, oxytocin is, Zak says, "the 'social glue' that adheres families, communities, and societies while simultaneously acting as an 'economic lubricant' that enables us to engage in all sorts of transactions."[5] It is, as another scientist has described it, the "grease of the social brain."[6] Oxytocin is produced mainly in the hypothalamus, where it is either released into the blood via the pituitary gland or to other parts of the brain and spinal cord, where it binds to oxytocin receptors. The hormone is ultimately what facilitates the bonds we make with other people and our pets, helps us be less selfish, and even encourages us to think and act for the benefit of a larger social group. It is a polymath of a hormone that is now recognized for having diverse roles in the body, from social and sexual function to regulation of appetite and body weight, immune and nervous function, and bone mass. Newer research is even cluing us in to how the molecule is indispensable for healthy muscle maintenance and repair as we age. It may be the key to helping muscles work like new, improving their regeneration by enhancing aged muscle stem cell proliferation.[7] It also has been shown to stave off osteoporosis. In fact, oxytocin could become an antiaging drug that older folks use in the form of a nasal spray to exert positive effects on some of the symptoms of aging. According to a recent dermatology study, for example, people with high oxytocin levels were shown to have significantly lower skin age scores—more youthful-looking skin—than expected, even among people with strong histories of lifetime sun exposure.

Unfortunately, it's not easy to measure levels of oxytocin directly—especially when it comes to oxytocin in the brain. In most studies, scientists collect samples from other fluids, such as blood, urine, and saliva, to serve as proxies for oxytocin activity in the brain. But this is far from an exact science, and debates loom large in how we quantify and qualify oxytocin levels in a given body. The feverish interest in studying oxytocin's wide-ranging effects in human health, however, will no doubt lead to better methods of measuring and defining this hormone's roles in our lives.

To say Paul Zak has been devoted to spreading the love about this important hormone is an understatement. From his perspective, oxytocin is the "moral molecule" behind all human virtue that keeps us as a society together. Morality is uniquely human, but oxytocin is not. As I hinted, it's in all mammals and is part of an ancient group of chemicals found throughout the animal kingdom. Octopuses have their own biochemical version that works with their physiology, as do birds, reptiles, and fish. But in us, oxytocin serves unique purposes and has been bathing our brains at a higher rate since about two hundred thousand years ago when a mutation conferred more of its production. This was about the time our species launched out of Africa, and by then, our brains had evolved and grown to be big, complex organs. Perhaps more oxytocin helped us conquer the planet and form complex societies, as it paved the way for us to forge the kind of social bonds we needed to survive and "civilize" as peoples.

Unfortunately, we can't force its release from the brain to benefit from its positive, affectionate effects at will. We have to give to get, as it were. Oxytocin is a gift you have to bestow on—or, more precisely, spark within—someone else; it's virtually impossible to conjure it all on your own. And as we age, our production of oxytocin can decline if we're not proactive in ushering its release to benefit from its effects.

Hold that thought while we take a scenic byway through some labs that have been learning from voles how to love and connect with others. We are not the only animals that bond and form monogamous social alliances that last a lifetime. Fully 97 percent of mammals do not pair up to rear their young. But we do, and so do voles. These little creatures give us a peek into oxytocin's remarkable sway over our relationships, the interpersonal connectivity that's so vital to life and longevity, and our capacity to love.

Vole Is an Anagram of L-O-V-E

A vole looks as if it could be a rat mixed with a hamster or mole, or maybe a new type of field mouse with some gerbil and gopher genes. Small rodents you could easily hold in your hand, voles are relatives of mice and closely related to lemmings, with coarse grayish-brown fur, hairy tails, and small heads and ears. Although there are approximately 155 vole species, the prairie vole gets the attention of people who study the science of monogamy because these voles are famous for the nature of their bonds; they hold clues to why we share the same urge to care for our partners, coddle our children, comfort mistreated friends and family members, and express empathy and mourn our dead.

Voles live throughout the grasslands of the United States and Canada, where they reside in short burrows in nests made of grass and leaves. A handful of them take up residence in Larry Young's domain in Atlanta's Yerkes National Primate Research Center, which is part of Emory University, where Young is director of the Center for Translational Social Neuroscience. This is where Young, who also heads the Division of Behavioral Neuroscience and Psychiatric Disorders at the Yerkes Center, focuses on the evolution of the brain's neural circuitry underlying social relationships. He also aims to not only understand the root causes—and drives—of our social bonds but also to translate his findings into treatments to improve social behavior in people with psychiatric disorders such as autism, social anxiety disorder, bipolar disorder, and schizophrenia. Voles are his prime subjects. They are remarkably humanlike in their pair bonding, which happens largely because of oxytocin. Like us, their brains house receptors for this hormone. The resulting pleasurable feeling is mutual, and chemical, leading a bond to form.

The bond making is straightforward. The male and female meet; the male courts the female using sexual chemosignals in his urine that she licks and prompt her to go into estrus (heat), which means she becomes sexually receptive and active within a day or so (female prairie voles do not enter puberty at a specific age; it's all about exposure to this chemical). The two mate and soon after, they forge an unbreakable bond that dictates the couple's destiny, as they now prefer to stay together forever. They will cuddle and groom each other, sharing parental duties in raising up to four litters a year. The *Smithsonian Magazine* described laboratory experiments in which "a female prairie vole receives an oxytocin injection into her brain, she huddles with her partner more and forms stronger bonds."[8] If one member of the pair dies, the survivor shuns all other voles as if in permanent mourning.

Larry Young is another scientist who exudes enthusiasm for his work when he talks about his observations and discoveries as an animal researcher.[9] Charismatic and avuncular, Young is someone who looks like he came from rural roots that left him with a love for nature. He has a cherubic round face, neatly trimmed salt-and-pepper beard, and wide brown eyes. After growing up in small-town Georgia a mile down a dirt road, he eventually made it to the University of Georgia for his bachelor's degree in biochemistry before moving on to his PhD in neuroscience at the University of Texas at Austin. He admits that his interest in brain chemistry and, in particular, the science of connection may have partly stemmed from his own experience through a young marriage, children, divorce, marriage again, and more children. He says he didn't know about DNA until he reached college and fell in love with molecular biology.

His first glimpse of vole behavior that would set the path of his career was during a postgraduate research stint in a Texas lab studying whiptail lizards. These are no average lizards. They can shift gender between female and male through hormone fluctuations. Young found he could inject certain hormones related to mating and change their sexual behavior too. And when he moved on to Yerkes Center, he delved into understanding the genetic underpinnings to this behavior. Because meadow voles, a close cousin of prairie voles, do not mate for life, Young wanted to answer this question: Can we turn the socially promiscuous meadow vole into a faithful prairie-like vole? And indeed, he did. By injecting a prairie vole gene that codes for a vasopressin receptor into a virus, which acts as a transporter, and then injecting the virus into the reward centers of a young, sexually naive meadow vole brain, he essentially transformed the meadow vole into a bond-craving prairie vole.[10] (Vasopressin is another hormone under the same umbrella as oxytocin; it promotes pair bonding in males.) Young's thought process was that if the hormones responsible for maternal behavior in females (oxytocin) and territoriality in males (vasopressin) were released during sex, the powerful hormones would augment the male-female bond.[11] Although territoriality may not seem to be related to bonding, it's one of the features for establishing that inexorable connection. The amount of time a pair spends in the same territory is indicative of the pair bond's strength, and Young seems to have been right.

The difference between the disloyal meadow vole and the loyal prairie vole is that the prairie voles have both oxytocin and the vasopressin receptors in specific areas of their brains, the area responsible for reward and addiction, and meadow voles do not.[12] That is an important point to remember: the areas in the brain that facilitate our capacity to connect, bond, and love are the same centers associated with addiction to harmful substances like mind-altering drugs and alcohol.* (And if you're wondering if oxytocin and the highly addictive drug OxyContin are related, the answer is no: OxyContin, a long-acting form of oxycodone, gets its name from the drug's continuous action to dull pain.) Mind you, these are primitive areas of the brain

*Apparently we're not the only animals to enjoy alcohol. In addition to bats, birds, bees, and tree shrews getting drunk on fermented tree nectar, voles love booze too and can drink the equivalent of fifteen bottles of wine in a day. In a wild experiment done by Andre Walcott and Andrey Ryabinin from the University of Oregon, they looked at the effects of alcohol consumption on prairie vole relationships and discovered that they experience similar problems as humans do when one mate overindulges: they decouple. A 2003 study found that "drinking or drug use" has been shown to be the third most common reason for divorce in the United States.

that have long held sway over our behaviors to keep us reproducing and enjoying pleasurable experiences, even if some of those experiences could be harmful. Such a phenomenon dovetails with what we explored earlier: the line between pleasure and pain is blurry. And a strong craving for the same sexual partner and a bona fide sex addiction are not poles apart, as they share some of the same underlying chemistry.

Young emphasizes that he's not necessarily observing humanlike love between voles but rather a special bond between the animals that is similar to what we humans experience, especially within the context of child-rearing and feeling a commitment to care for and protect our progeny. He does, however, think we should see ourselves as part of a continuum—the neurochemical bond between voles and the romantic bonds we keep in our human relationships in which we use terms like *love* may not be far apart from a chemical standpoint. He also says that voles may be monogamous for purposes of family life, but promiscuous sexual exploits are not beneath them (sexual monogamy is rare in nature). Similar to what happens in human relationships, the pairing off of voles doesn't stop what researchers call "opportunistic infidelity." Many males stray from their main squeezes for a tryst with hot tail, so to speak, and can end up fathering offspring outside the nest and accidentally end up raising other voles' babies if the female strays. About 10 percent of young voles are from a father that is not their mother's primary partner.[13]

And similar to the dating experience among humans, some males don't end up finding a mate to pair with and are named "wanderers" (female voles are not likely to become spinsters). A closer look at these footloose bachelors finds something else intriguing: Young has discovered a genetic difference between the two. The gene that codes for the vasopressin receptor gene is slightly different in the devotees than in the strayers. And loyalists have been demonstrated to have more receptors for vasopressin in targeted areas of the brain.[14]

This brings up another salient inquiry: Does this help explain human disparities in who stays and who strays? Is there a fidelity or, conversely, an infidelity gene? That's currently under debate, but studies have shown that variations in the genes that code for oxytocin and vasopressin receptors may affect how individuals behave and bond with others. What's more, studies also show that males that have pups out of a committed relationship could owe their adultery to having inherited variants of another gene that affect a part of the brain involved in remembering images and location, making them more likely to roam and meet other potential partners.[15] In other words, they are genetically programmed to have bad spatial memory, so they don't remember the exact locations of their established social encounters. Which means they are more likely to meander out of their own territories and hook up with other females.

Adding depth to this story is the fact that a vole's early life experiences, such as trauma or neglect, seem to affect its future bonding. Male prairie voles, for example, that experience stress in early life indiscriminately huddle with both their partner females and other females; they cannot commit to a monogamous bond. Research has shown that "the baby voles isolated from the licking and grooming of parents, an important bonding activity that also stimulates oxytocin production, have trouble bonding with future mates—but only if the isolated voles also have a relatively low density of oxytocin receptors in reward areas of the brain."[16] This again mimics what we see in humans: early life trauma can have lifelong impacts on a person's ability to connect with, trust, and form lasting bonds with others. The next question to answer is whether we can correct for these unfortunate outcomes using doses of oxytocin. If only a squirt of oxytocin could heal a traumatic past and bestow on someone a greater capacity to interact with others, to bond, and to love.

The devotion of most male voles to their progeny—and the mothers of their progeny—is what continues to intrigue scientists. Unlike the vast majority of male mammals, male voles stick around to help raise their children, and the moms don't take no for an answer.

A female will physically pull on her partner by the scruff of his neck if he's not doing his part. Most astonishing of all, and which I've also already mentioned, when a vole dies, the established partner experiences something similar to grief.[17]

Here's where some of the experiments have been breathtaking.[18] What happens when you take a vole that has just lost a partner and drop it into a bucket of water? It sounds like a horrible experiment but it's how researchers observe vole behavior under stressful circumstances, and it does not harm them. (Researchers are sure to rescue the creatures before they come to any danger.) The dunked vole will passively float and not struggle nearly as much as a dunked vole that has not lost its partner. In other words, the vole that lost its spouse will act depressed, not caring whether it lives or dies. Is such an observation a sign of depression? Young thinks the behavior is akin to drug withdrawal—the vole has lost its source of addiction, leading to "love sickness." Furthering this research, the scientists looked into the brains of the animals that lost their partner and demonstrated elevated levels of corticotropin-releasing factor (CRF), one of the stress hormones that in humans has been associated with depression, sleep issues, and anxiety. Next, the scientists blocked the receptors in the brain for CRF, and, amazingly, the bereaved voles fought vigorously in the water, like voles that hadn't lost their mates. As Young said in *Smithsonian Magazine*, "It helps us understand the neurocircuitry that may be involved in depression in general.[19] Studies are currently underway to look for ways we can use drugs to target the CRF pathway for treating anxiety and depression.

Another surprising finding from the voles is that they show empathy. Not until 2016 did Larry Young's group find that prairie voles console friends and family members in distress, proving that humans and other large-brained animals are not the only species to recognize and help others in need.[20] This illustrates another important lesson and case for friendship: we need one another to get through tough times in life. Young has shown that voles not only proceed to touch and groom their partners who are stressed, but caring for a distressed partner can leave the caregiver stressed also. This leads the scientists toward thinking that empathy is driving the consoling activity. And further work showed this activity, similar to us, was controlled by the anterior cingulate cortex area of the brain. Young said in a *Popular Science* article, "This does not mean animals experience empathy in the same way we do, but the basic foundation for empathy and consolation may be present in many more species than once thought." Behaviors once considered to be uniquely human may not be so; animals without complex cognitive abilities on par with ours can harbor the same behavior for survival. And it goes without saying that if empathy is a survival mechanism conserved by evolution in many species, then we would do well to work on our empathic behaviors as well—with those we already love and those we casually meet.

I must also pay tribute to Tom Insel, whose early work with voles in the late 1980s and collaborations with Young in the 1990s laid the foundation for understanding the neurobiology of social attachments and monogamous pair bonding.[21] Now in his early seventies but still runner-trim and as ambitious as ever, Insel, who was once dubbed the "nation's psychiatrist," is the former director of the National Institute of Mental Health (NIMH) and continues his mission

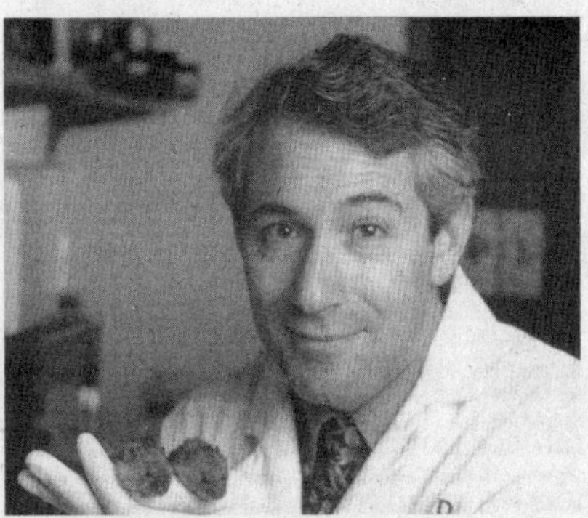

Tom Insel and his voles. Insel's early work with these cute creatures led to profound insights about the love and trust hormone oxytocin.

to change how we address mental health. His frustrations at the lack of progress in our mental health crisis are raw and real, but Insel remains eternally optimistic.

Prior to his NIMH post, which he held for thirteen years, Insel was the founding director of the Center for Behavioral Neuroscience at Emory University, where he helped lead revolutionary studies on vole behavior alongside Young and another scientist, Zuoxin Wang, whose career has also been built on work with voles. Their revelations came at a time when the field of psychiatry was at an inflection point—it desperately needed new insights with biological underpinnings to behavior and that studied the interplay of biology and environment.

When Insel first dallied in the world of neurobiology as a young fellow at the National Institutes of Health in the mid-1980s, scientists didn't know nearly as much about the biology of attachment as they do today. He fondly recalls the day Marianne Wamboldt, a postdoc, joined his lab after taking a six-month maternity leave following her psychiatry residency. After her first day back at work, where she was charged with studying baby cries from rats separated from their mothers, she found herself sobbing, for she had just left her own child behind. At the time, Insel was trying to understand the neurobiology of anxiety. Wamboldt protested, declaring that she was now going to study maternal behavior instead.

"I don't think there's any science there," Insel responded. He now laughs with some embarrassment at that comment.

"Give me a week," she replied, and came back with a stack of papers that became his metaphorical launchpad. The investigations began, and Insel soon found himself immersed in oxytocin's alchemy in human behavior, eventually teaming up with Young and Wang for experiments that ultimately changed the medical textbooks and how we appreciate the bonds we keep in fellowship and familial relationships. "I was a vole as a teenager," he quips. Soon after his eighteenth birthday, he married his wife and was about to celebrate their fiftieth anniversary when we spoke. His own children, now in their forties, taught him the power of having children on one's psychology and biology. Now an empty nester, Insel enjoys the daily oxytocin doses from his wife and dog, Teddy.

The concept of a daily oxytocin dose has real-world applications. One case in point comes from scientists at the University of Minnesota who did a remarkable experiment to promote conservation efforts: they administered oxytocin to lions on a wildlife reserve in Dinokeng, South Africa.[22] These lions are incredibly social animals but can be ferociously aggressive to other lions outside their circle of friends and family—to the point of death. When the researchers spritzed oxytocin up their noses in a groundbreaking study, they turned a group of twenty-three captive lions into friendlier versions of themselves who acted nicer to strangers of their own kind.

I should temper the cheerleading around oxytocin with a warning that we're not yet at a point we can freely prescribe the molecule the way we can other drugs to target a symptom or biological problem in humans. Context appears to matter when it comes to the benefits of oxytocin. Yes, it's linked to positive outcomes like increased trust, social bonding, and even a tendency to act more charitably financially, but like most other hormones, it can have unintended consequences. Some studies suggest that it can have a dark side, decreasing trust and sociability in certain people depending on the context.[23] Women, for example, whose relationships are in peril can harbor high levels of this hormone. And new research shows that this hormone can strengthen bad memories and lead to increased fear and anxiety in future stressful situations.[24]

Clearly oxytocin is a complicated hormone enmeshed with our ever-more-complicated emotions that begs further research for medical solutions. The work of people like Larry Young may one day help us tackle serious psychiatric disorders by harnessing oxytocin's benefits. It's also important to keep in mind that most hormones don't directly influence behavior; they affect our thinking and emotions, and it's *those* that influence our behavior. Young himself shies away from calling oxytocin the love hormone. He's the scientist who prefers to use the phrase "grease of the social brain"; it acts as a lubricant to help us fortify our connections. So while we're not going to casually add oxytocin to our morning cup of coffee (yet), we could do well with boosting it naturally in our lives to reap its positive rewards in our everyday connections. And this brings me back to Paul Zak.

Eight Hugs a Day

When you ask Paul Zak about oxytocin, his affinity for the molecule is palpable. He explains it simply: When someone interacts with you in a positive way, your brain releases oxytocin, which will reduce your stress. The oxytocin boost motivates you to return the favor and act similarly toward the other person; it is chemical.[25] Sounds biblical—the Golden Rule about treating others as you want to be treated. And he may be on to something. Zak sees oxytocin as one of our survival mechanisms and explains that among the underappreciated realities of daily life is the fact we encounter strangers every day. How do we know who is safe to approach versus those we should avoid? Oxytocin, Zak proudly claimed, is a critical component of training our brains to know the difference. When we see someone we recognize or someone we deem "safe" to interact with, it's oxytocin that facilitates that connection.

In a 2022 study led by Zak, he and colleagues at Claremont and USC found that release of oxytocin can increase with age, especially after middle age, and is associated with greater satisfaction with life and prosocial behaviors.[26] In other words, it's not inevitable that oxytocin declines with age, but we have to work at sustaining healthy levels. That's a good, motivating force, because as we get older, we're more likely to encounter loneliness as friends and family members die before us or we naturally lose connections with people as we become less able-bodied, agile, and mobile. Many things can alter our social networks as we age, including illness, retirement, and lack of mobility. Perhaps evolution is trying to persuade us—through more oxytocin—to sustain social relationships because it's essential to a longer life.

Such an idea makes sense when you consider other studies about the "best practices" for aging well and feeling happy as the years tick by. Surprise: Money and fame have been shown in study after study to not sustain people's happiness throughout life. Although a certain amount of money supports a happier life, it takes far less than you'd imagine (at least $85,000 a year for an individual in 2021).[27] And being rich is not an antidote to unhappiness. Social relationships and networks are excellent predictors of living a long and healthy life—many times better predictors than even genetics or your finances. The support these relationships can give us has tremendous impacts on our health.[28]

If that sounds absurd, the Harvard Study of Adult Development has been tracking how health is influenced by our social connections. This is the longest-running study on health and happiness ever conducted, with much of the data going back over eighty years, starting with data collected during the Great Depression. The study is now led by Robert Waldinger, a psychiatrist at Massachusetts General Hospital and a professor of psychiatry at Harvard Medical School (and a Zen priest).[29] Waldinger's 2015 TED Talk on the subject, "What Makes a Good Life?," has been viewed more than 42 million times.[30]

In addition to following participants in the ongoing study through the years using medical records and questionnaires, the researchers have conducted blood tests and brain scans and have interviewed family members. What stood out time and time again was the vital importance of good social connections. As Waldinger recounted in his TED Talk, "People who are more socially connected to family, friends, and their communities are happier, and physically healthier, and they live longer than people who are less well connected."[31] People's level of satisfaction with their relationships at age fifty, for example, has been shown to be a better predictor of physical health at age eighty than their cholesterol levels at midlife. Waldinger also said, "And the experience of loneliness turns out to be toxic. People who are more isolated than they want to be from others find that they are less happy, their health declines earlier in midlife, their brain functioning declines sooner and they live shorter lives than people who are not lonely."[32] The study has also revealed that it's not the number of friends you have that counts. As Waldinger explained in his TED Talk, neither is whether you're in a committed relationship. Much to the contrary, what matters is the quality of your close fellowships. When you experience a securely attached relationship in older age, one in which you can rely on another person, you're supremely protected from cognitive decline and more likely to preserve your memory. That's not to say you won't have your arguments, but if the ties that bind are intact and unshakable, good relationships will help lead you to better health and well-being. The biology behind the power of our bonds to support health is multifaceted and likely involves a lot of chemical pathways beyond molecules like oxytocin. Many factors are at play, from those that affect our levels of inflammation to epigenetic forces that translate to better gene activity and cellular renewal to bolster the body's resiliency.

Waldinger pushes people to spend time developing their relationships with family, friends, and community, and surely Zak would agree that the more enriching our relationships are, the more we stand to gain all the way down to how our bodies' chemistry works to keep us alive and well. Making connections can be as rudimentary as increasing the time with your loved ones, to going out and making new and enduring relationships in your community, no matter your age. Talk to strangers. Aim for eight hugs a day (and pets count) because physical touch is powerful in pumping out oxytocin. And seek group movement, as Zak calls it: dance together, engage in group exercise, share stories, go to the movies, enjoy concerts. And of course sex and mutual gazing can also support connection, as these activities get those oxytocin juices flowing naturally. Even the often pleasurable act of gossiping can prime the oxytocin pump.[33] Gossip may have negative connotations, but it's among our most pervasive social behaviors that can encourage bonding in a positive light.

In a *Science of People* interview Zak took his oxytocin-pumping activities even further, using memory of events, when he said, "Our brains use our memories to activate specific patterns for our interactions with people." If Dr. Zak hugs someone in person, then uses *hugs* in an email the following week to that same person, the brain will activate the memory of the in-person hug just by reading that word. This triggers oxytocin.[34]

Zak has uncovered some unexpected incidental findings in his research. One of the most important he thinks is that none of us are "average." When you look at data, he said, there are normal ranges, and averages, but we each are unique. He continued, "I'm super accepting of weirdness. I don't expect consistency with people. I expect variety. And that's okay because it makes us interesting!"[35]

One of Zak's quirks is to call out the emotions he sees in others in the hope of making his interactions as valuable as possible. Rather than assume that someone is "fine," he'll say, "You look happy" or "You look agitated." This creates immediate impact, as the person he's interacting with will often be grateful for his attention to their emotional state, which creates a cycle of empathy and authentic connection.[36]

That may not be your style of interacting, but no matter how you choose to authentically connect, the biggest hurdle we all have to clear is making the effort to create quality bonds through communication free from the confines of impersonal screens and digital distractions. We humans are creatures built to experience the full spectrum of nature's beauty and other people in the material world—not always in a technological one. And it's this final lesson that brings us full circle in the nature of a good, long life.

Touchy-Feely

Technology has no doubt changed our world—including matters of health and medicine—for the better. But as with so many things in life, technology has its downsides when used or consumed too much, at the wrong time, or with ill intentions. Modern technology has been a slow burn on our ancient ways of socializing and communicating. We now spend nearly half of our waking hours fixed on a screen, which amounts to about twenty-two years over the course of a typical life span.

Although we were initially sold, for example, on social media being a connector, it's had the opposite effect for many people—promoting more loneliness, feelings of isolation, and the "I'm not good enough" sentimentality that sabotages our well-being. Social media has also led to deeper divides between people's ideas and ideologies, which further casts us apart from one another and prevents us from making and strengthening those life-preserving bonds. And as we become more addicted to our devices and virtual worlds, we simultaneously become less immersed in nature and less attached to the beauty and gifts of nature. Nature can heal, however, and we are made to enjoy its boundless health-promoting powers.

For the first time ever, we're witnessing doctors "prescribe" walks in the woods and time outside—what's called nature therapy—to help individuals treat disorders as diverse as depression, anxiety, attention deficit disorder, hypertension, obesity, diabetes, PTSD, autoimmune disorders, and chronic pain. Nature therapy, guided by and practiced in nature, has many names, including *earthing*, *ecotherapy*, and *Shirin-yoku* (the Japanese term for "forest bathing," or taking in the forest). Shirin-yoku is a key part of health and medicine in Japan and is now being practiced around the world. At the Sensei Wellness retreat I helped put together on the Hawaiian island of Lanai, Shirin-yoku is one of the most popular items on its menu of activities.[37]

Studies now abound proving the power of nature in combating many ills, from behavioral issues and myopia in youths to serious mental health challenges and crippling stress in adults (and their myopic perspectives).[38] It has even been demonstrated to help people recover from medical procedures and surgery, as studies show postoperative patients recover faster when they have a window to green space in their room.[39] Through many biological events that recruit, among other things, the nervous and endocrine systems to exert calming effects, nature therapy offers a long list of benefits. Among the other ones documented in the scientific literature, nature therapy supports immune function; improves performance on working memory, cognition, focus, and concentration; lowers stress and blood pressure; increases self-esteem, energy, and motivation; boosts mood; and lowers pain. These benefits, which had long been anecdotal, have been officially measured from psychological and physiological markers in scientific settings. I don't know anything else that can check off all those boxes.

We are the only creatures on this earth that have purposefully veered away from nature therapy in our habits. And what's shocking to me is how long it has taken for us to appreciate nature's role in our health and happiness. Thousands of years after Cyrus the Great planted a garden in the middle of a Middle Eastern city (now part of Iran) to increase human health in the sixth century BCE, we finally have bona fide prescriptions for nature. You can't put ecotherapy in a bottle, but you can step outside to partake of its magic and feel an increased meaningfulness in life. And it needn't take all day, though a full day spent in nature without any digital device is a good idea once in a while. When one group of people ranging in age from eighteen to seventy-two ditched social media for a full week for a study, they reported dramatic improvements in well-being and drops in depression and anxiety.[40] But for everyday exposure therapy in nature, a few minutes can do the trick. An ideal commitment that has been scientifically backed is 120 minutes per week, which amounts to roughly seventeen minutes a day. You can break that up into three six-minute intervals—morning, midday, and evening. As with exercise, it's ideal to enjoy those snippets of nature throughout the day rather than in one fell swoop on the weekend. And you don't have to find a lush forest or sprawling beach. Any contact with nature will do, be it a backyard, local park, or hillside path.

Nature therapy is completely drug-free, but it can be combined with medications. For addressing mental health matters, for example, you can combine nature therapy with traditional talk therapy, certain medications, and calming activities like painting, exercising, or gardening. And you can amplify nature therapy's effects by bringing along another person (and maybe a dog or two) to share the experience (and talk about your problems). It's a win-win that boosts that oxytocin and secures those vital bonds. They key is to lose the love affair with mindless technology (at least for defined periods of time) and gain a mindful love affair with nature.

Be creative, intentional, and diverse with your nature immersions whenever you can. Some data suggest that diverse natural environments may offer some benefits, so go to different places for your excursions.[41] Mix up your nature settings as best you can, which can simply mean taking different routes for your evening strolls in the neighborhood. Pay close attention to the plants around you (and bring some greenery inside to have around your living and work spaces), go barefoot on soft soil, listen to birds, feel the wind, and try visiting an animal sanctuary to interact with a wider array of animals than you're used to. Another idea is to consider getting an aquarium. Watch what the natural world around you is doing, and bring others with you. Those two things—nature and people—are what make the world go around.

There's no substitute for authentic connections made in the real world with real people physically in our presence, and by the same token, there's no substitute for nature in any virtual or online experience. You have to get outside and use all your senses—touching, seeing, smelling, tasting, and hearing. This not only triggers the optimal release of happy hormones but also taps into our deepest needs as humans who have roamed the planet's nature for centuries. Evolution has made us creatures of nature, and we cannot negate or evade this need. Just as we can't live off processed junk food alone, we can't live off technology alone either. No apps will do the walking or running for you. No social media account will do the love- or friendship-making for you. Heartbeats, hands, faces, hugs, and kisses are meant to be experienced in the physical world. Go there—to the natural world of wonderment and the human world of wonderful people—and you will likely live better and for a good long time.

Creature Cheat Sheet

We are all bound by nature, just as we are bound to one another in fellowship and love. These bonds are chemical and real, and essential to survival. The more we can spend time with and love other people, form lasting bonds, and enjoy nature's contributions to wellness, the more we stand to gain more vibrant years to life. And the keys to this kingdom of optimal well-being are attainable by all who dare to walk in the wild; be openhearted and strike up conversations with strangers (even if you're an introvert); hug those they love (aim for a solid twenty seconds) and use written forms of oxytocin in correspondence with them; embrace people's weirdness; gossip for good; be nice to people and make friends; create memories in group settings like dancing and going to the movies (even taking one friend to the movies is better than going solo); think about how to be of service to others and act accordingly; be as good of a neighbor as a lover; and tune in to the calls from the crickets at night and the birds by day.

Whenever people ask me to prescribe something to make them feel better, I often joke: "Seventeen milligrams twice a day." It's my way of saying there's no cure-all or pill that will make you feel better or live forever. The path to improvement is not finding the one thing you are lacking. It's following a collection of rules, a collection of which you've now amassed from this book. To which I'll add my final rule: seventeen minutes a day. Remember, Mother Nature knows best. So let the rewilding begin again and again.

Epilogue

I hope you've enjoyed this journey and picked up a few new strategies to apply to your life today as you pursue a long and happy one. I also hope the incredible creatures we've encountered in these pages have sparked in you a renewed desire to observe, respect, and conserve this amazing planet of ours.

Mother Nature is the best mentor. And she'll be in your life for as long as you roam this world. Here's her ultimate cheat sheet for you to carry wherever you go:

- Our collective zoo is filled with a wondrous diversity of peoples, habitats, and opportunities to play. So stand tall and sit up straight, respect your inner fish as I covered in chapter 1, and move through the world with curiosity and a willingness to adapt. While we are all sheltered zoo animals in our own way, we have the uniquely human ability to optimize our habits to improve our health and, in turn, our productivity.
- Companionship comes in many forms, and our canine comrades can be our best friends. Welcome a dog or two (or any other pet) into your life, even if that pet belongs to a neighbor or a friend. Pets will help you stay calm and connected and to live more in the moment.
- Pay attention to patterns in your world like a pigeon does to

build better, stronger memories. And don't always take the same routes on your way to work, home, or the market; mix it up to exercise your brain's navigational skills. Write down encounters you want to remember, and sleep on important decisions.

- You're not a giraffe, so keep your blood pressure in check by maintaining cardiovascular fitness and leanness, not smoking, sleeping soundly in a flat position, maintaining dental hygiene, and moving frequently throughout the day. Take medications if you cannot get your blood pressure under control; they can save your life.
- Protect your DNA. Unlike those lucky elephants, whose bodies can correct cancer-causing mutations, we must be more proactive in our anticancer habits. Avoid dangerous exposures to chemicals and radiation (including UV light), skip extraneous vitamins and supplements, and keep inflammation under control. Certain medications (e.g., statins, aspirin) can help when you cannot control inflammation through lifestyle choices.
- Eat a diverse diet, but stay as close to nature as possible. Enjoy meals with others; shared food can be currency for connection, as it is for our cousin chimps. And like chimp parents, teach children to take some risks, explore on their own, and learn through trial and error.
- Teamwork, community building, and helping others in distress like warrior ants do is always a good thing. But so is choosing to work in a setting that's safe and supports your well-being. Does your job help you stay healthy and happy? Or is it time to explore new opportunities? Like an ant, the role you play has a great effect on your behaviors and risk factors.
- Reshape your DNA's expression through your habits. Your environment—and how you interact with it—plays heavily

into how you age. As the rhinos teach us, something as simple and subtle as a single ingredient can have a life-changing effect on our biology. And don't forget to keep a workout routine that includes interval training and social engagement.

- Like the octopus, we all want to die fast. But unlike the nine-brained octopus, we want to live long lives first. One of the key ways we can achieve this is by caring for our insulin-signaling systems, especially after our childbearing years. This means maintaining optimal blood sugar balance, body mass index, and overall bodily homeostasis. And we shouldn't forget to work on both our emotional and social intelligence too. We are empathic, social creatures.
- Respect your inner stardust. We are complex metaorganisms comprising more than just human cells. Microbes and viruses have shaped our existence, evolution, and survival for eons. Nurture your inner microbial comrades that collaborate with your physiology and have a big influence on your well-being all the way up to your brain. This means protecting a healthy microbiome via gut-friendly foods in the form of prebiotics.
- Pain is a pain, but pigs, squirrels, and albatrosses can tell us a lot about subduing Poena. Our attitudes, personalities, and memories all play a role in our experience of pain. Sometimes simple acts of altruism, bold sociality, and imagining a more painless future can be enough to dial that agony back a notch or two.
- Love makes the world go round. Around five hundred million years ago, long before voles started to pair-bond and humans waved hello, oxytocin made its earthly debut in a group of ancient vertebrates that later became jawless fish. It's an incredible hormone that helps us connect, trust, look younger, and live a longer life. Keep it pumping: be friendly and openhearted (talk to strangers!), look people (and creatures) in

the eye, give more hugs (aim for eight a day!), and get out into nature as often as possible.

Mother Nature lives in all of us and can be a source of inspiration and delightfully surprising. When artificial intelligence expert Eric Bonabeau studied swarm intelligence many years ago, he focused on the limits of human decision-making in an unpredictable world. When I spoke to him about his early work, we had a captivating conversation about the nature of creativity and the power of serendipity, or what he called “happy accidents.” We can plan out our lives and try to follow our doctors’ rules and recommendations but still be at the whim of nature’s unpredictability. And that’s okay. Human nature may crave certainty, but once in a while, it also loves a little surprise (and a safe scare). Happy accidents can take you to places you’ve never thought to go but where you’re meant to be—perhaps the savannas of East Africa or the deep-sea depths of the Gulf of Mexico, or your backyard.

Seize your rewilding.

Acknowledgments

In early 1992, I tried to write my first book. Aptly titled *MS to MD*, the book was supposed to be about life as a medical student (hence the initials "MS"). Medical school was the most exciting thing to me, and I was excited to demystify the experience. As often as I could, I hopped on the train from Washington, DC's Union Station for the six-and-a-half-hour ride to visit Amy in New Haven, Connecticut, where she was earning her master's degree in drama at Yale. I'd sit on the back porch of the house she'd rented in nearby Milford and write about the happenings in medical school, from helping to care for patients to explaining how we were taught medicine. I'd recently been given my first laptop and eagerly used it on my travels back and forth. It was a Toshiba T3300SL, with a whopping 2 MB of RAM and an 80 MB hard drive. State of the art. The monochrome computer cost $5,299 at launch and weighed almost six pounds. I didn't have that kind of money back then, so I was grateful for the loan.

I eventually abandoned the writing process, a fool's errand. I still have a markup of the proposal I'd sent to an agent, who clearly took time indicating its shortcomings: "I'd like more detail here. . . . This section needs to be fleshed out. . . . Is this worthy of a whole chapter?" Before I could say anything to merit an entire book, I'd have to learn a lot of lessons—some of them hard-won, many of them unexpected, and all of them necessary.

One of my most influential mentors, whom I've written about

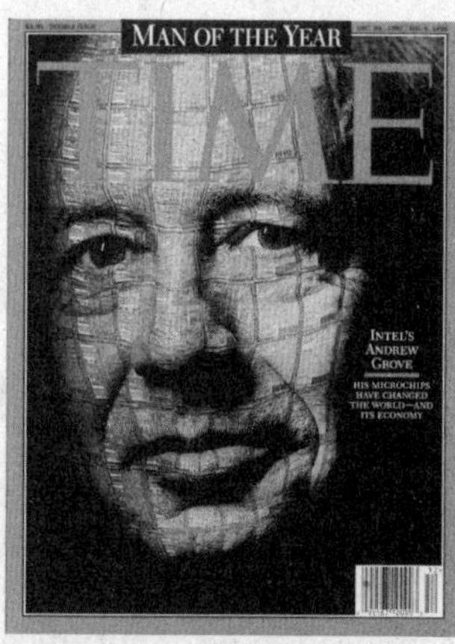

Andy Grove, "Man of the Year," gracing *Time* magazine's cover in 1997.

before, was Andy Grove, one of the founders and CEOs of Intel, the world's most successful microchip company. He shifted my life and my approach to medicine, starting one day in 1997 when he knocked on my door in the Rockefeller Research Labs in New York City while visiting my institution after recently being diagnosed with cancer. I was a newly minted independent scientist at Memorial Sloan Kettering, and my laboratory was a tiny room barely big enough for me and two research assistants. I was studying and treating lymphoma at the time, a cancer of the immune cells. But Andy had other visions for me.

I saw my grandfather in him, Jacob Agus, a rabbi from Baltimore. Andy may have been gruff and lacked the social graces to compliment anyone even when it was warranted, but he had an indelible influence on me. I owe him thanks for helping me become a better communicator. "David, you're a horrible public speaker!" Andy once scolded me, and then helped me set up daily speaking gigs after my long workday at Sloan Kettering for practice.

Hyatt Rickey's used to be a landmark in the heart of Silicon Valley. The hotel served presidents, athletes, celebrities, and the next darling in tech. The *Palo Alto Weekly* reported that it has hosted "gay rodeo riders and string-picking banjo players to knife collectors and law librarians. More than a mere meeting place, the hotel represented friendships formed and relationships cultivated."[1] When I entered Hugo's Cafe inside Hyatt Rickey's at 8:30 a.m. in May 1999, Andy was already seated. He asked me what I wanted for breakfast, and I ordered two eggs over easy and wheat toast. He ordered a cup of milk. I quickly asked him if that was all he was going to have, and he looked at me like I was crazy.

"No, I'm having cereal," he said. "They charge twelve dollars for a bowl of cereal." He ceremoniously took out a plastic bag filled with Chex that he'd ferried from home, along with some dates, oat bran, and soy powder.

I sensed we were about to have "the Conversation," the one that would change my life. Andy told me that my career would stagnate on the East Coast. He said people hit singles there all the time, but in California, people swung for the fences. And if I struck out? No problem. He assured me that I could just start again. He later helped me decide to go to Cedars-Sinai/UCLA, telling me that the system of universities on the West Coast was not as hierarchical as those in the East. My chances of making an impact early in my career would be greater out West. California has been my home ever since.

One of the most profound ways Andy shifted my perspective is in how I appreciate the body. Early in my career, I'd been looking at science and medicine in a reductionist way. My research was studying how molecule A signaled to molecule B. While this basic science is important, it doesn't take a step back to look at the whole as a complex biological system. A talk that Andy gave once at a cancer biology meeting has always stayed with me. I remember him saying that while he was CEO, Intel bet the entire company on each new generation of computer processor chips. Everyone in the company and every company asset was used to make the next generation—and if the chip failed, so would Intel. In science and medicine, he said, we are so focused on one experiment at a time—trying to get our next publication or a new grant—that we don't take risks and try big experiments. The big bet would take too long or require too many resources, and if the direction proved a dead end, the scientist would have to shut down the laboratory because there would no longer be financial support. Scientists, Andy stated, want small incremental gains so they can keep on doing what they are doing.

Andy mocked the idea of doing "good science," noting how little that term meant. In grant reviews for foundations, he would hear reviewers say over and over, *This is excellent science*, which was put forward as a reason to fund a grant. What he wanted to hear was how science or medicine would be changed by the results of the experiment. How would the results affect the treatment of a cancer or the lives of patients?

Andy also believed in different disciplines working together. I vividly recall visiting him at Intel in Santa Clara. As he showed me around, he pointed out how all the departments were represented on that floor: marketing, research, development. He wanted members of them all to meet at the central coffee station regularly to discuss the work each department was doing. This idea would influence me greatly in designing the floor plans of the Ellison Institute building in Los Angeles.

A few years ago, when another tech giant, Oracle founder Larry Ellison, and I were having breakfast at his house in Malibu, I thought of Andy. Larry had asked me what my dream was, and I told him that I wanted people to collaborate, not wall themselves off into different silos. One building for the physics department, one for math, and one for biology made no sense. All the disciplines needed to be together, and I wanted them all to apply their expertise to cancer. I wanted patients to walk by a lab and see where groundbreaking science was taking place, to see where people were working to cure them and be able to interact with the researchers. To the patient, the researchers would be hope personified, and to the researchers, the patient would be their motivation to keep working through the night. The separation of the lab and clinic made no sense. This idea crystallized for me the day I introduced Lorna Luft to the head of my laboratory, Shannon Mumenthaler. Lorna, an actress and the daughter of Judy Garland, had metastatic breast cancer that responded well to immunotherapy. The look on Lorna's face when she met the people working behind the scenes to develop therapies to save her life was indescribable. She and Shannon became fast friends. So when Larry asked how much I'd need to build that dream, it was my turn to not mince words. I threw out a number I had quickly calculated in my head—two hundred million dollars—and he said "Done."*

With the opening of the Larry Ellison Institute for Transformative Medicine in the middle of the pandemic in 2021, my hope was to break down those silos and make quicker headway with lifesaving research. We have a lot of problems to solve in health. But with medical researchers and evolutionary biologists like the ones I've featured in this book together exploring the world from various perspectives, I think we're on the way to some exciting progress.

Now on to the specific people who made this book happen:

As I did in my first three books, I thank my patients for allowing me to hone my message with them and, most important, for the privilege of being involved with their care. You teach me every day. I see the progress in science and medicine manifest as hope in your eyes every time we speak.

*As an aside, Andy sent me an email after Larry had purchased a 98 percent share of the Hawaiian island of Lanai, saying, "Saw Larry bought Lanai. He finally realized there is more value in hardware than software." Larry's interactions with Andy were equally memorable. Larry once told me the story of going with Steve Jobs to Andy's house for dinner. Larry and Steve were not known for on-time arrivals, but for dinner at Andy's, they were sure to be prompt. They even had time to stroll through the neighborhood first. When they all sat down at the table, Larry triumphantly told Andy that he and Steve had decided that Andy was the only one either entrepreneur would work for in Silicon Valley. After a long pause, Andy replied, "Neither of you is good enough to work for me."

One person I especially thank (again) is Larry Ellison, as our partnership has been one of the great highlights of late. Over the past two decades, our friendship has grown closer, and your mentorship of me has affected all aspects of my life. I am privileged to work in an institute with your name on the door, and I'm excited for many more decades of meaningful work together. As we worked closely during the pandemic, I gained a new appreciation for your deep knowledge and passion to make a significant difference in the world and share your fervent belief that technology will improve the human condition for all.

I feel so lucky to be able to write and educate about health and science. I have many to thank for enabling the work I do and for their love and support over the years. This book reflects the culmination of not just my lifetime work in science and medicine but also my ongoing collaboration with many individuals and teams of people.

To Robert Barnett, who has expertly and caringly represented, protected, and guided me through all of my books and media relationships: your mentorship, wisdom, and friendship have meant much to me. I couldn't have done any of this without you.

I have been with the same publishing house for all the books I have written, and I couldn't imagine a better and more supportive environment. I thank the crew at Simon & Schuster, led by Megan Hogan and Priscilla Painton, whose support, faith, and skill made this book possible. Megan's and Priscilla's exquisite editorial stewardship made this a much better, clearer, and focused book. Thanks also to their fantastic colleagues who each served a signature role from their various departments: Larry Hughes, Elizabeth Venere, Alison Forner, Paul Dippolito, Yvette Grant, Beth Maglione, Amanda Mulholland, Maxwell Smith, Marie Florio, and their fearless leader and my friend, Jonathan Karp. Thank you for putting up with me (I know it isn't easy) and for your faith in my work.

I am indebted to the team at the Ellison Institute for Transformative Medicine, who enable me to wear multiple hats—to be a physician, teacher, policy advocate, and researcher and find the time to write. I particularly thank my fantastic leadership team: Anna Barker, Katrina Barron, Olga Castellanos, Jonathan Katz, Jerry Lee, Shannon Mumenthaler, Kelly Santoro, Gabriel Seidman, and the leader of the leaders—my partner in the institute, Lisa Flashner. *Thank you each for the work you do* to make a meaningful impact on our patients' lives. Thank you for your loyalty and friendship and for the caring you give to the patients we are honored to treat. Thanks also for your work in figuring better ways to understand and manage disease. To the team of Reva Basho, Jacqueline Chu, Mary Duong, Mitchell Gross, Caitlin Hastings, Beverly Ikwueme, Jillian Infusino, Jackie Lopez, Melissa Melgoza, Sharon Orrange, and Trish McDonnell. To the teams at Project Ronin, Sensei Retreats, Sensei Ag, Global Health Security Consortium, Global Pathogen Analysis Service, and Imagene, I am excited every time we meet; the work we do together will increasingly have meaningful impact on the lives of so many.

I have the privilege of seeing breaking health and technology information daily through my involvement with CBS News. The outstanding leadership at CBS News—Shawna Thomas, Neeraj Khelani, and Susan Zirinsky—empowers me to educate and inform, and Angelica Fusco and Leigh Ann Winick collaborate with me on every story and are excellent at distilling the essence and truth from science news, an extremely difficult task! Your collective passion to understand and enlighten comes through every day. I am lucky to be a part of such a program.

To my friends who have helped me these past years, not just with the book, but also with other meaningful projects, Sir John Bell, Marc Benioff, Sir Tony Blair, Rick Caruso, Amy Coleman, John Doerr, Michael Dell, David Ellison, Lord Norman and Lady Elena Foster, Miles Gilburne, Al Gore, Davis Guggenheim, Danny Hillis, Matthew Hiltzik, Arianna Huffington, Peter Jacobs (and the CAA team), Gayle King, Mila Kunis, Ashton Kutcher, Clifton Leaf, Eric Lefkofsky, Jimmy Linn, Dan Loeb, Paul Marinelli, Fabian Oberfeld, Guy Oseary, Robin

Quivers, Linda Ramone, Shari Redstone, Haim Saban, Joe Schoendorf, Dov Seidman, Greg Simon, Elle and Paul Stephens, Howard Stern, Meir Teper, David N. Weissman, Sakiko Yamada, and Yoshiki: I appreciate your mentorship, friendship, and advice beyond measure. To friends and mentors who have passed in these recent years, always too soon: Eli Broad, Bill Campbell, Robert Dole, Bob Evans, Murray Gell-Mann, Ruth Bader Ginsburg, Brad Grey, Mark Hurd, John McCain, Shimon Peres, Colin Powell, and Sumner Redstone. To my personal exercise guru, Char Kane, thank you for helping me to practice what I preach.

I give deep thanks to the amazing scientists who spent time with me and gave me an understanding and deep appreciation for their work. Their passion was contagious:

- Piero Amodio, PhD, postdoctoral researcher, Department of Biology and Evolution of Marine Organisms, Stazione Zoologica Anton Dohrn
- Eric Bonabeau, PhD, professor of practice, SFI-ASU Center for Biosocial Complex Systems, professor of practice, Arizona State University
- Prosanta Chakrabarty, PhD, professor of ichthyology, evolution and systematics, curator of fishes, Louisiana State University
- Barbara Durrant, PhD, Henshaw Endowed Director of Reproductive Sciences, San Diego Zoo Wildlife Alliance
- David Allan Feller, PhD, JD, senior contracts manager, Judge Business School, University of Cambridge
- Erik Thomas Frank, PhD, group leader, Evolution of Social Wound Care, Department of Animal Ecology and Tropical Biology, University of Würzburg
- Alan R. Hargens, PhD, professor and director of the Orthopaedic Clinical Physiology Lab at the University of California, San Diego

- Tom Insel, MD, cofounder of Mindstrong Health and Vanna Health and former director of the National Institute of Mental Health
- Elinor K. Karlsson, PhD, director of the Vertebrate Genomics Group at the Broad Institute of MIT and Harvard, and professor in bioinformatics and integrative biology at the University of Massachusetts Medical School
- Michael Kent, DVM, professor of surgical and radiological sciences, University of California, Davis School of Veterinary Medicine
- Judith Korb, PhD, professor of evolution and ecology, Institute of Biology 1, University of Freiburg
- Joshua D. Schiffman, MD, professor of pediatrics (hematology/oncology), investigator, Huntsman Cancer Institute, University of Utah
- Craig Stanford, PhD, professor of biological sciences and anthropology, University of Southern California, and codirector, USC Jane Goodall Research Center
- Larry J. Young, PhD, professor of psychiatry, division chief, Behavioral Neuroscience and Psychiatric Disorders, Emory National Primate Research Center and Director of the Center for Translational Social Neuroscience, Emory University
- Paul Zak, PhD, professor of economic sciences, psychology and management, and director, Center for Neuroeconomics Studies, Claremont Graduate University, and member of the Neurology Department at Loma Linda University Medical Center

To my family for their unwavering support and love; thank you to my amazing, beautiful, and inspiring wife, Amy, and our two fantastic children (now adults), Sydney and Miles. To my mother and father, Sandy and Zalman, who motivate and inspire me, by example, to help others through science and medicine. And to the rest of the

Povich and Agus gang, led by Phyllis Baskin, Maury Povich, and Connie Chung, and my two younger brothers, Joel and Michael, I thank you and love you.

And finally, to Mother Nature, thank you for all the lessons and the privilege of being on this incredible planet with all of your creatures. I hope we can be good stewards of your work.

I'll leave you with one more gem from Andy Grove: "Success breeds complacency. Complacency breeds failure. Only the paranoid survive." My understanding of that last line is to be perpetually fierce, curious, and adaptable; don't sit idly or complacently. Expose yourself to change and challenges that can be uncomfortable, and embrace the ride with resolve. After all, that's what nature does. You're just as much a part of it as that tree, bee, and breath of wind outside.

Endnotes

A comprehensive list of notes to accompany statements made in this book would be a tome in itself due to the volume of sources and scientific literature I could cite. Most sentences could contain ten references. For general statements, I trust you can find a wellspring of sources and evidence yourself online with just a few taps of the keyboard, assuming you visit reputable sites that post fact-checked, credible information that's been vetted by experts. This is especially important when it comes to matters of health and medicine.

The best medical journal search engines do not require a subscription. Many listed in the notes include pubmed.gov (an online archive of medical journal articles maintained by the US National Institutes of Health's National Library of Medicine); sciencedirect.com and its sibling, SpringerLink; the Cochrane Library at cochranelibrary.com; and Google Scholar at scholar .google.com, a great secondary search engine to use after your initial search. The databases accessed by these search engines include Embase (owned by Elsevier), Medline, and MedlinePlus and cover millions of peer-reviewed studies from around the world. Studies often get published in advance online before being formally released in peer-reviewed journals. I've done my best to include all the studies specifically highlighted and added more in places to round out conversations. I've also moved a few lengthier notes and additional memos to the end here rather than clutter up the main pages with distracting footnotes. Use the entries as launchpads for further inquiry, and don't forget to check out my website at www.davidagus.com for updates.

INTRODUCTION

1. In his *Zoonomia; or, The Laws of Organic Life*, Erasmus Darwin wrote, "Would it be too bold to imagine, that in the great length of time, since

the earth began to exist, perhaps millions of ages before the commencement of the history of mankind, would it be too bold to imagine, that all warm-blooded animals have arisen from one living filament, which the great First Cause endued with animality, with the power of acquiring new parts attended with new propensities, directed by irritations, sensations, volitions, and associations; and thus possessing the faculty of continuing to improve by its own inherent activity, and of delivering down those improvements by generation to its posterity, world without end!"

CHAPTER 1: Living in a Zoo Cage

1. R. M. Sapolsky, *Why Zebras Don't Get Ulcers: The Acclaimed Guide to Stress, Stress-Related Diseases, and Coping* (New York: Freeman, 1994).
2. Michael S. Kent, "Association of Cancer-Related Mortality, Age and Gonadectomy in Golden Retriever Dogs at a Veterinary Academic Center (1989–2016)," *PloS One*, February 6, 2018, https://www.ncbi.nlm.nih.gov/pmc/articles/PMC5800597/.
3. N. E. Klepeis et al., "The National Human Activity Pattern Survey (NHAPS): A Resource for Assessing Exposure to Environmental Pollutants," *Journal of Exposure Science and Environmental Epidemiology*, 2001, 231–252.
4. United Nations, *2018 Revision of World Urbanization Prospects: The 2018 Revision*, https://population.un.org/wup/.
5. Firdaus S. Dhabhar et al., "Stress-Induced Redistribution of Immune Cells—from Barracks to Boulevards to Battlefields: A Tale of Three Hormones—Curt Richter Award Winner," *Psychoneuroendocrinology*, 2012, 1345–1346.
6. Margee Kerr, Greg J. Siegle, and Jahala Orsini, "Voluntary Arousing Negative Experiences (VANE): Why We Like to Be Scared," *Emotion* 19, no. 4 (2019): 682–698. Also see Kerr's book *Scream: Chilling Adventures in the Science of Fear* (New York: Public Affairs, 2015), and Margee Kerr, "Why Is It Fun to Be Frightened?," *Conversation*, October 12, 2018, https://theconversation.com/why-is-it-fun-to-be-frightened-101055.
7. Kerr, "Why Is It Fun to Be Frightened?"
8. George Fink, "Stress: The Health Epidemic of the 21st Century," *SciTech Connect*, 2016, http://scitechconnect.elsevier.com/stress-health-epidemic-21st-century/.
9. Quinton Wheeler and Mary Liz Jameson, "Scientists List Top 10 New

Species," *ASU News*, May 23, 2011, https://news.asu.edu/content/scientists-list-top-10-new-species.

10. See Prosanta Chakrabarty's TED Talks at https://www.ted.com/speakers/prosanta_chakrabarty.
11. Carsten Niemitz, "The Evolution of the Upright Posture and Gai: A Review and a New Synthesis," *Die Naturwissenschaften*, 2010, 241–263, https://www.ncbi.nlm.nih.gov/pmc/articles/PMC2819487.
12. Elisabeth Stephanie Smith and Herbert Riechelmann, "Cumulative Lifelong Alcohol Consumption Alters Auditory Brainstem Potentials," *Alcoholism: Clinical and Experimental Research*, March 2004, https://pubmed.ncbi.nlm.nih.gov/15084909/.
13. Michael Fetter et al., "New Insights into Positional Alcohol Nystagmus Using Three-Dimensional Eye-Movement Analysis," *Annals of Neurology*, 1999, 216–223, https://doi.org/10.1002/1531-8249(199902)45:2%3C216::aid-ana12%3E3.0.co;2-f.
14. Carissa Wilkes et al., "Upright Posture Improves Affect and Fatigue in People with Depressive Symptoms," *Journal of Behavior Therapy and Experimental Psychiatry*, March 2017, https://pubmed.ncbi.nlm.nih.gov/27494342/.
15. Kim Acosta, "How Your Posture Affects Your Health." *Forbes Health*, August 4, 2021, https://www.forbes.com/health/body/how-to-fix-bad-posture/.
16. Daniel E. Lieberman, *The Story of the Human Body: Evolution, Health and Disease* (New York: Pantheon, 2013).
17. GBD 2017 Diet Collaborators, "Health Effects of Dietary Risks in 195 Countries, 1990–2017: A Systematic Analysis for the Global Burden of Disease Study 2017," *Lancet*, May 2019, 1958–1972.
18. Kevin D. Hall et al., "Ultra-Processed Diets Cause Excess Calorie Intake and Weight Gain: An Inpatient Randomized Controlled Trial of Ad Libitum Food Intake," *Cell Metabolism*, July 2019, 67–77.
19. Ibid.
20. "Research News in Brief," InSight+, June 3, 2019, https://insightplus.mja.com.au/2019/21/research-news-in-brief-99/, and G. Calixto Andrade et al., "Consumption of Ultra-Processed Food and Its Association with Sociodemographic Characteristics and Diet Quality in a Representative Sample of French Adults," *Nutrients*, 2021, 682. Also see Anaïs Rico-Campà et al., "Association between Consumption of Ultra-Processed Foods and All-Cause Mortality: SUN Prospective Cohort Study," *BMJ*, May 2019, l1949.

21. Rico-Campà et al., "Association between Consumption of Ultra-Processed Foods and All-Cause Mortality."
22. M. Bonaccio et al., "Joint Association of Food Nutritional Profile by Nutri-Score Front-of-pack Label and Ultra-processed Food Intake with Mortality: Moli-sani Prospective Cohort Study," *BMJ*, 2022, e070688. Also see L. Wang et al., "Association of Ultra-Processed Food Consumption with Colorectal Cancer Risk Among Men and Women: Results from Three Prospective US Cohort Studies," *BMJ*, 2022, e068921.
23. Joana Araújo, Jianwen Cai, and June Stevens, "Prevalence of Optimal Metabolic Health in American Adults: National Health and Nutrition Examination Survey 2009–2016," *Metabolic Syndrome and Related Disorders*, February 2019, 46–52.
24. Meghan O'Hearn et al., "Trends and Disparities in Cardiometabolic Health among U.S. Adults, 1999–2018," *Journal of the American College of Cardiology*, July 2022, 138–151.
25. Daniel E. Lieberman, *The Story of the Human Body: Evolution, Health, and Disease* (New York: Pantheon Books, 2013).

CHAPTER 2: Oh My Dog!

1. David Allan Feller, "Heir of the Dog: Canine Influences on Charles Darwin's Theories of Natural Selection," MA thesis, University of Hawaii, 2005, https://scholarspace.manoa.hawaii.edu/server/api/core/bitstreams/311ed156-ceab-4d1a-b84f-b65047ba3f72/content.
2. Maria Lahtinen et al., "Excess Protein Enabled Dog Domestication during Severe Ice Age Winters," *Scientific Reports*, January 2021, 7.
3. Brian Hare and Vanessa Woods, *The Genius of Dogs: How Dogs Are Smarter Than You Think* (New York: Dutton, 2013).
4. Lee Alan Dugatkin, "Jump-Starting Evolution," *Cerebrum*, April 2020, cer-03-20.
5. Bridgett M. von Holdt et al., "Structural Variants in Genes Associated with Human Williams-Beuren Syndrome Underlie Stereotypical Hypersociability in Domestic Dogs," *Science Advances*, July 2017, e1700398.
6. Juliane Kaminski et al., "Evolution of Facial Muscle Anatomy in Dogs," *Proceedings of the National Academy of Sciences*, June 2019, 14677–14681.
7. Brian Hare and Vanessa Woods, "Humans Evolved to Be Friendly," *Scientific American*, August 1, 2020, https://www.scientificamerican.com/article/humans-evolved-to-be-friendly/.
8. Usha Lee McFarling, "How Beagles and Goldens Could Help Researchers

Find the Next Cancer Therapy for Humans," *STAT*, August 29, 2022, https://www.statnews.com/2017/10/04/dogs-cancer-treatment-humans/, and "One Health Basics," Centers for Disease Control and Prevention, November 5, 2018, https://www.cdc.gov/onehealth/basics/index.html.

9. Aryana M. Razmara et al., "Natural Killer and T Cell Infiltration in Canine Osteosarcoma: Clinical Implications and Translational Relevance," *Frontiers in Veterinary Science*, November 16, 2021, https://www.frontiersin.org/articles/10.3389/fvets.2021.771737/full.
10. W. C. Kisseberth and D. A. Lee, "Adoptive Natural Killer Cell Immunotherapy for Canine Osteosarcoma," *Frontiers in Veterinary Science*, June 2021, 672361.
11. "Dog Genome Project," Broad Institute, October 4, 2016, https://www.broadinstitute.org/scientific-community/science/projects/mammals-models/dog/dog-genome-links.
12. See Karlsson's papers listed on her site: https://karlssonlab.org/about/people/elinor-karlsson/.
13. Jeff Akst, "OCD-Linked Canine Genes," *Scientist*, February 19, 2014, https://www.the-scientist.com/the-nutshell/ocd-linked-canine-genes-37939.
14. Ibid.
15. Cross-Disorder Group of the Psychiatric Genomics Consortium, "Genomic Relationships, Novel Loci, and Pleiotropic Mechanisms across Eight Psychiatric Disorders," *Cell*, December 2019, 1469–1482.
16. Bru Cormand and Raquel Rabionet, "International Study Completes the Largest Genetic Map of Psychiatric Disorders So Far," *Actualitat*, September 3, 2020, https://web.ub.edu/en/web/actualitat/w/international-study-completes-the-largest-genetic-map-of-psychiatric-disorders-so-far-.
17. Daphne Miller, "A New Meaning for 'Sick as a Dog'? Your Pet's Health May Tell You Something about Your Own," *Washington Post*, July 1, 2019.
18. C. R. Bjørnvad et al., "Neutering Increases the Risk of Obesity in Male Dogs But Not in Bitches—A Cross-Sectional Study of Dog- and Owner-Related Risk Factors for Obesity in Danish Companion Dogs," *Preventive Veterinary Medicine,* October 2019, 104730. Also see "Obesity in Children and Teens," *American Academy of Child and Adolescent Psychiatry, Facts for Families,* April 2017, https://www.aacap.org/AACAP/Families_and_Youth/Facts_for_Families/FFF-Guide/Obesity-In-Children-And-Teens-079.aspx.
19. Jenni Lehtimäki et al., "Skin Microbiota and Allergic Symptoms Associate

with Exposure to Environmental Microbes," *Proceedings of the National Academy of Science USA*, May 2018, 4897–4902.

20. Clara Wilson et al., "Dogs Can Discriminate between Human Baseline and Psychological Stress Condition Odors," *PLoS One*, September 2022, e0274143.
21. Molly K. Crossman et al., "The Influence of Interactions with Dogs on Affect, Anxiety, and Arousal in Children," *Journal of Clinical Child and Adolescent Psychology*, 2020, 535–548.
22. Mwenya Mubanga et al., "Dog Ownership and the Risk of Cardiovascular Disease and Death: A Nationwide Cohort Study," *Scientific Report*, November 17, 2017, https://doi.org/10.1038/s41598-017-16118-6.
23. "Get Healthy, Get a Dog," Harvard Health Publishing, January 2015, https://www.health.harvard.edu/promotions/harvard-health-publications/get-healthy-get-a-dog-the-health-benefits-of-canine-companionship.
24. Robert DiGiacomo, "Should I Let My Dog Sleep Late Every Day?," American Kennel Club, August 23, 2016, https://www.akc.org/expert-advice/health/why-do-dogs-sleep-so-much/.
25. E. Sanchez et al., "Sleep Spindles Are Resilient to Extensive White Matter Deterioration," *Brain Communications*, June 2020, fcaa071. Also see Z. Fang et al., "Brain Activation Time-Locked to Sleep Spindles Associated with Human Cognitive Abilities," *Frontiers in Neuroscience*, February 2019, 46.

CHAPTER 3: Take the Long Way Home

1. Society for Personality and Social Psychology, "How We Form Habits, Change Existing Ones," *ScienceDaily*, August 8, 2014, www.sciencedaily.com/releases/2014/08/140808111931.htm. Also see D. T. Neal et al., "The Pull of the Past: When Do Habits Persist Despite Conflict with Motives?," *Personality and Social Psychology Bulletin*, November 2011, 1428; Sarah Stark Casagrande et al., "Have Americans Increased Their Fruit and Vegetable Intake? The Trends between 1988 and 2002," *American Journal of Preventive Medicine*, April 2007, 257.
2. Adam Gazzaley et al., "Video Game Training Enhances Cognitive Control in Older Adults," *Nature*, September 2013, 97–101.
3. T. L. Harrison et al., "Working Memory Training May Increase Working Memory Capacity But Not Fluid Intelligence," *Psychological Science*, December 2013, 2409–2419. Also see Anne Cecilie Sjøli Bråthen et al.,

"Cognitive and Hippocampal Changes Weeks and Years after Memory Training," *Scientific Reports*, May 2022, 7877.

4. Richard M. Levenson et al., "Pigeons (*Columba livia*) as Trainable Observers of Pathology and Radiology Breast Cancer Images," *PLoS One*, November 2015, e0141357.
5. Parrots have long been admired for their longevity and intelligence, the latter of which gives them highly developed cognitive abilities and an impressive talent for talking. But we didn't know what their secret was until 2018, when neuroscientists at Carnegie Mellon University and Oregon Health and Science University published findings that the parrot's genome contains a set of 344 genes that are likely involved in various processes that affect life span, including how the parrot can repair faulty DNA and control cellular growth (and prevent cancer). The authors point out how two different species—parrots and humans—can find similar solutions to problems via evolution. What's most remarkable is that the scientists found changes in parts of the parrot genome that are strikingly similar to those that set us apart from other primates. And this part of the genome controls the expression of nearby genes that play a role in brain development and cognition. That is, the set of genes that relate to intelligence is also physically close to genes that relate to longevity in the DNA of both humans and parrots—a phenomenon called convergent evolution, whereby different organisms independently evolve similar traits. Both humans and parrots evolved similar methods for developing higher cognitive abilities.

   Parrots could be useful models for studying certain brain-related disorders such as autism and schizophrenia. While this area of research remains controversial, the thinking is that because parrot genomes share genetic changes related to genes critical for brain function, when those genes go awry from mutations, cognitive deficits can result. If we can learn more about those genes, then maybe future gene therapies can lead to better treatments and cures for these complex neurocognitive challenges.
6. Mark Mancini, "15 Incredible Facts about Pigeons," *Mental Floss*, March 13, 2023, https://www.mentalfloss.com/article/535506/facts-about-pigeons.
7. Donnie Zehr, "Homing Pigeons in the Military," ClayHaven Farms, January 8, 2021, https://www.clayhavenfarms.com/blog/homing-pigeons-in-the-military.
8. Ibid.

9. Robert W. de Gille et al., "Quantum Magnetic Imaging of Iron Organelles within the Pigeon Cochlea," *Proceedings of the National Academy of Sciences USA*, November 2021, e2112749118.
10. David Simpson, "How Do Pigeons Find Their Way Home? We Looked in Their Ears with a Diamond-Based Quantum Microscope to Find Out," *Conversation*, November 17, 2022, https://theconversation.com/how-do-pigeons-find-their-way-home-we-looked-in-their-ears-with-a-diamond-based-quantum-microscope-to-find-out-171738.
11. C. X. Wang et al., "Transduction of the Geomagnetic Field as Evidenced from Alpha-Band Activity in the Human Brain," *eNeuro*, March 2019. Also see Eric Hand, "Maverick Scientist Thinks He Has Discovered a Magnetic Sixth Sense in Humans," *Science*, June 23, 2016, https://www.science.org/content/article/maverick-scientist-thinks-he-has-discovered-magnetic-sixth-sense-humans, and see Climate.nasa.gov.
12. Kelly Servick, "Humans—Like Other Animals—May Sense Earth's Magnetic Field," *Science*, March 18, 2019, https://www.science.org/content/article/humans-other-animals-may-sense-earth-s-magnetic-field.
13. See Climate.nasa.gov.
14. Servick, "Humans—Like Other Animals."
15. Connie X. Wang et al., "Transduction of the Geomagnetic Field as Evidenced from Alpha-Band Activity in the Human Brain," *eNeuro*, March 18, 2019, https://doi.org/10.1523/eneuro.0483-18.2019.
16. Ibid.
17. Sergio Vicencio-Jimenez et al., "The Strength of the Medial Olivocochlear Reflex in Chinchillas Is Associated with Delayed Response Performance in a Visual Discrimination Task with Vocalizations as Distractors," *Frontiers in Neuroscience*, December 2021, 759219.
18. Ed Yong, "Pigeons Outperform Humans at the Monty Hall Dilemma," *Discover Magazine*, April 2, 2010.
19. Walter Herbranson and Julia Schroeder, "Are Birds Smarter Than Mathematicians? Pigeons (*Columba livia*) Perform Optimally on a Version of the Monty Hall Dilemma," *Journal of Comparative Psychology*, February 2010.
20. Ibid.
21. Herbranson and Schroeder, "Are Birds Smarter Than Mathematicians?"
22. Louisa Dahmani and Véronique D. Bohbot, "Habitual Use of GPS Negatively Impacts Spatial Memory during Self-Guided Navigation," *Scientific Reports*, April 2020, 6310.

CHAPTER 4: The Giraffe Paradox

1. Walter Isaacson, "Anatomy, Round Two," *Medium*, October 31, 2017, https://medium.com/s/leonardo-da-vinci/anatomy-round-two-aaff3e296549.
2. Ibid.
3. Ibid.
4. Philippa Roxby, "What Leonardo Taught Us about the Heart," *BBC News*, June 28, 2014, https://www.bbc.com/news/health-28054468.
5. Malenka M. Bissell, Erica Dall'Armellina, and Robin P. Choudhury, "Flow Vortices in the Aortic Root: In Vivo 4D-MRI Confirms Predictions of Leonardo da Vinci," *European Heart Journal*, May 2014, 1344.
6. Hannah V. Meyer et al., "Genetic and Functional Insights into the Fractal Structure of the Heart," *Nature*, August 2020, 589–594.
7. Marco Cambiaghi and Heidi Hausse, "Leonardo da Vinci and His Study of the Heart," *European Heart Journal*, June 19, 2019, 1823–1826, https://doi.org/10.1093/eurheartj/ehz376.
8. Cold Springs Harbor Laboratory, "Understanding the Inner Workings of the Human Heart," *ScienceDaily*, August 19, 2020, http://www.sciencedaily.com/releases/2020/08/200819110925.htm.
9. Hannah V. Meyer, "Genetic and Functional Insights into the Fractal Structure of the Heart," *Nature*, August 19, 2020, 589–594, https://doi.org/10.1038/s41586-020-2635-8.
10. "Critical Reasons for Crashes Investigated in the National Motor Vehicle Crash Causation Survey," National Highway Traffic Safety Administration, February 2015, https://crashstats.nhtsa.dot.gov/#!/.
11. Randall C. Thompson et al., "Atherosclerosis across 4000 Years of Human History: The Horus Study of Four Ancient Populations," *Lancet*, April 2013, 1211–1222.
12. James E. Dalen, "The Epidemic of the 20th Century: Coronary Heart Disease," *American Journal of Medicine*, May 5, 2014, 807–812, https://doi.org/10.1016/j.amjmed.2014.04.015.
13. For facts about smoking and its effects on risk factors for disease and death, see the Food and Drug Administration's site (www.fda.gov) and that of the Centers for Disease Control and Prevention (www.cdc.gov).
14. J. Fay and N. A. Sonwalkar, *Fluid Mechanics Hypercourse CD-ROM* (Cambridge, MA: MIT Press, 1996).

15. "Gravity Hurts (So Good)," NASA, August 2, 2001, https://science.nasa.gov/science-news/science-at-nasa/2001/ast02aug_1.
16. Karl Gruber, "Giraffes Spend Their Evenings Humming to Each Other," *New Scientist,* September 17, 2015, www.newscientist.com/article/2058123-giraffes-spend-their-evenings-humming-to-each-other.
17. H. Kasozi and R. A. Montgomery, "How Do Giraffes Locate One Another? A Review of Visual, Auditory, and Olfactory Communication among Giraffes," *Journal of Zoology*, 139–146, https://doi.org/10.1111/jzo.12604.
18. "Looking Forward to the Space Station," NASA, August 2000, https://science.nasa.gov/science-news/science-at-nasa/2000/ast02aug_1.
19. "Space Travel Can Affect Astronauts' Sense of Taste and Smell," *Physics Today*, February 24, 2012, https://physicstoday.scitation.org/do/10.1063/PT.5.025900/full/.
20. Kelly Young, "Noisy ISS May Have Damaged Astronauts' Hearing," *New Scientist*, June 21, 2006, https://www.newscientist.com/article/dn9379-noisy-iss-may-have-damaged-astronauts-hearing/.
21. Charles Spence and Heston Blumenthal, *Gastrophysics: The New Science of Eating* (New York: Penguin Books, 2018).
22. "Looking Forward to the Space Station."
23. Bob Holmes, "The Cardiovascular Secrets of Giraffes," *Smithsonian Magazine*, May 21, 2021, https://www.smithsonianmag.com/science-nature/cardiovascular-secrets-giraffes-180977785/.
24. Bob Holmes, "How Giraffes Deal with Sky-High Blood Pressure," BBC, August 4, 2021, https://www.bbc.com/future/article/20210803-how-giraffes-deal-with-sky-high-blood-pressure.
25. Morris Agaba et al., "Giraffe Genome Sequence Reveals Clues to Its Unique Morphology and Physiology," *Nature Communications*, May 2016, 11519, and Chang Liu et al., "A Towering Genome: Experimentally Validated Adaptations to High Blood Pressure and Extreme Stature in the Giraffe," *Science Advances*, March 2021.
26. Barbara N. Horowitz et al., "The Giraffe as a Natural Animal Model for Resistance to Heart Failure with Preserved Ejection Fraction," Preprint, doi: 10.20944/preprints202010.0625.v1, October 2020.
27. Holmes, "The Cardiovascular Secrets of Giraffes."
28. Christian Aalkjær and Tobias Wang, "The Remarkable Cardiovascular System of Giraffes," *Annual Review of Physiology*, February 2021, 1–15.
29. Q. G. Zhang, "Hypertension and Counter-Hypertension Mechanisms in

Giraffes," *Cardiovascular & Hematological Disorders-Drug Targets*, March 2006, 63–67.

30. Alan R. Hargens, "Gravitational Haemodynamics and Oedema Prevention in the Giraffe," *Nature*, September 3, 1987, 59–60, https://doi.org/10.1038/329059a0.
31. Anna Lena Burger, "Nightly Selection of Resting Sites and Group Behavior Reveal Antipredator Strategies in Giraffe," *Ecology and Evolution*, February 14, 2020, 2917–2927, https://doi.org/10.1002/ece3.6106.

CHAPTER 5: "Yo, Elephant Man"

1. "Animals Affected by Humans," *BBC Earth*, August 11, 2021, https://www.bbcearth.com/news/animals-affected-by-humans.
2. James Ritchie, "Fact or Fiction?: Elephants Never Forget," *Scientific American*, January 12, 2009, https://www.scientificamerican.com/article/elephants-never-forget.
3. Andrew C. Halley, "Brain at Birth," *Encyclopedia of Evolutionary Psychological Science*, August 7, 2018, 1–8, https://doi.org/10.1007/978-3-319-16999-6_802-1.
4. Joshua M. Plotnik, Frans B. M. de Waal, and Diana Reiss, "Self-Recognition in an Asian Elephant," *Proceedings of the National Academy of Sciences USA*, November 2006, 17053–17057.
5. Karin Brulliard, "Watch Female Elephants Stage a Dramatic Rescue of a Drowning Baby Elephant," *Washington Post*, October 28, 2021, https://www.washingtonpost.com/news/animalia/wp/2017/06/22/watch-female-elephants-stage-a-dramatic-rescue-of-a-drowning-baby-elephant/.
6. Joshua M. Plotnik and Frans B. M. de Waal, "Asian Elephants (*Elephas maximus*) Reassure Others in Distress," *PeerJ*, February 2014.
7. Laura Parker, "Rare Video Shows Elephants 'Mourning' Matriarch's Death," NationalGeographic.com, August 31, 2016, https://www.nationalgeographic.com/animals/article/elephants-mourning-video-animal-grief?loggedin=true.
8. Gordon L. Flett and Marnin J. Heisel, "Aging and Feeling Valued Versus Expendable during the COVID-19 Pandemic and Beyond: A Review and Commentary of Why Mattering Is Fundamental to the Health and Well-Being of Older Adults," *International Journal of Mental Health and Addiction*, 2021, 2443–2469.

9. Charles Foley, Nathalie Pettorelli, and Lara Foley, "Severe Drought and Calf Survival in Elephants," *Biology Letters*, October 2008, 541–544.
10. "Elephant Elders Know Better," Wildlife Conservation Network Newsroom, August 21, 2008, https://newsroom.wcs.org/News-Releases/articleType/ArticleView/articleId/4981/Elephant-Elders-Know-Better.aspx.
11. Leonard Nunney, "Size Matters: Height, Cell Number and a Person's Risk of Cancer," *Proceedings of the Royal Society B: Biological Sciences*, 2018, 20181743, https://doi.org/10.1098/rspb.2018.1743.
12. R. Peto et al., "Cancer and Ageing in Mice and Men," *British Journal of Cancer*, October 1975, 411–426.
13. Daniel E. Koshland, "Molecule of the Year," *Science*, December 24, 1993, 1953, https://doi.org/10.1126/science.8266084.
14. M. Oren, "p53: Not Just a Tumor Suppressor," *Journal of Molecular and Cell Biology*, July 2019, 539–543.
15. Alexander Nazaryan, "Why Elephants Don't Get Cancer—and What That Means for Humans," *Newsweek*, October 8, 2015, https://www.newsweek.com/2015/10/16/researchers-studying-elephants-improve-cancer-treatment-380822.html.
16. Carrie Simonelli, "Their Biggest Role Yet," *Providence Journal*, April 25, 2016, https://www.providencejournal.com/story/lifestyle/health-fitness/2016/04/25/elephants-may-play-role-in-preventing-cancer-says-brown-graduate/29794497007/.
17. Phoebe Hall, "Think Big," *Medicine @ Brown*, October 18, 2016, https://medicine.at.brown.edu/article/think-big/.
18. Ibid.
19. Nazaryan, "Why Elephants Don't Get Cancer."
20. "Why Care?," Worldelephantday.org, 2019, https://worldelephantday.org/about/elephants.
21. Iñigo Martincorena et al., "Somatic Mutant Clones Colonize the Human Esophagus with Age," *Science*, October 18, 2018, https://doi.org/10.1126/science.aau3879.
22. Wellcome Trust Sanger Institute, "Mutated Cells Drive out Early Tumors from the Esophagus," *ScienceDaily*, October 13, 2021, https://www.sciencedaily.com/releases/2021/10/211013122733.htm.
23. L. M. Abegglen et al., "Potential Mechanisms for Cancer Resistance in Elephants and Comparative Cellular Response to DNA Damage in Humans," *JAMA*, 2015, 1850–1860. Access and follow Joshua Schiffman's

work and papers at his lab's research hub online: https://uofuhealth.utah.edu/huntsman/labs/schiffman/.

24. Nazaryan, "Why Elephants Don't Get Cancer."
25. Ibid.
26. Leo Polansky, Werner Kilian, and George Wittemyer, "Elucidating the Significance of Spatial Memory on Movement Decisions by African Savannah Elephants Using State-space Models," *Proceedings of the Royal Society B: Biological Sciences*, April 2015.
27. Shuntaro Izawa et al., "REM Sleep-Active MCH Neurons Are Involved in Forgetting Hippocampus-Dependent Memories," *Science*, September 2019, 1308–1313.

CHAPTER 6: Carnivorous Males and Permissive Moms

1. Amy Hatkoff, *The Inner World of Farm Animals: Their Amazing Social, Emotional, and Intellectuals Capacities* (New York: Stewart, Tabori & Chang, 2019).
2. Craig B. Stanford, *The New Chimpanzee: A Twenty-First-Century Portrait of Our Closest Kin* (Cambridge, MA: Harvard University Press, 2018).
3. David R. Braun et al., "Earliest Known Oldowan Artifacts at >2.58 Ma from Ledi-Geraru, Ethiopia, Highlight Early Technological Diversity," *Proceedings of the National Academy of Sciences USA*, June 2019, 11712–11717.
4. Katherine D. Zink and Daniel E. Lieberman, "Impact of Meat and Lower Paleolithic Food Processing Techniques on Chewing in Humans," *Nature* 531, no. 7595, March 2016, 500–503. Also see Ambrosio Bermejo-Fenoll, Alfonso Panchón-Ruíz, and Francisco Sánchez Del Campo, "*Homo sapiens*, Chimpanzees and the Enigma of Language," *Frontiers in Neuroscience*, May 2019, 558.
5. Katherine D. Zink and Daniel E. Lieberman, "Impact of Meat and Lower Palaeolithic Food Processing Techniques on Chewing in Humans," *Nature*, March 9, 2016, 500–503, https://doi.org/10.1038/nature16990. And Lizzie Wade, "How Sliced Meat Drove Human Evolution," *Science*, March 9, 2016, https://www.science.org/content/article/how-sliced-meat-drove-human-evolution.
6. Zink and Lieberman, "Impact of Meat."
7. Nichols Wadhams, "Chimps Trade Meat for Sex—and It Works," *National Geographic*, April 7, 2009, https://www.nationalgeographic.com/animals/article/chimps-behavior-sex-news-animals.

8. University of Southern California, "Evolution's Twist: USC Study Finds Meat-Tolerant Genes Offset High Cholesterol and Disease," *ScienceDaily*, March 22, 2004, https://www.sciencedaily.com/releases/2004/03/040322081608.htm.
9. Ibid.
10. Kunio Kawanishi et al., "Human Species-Specific Loss of CMP-N-Acetylneuraminic Acid Hydroxylase Enhances Atherosclerosis via Intrinsic and Extrinsic Mechanisms," *Proceedings of the National Academy of Sciences USA* , August 2019, 16036–16045.
11. Kunio Kawanishi et al., "Human Species-Specific Loss of CMP-N-Acetylneuraminic Acid Hydroxylase Enhances Atherosclerosis via Intrinsic and Extrinsic Mechanisms," *Proceedings of the National Academy of Sciences*, 2019, 16036–16045, https://doi.org/10.1073/pnas.1902902116.
12. Ibid.
13. Harriëtte M. Snoek et al., "Sensory-Specific Satiety in Obese and Normal-Weight Women," *American Journal of Clinical Nutrition*, October 2004, 823–831.
14. Anahad O'Connor, "Is There an Optimal Diet for Humans?," *New York Times*, December 18, 2018, https://www.nytimes.com/2018/12/18/well/eat/is-there-an-optimal-diet-for-humans.html.
15. M. L. Kringelbach, "Activation of the Human Orbitofrontal Cortex to a Liquid Food Stimulus Is Correlated with Its Subjective Pleasantness," *Cerebral Cortex*, October 2013, 1064–1071, https://doi.org/10.1093/cercor/13.10.1064.
16. Tera L. Fazzino, Kaitlyn Rohde, and Debra K. Sullivan, "Hyper-Palatable Foods: Development of a Quantitative Definition and Application to the US Food System Database," *Obesity*, November 2019, 1761–1768.
17. Herman Pontzer et al., "Metabolic Acceleration and the Evolution of Human Brain Size and Life History," *Nature*, May 2016, 390–392. Also see Ann Gibbons, "Why Humans Are the High-Energy Apes," *Science*, May 2016, 639.
18. Leslie C. Aiello, "Brains and Guts in Human Evolution: The Expensive Tissue Hypothesis," *Brazilian Journal of Genetics* 20, no. 1 (March 1997).
19. Gibbons, "Why Humans Are the High-Energy Apes."
20. M. Arain et al., "Maturation of the Adolescent Brain," *Neuropsychiatry Disease Treatment*, 2013, 449–461.
21. Zhengguang Liu et al., "Leader Development Begins at Home: Over-Parenting Harms Adolescent Leader Emergence," *Journal of Applied Psychology*, October 2019, 1226–1242. Also see Christian Jarrett, "What

Leader Are You? It Depends on Your Parents," BBC, April 5, 2020, https://www.bbc.com/worklife/article/20200406-what-leader-are-you-it-depends-on-your-parents.

22. Shanta Barley, "Respect for Elders 'May Be Universal' in Primates," *New Scientist*, January 6, 2010, https://www.newscientist.com/article/dn18347-respect-for-elders-may-be-universal-in-primates/.
23. Janneke Nachtegaal et al., "The Association between Hearing Status and Psychosocial Health before the Age of 70 Years: Results from an Internet-Based National Survey on Hearing," *Ear and Hearing*, June 2009, 302–312.
24. National Institute on Aging's Research Highlights, "Social Isolation, Loneliness in Older People Pose Health Risks," April 23, 2019, https://www.nia.nih.gov/news/social-isolation-loneliness-older-people-pose-health-risks#:~:text=Research%20has%20linked%20social%20isolation%20Alzheimer's%20disease%2C%20and%20even%20death.
25. Frank R. Lin et al., "Hearing Loss and Cognitive Decline in Older Adults," *JAMA Internal Medicine*, February 25, 2013, https://doi.org/10.1001/jamainternmed.2013.1868.
26. Ibid. Also see Rochelle Sharpe, "Untreated Hearing Loss Linked to Loneliness and Isolation for Seniors," NPR, September 12, 2019, https://www.npr.org/sections/health-shots/2019/09/12/760231279/untreated-hearing-loss-linked-to-loneliness-and-isolation-for-seniors.

CHAPTER 7: Team Effort and Social Immunity

1. Edward N. Lorenz, *The Essence of Chaos* (Seattle: University of Washington Press, 1993).
2. Kenneth J. Locey and Jay T. Lennon, "Scaling Laws Predict Global Microbial Diversity," *Proceedings of the National Academy of Sciences*, May 2, 2016, https://doi.org/10.1073/pnas.1521291113.
3. Alan Burdick, "Monster or Machine? A Profile of the Coronavirus at 6 Months," *New York Times*, June 2, 2020, https://www.nytimes.com/2020/06/02/health/coronavirus-profile-covid.html.
4. Ann C. Gregory et al., "Marine DNA Viral Macro- and Microdiversity from Pole to Pole," *Cell*, May 2019, 1109–1123.
5. David M. Morens, Peter Daszak, and Jeffery K. Taubenberger, "Escaping Pandora's Box: Another Novel Coronavirus," *New England Journal of Medicine*, April 2, 2020, https://doi.org/10.1056/nejmp2002106.
6. Ahmed A. Zayed et al., "Science Cryptic and Abundant Marine Viruses

at the Evolutionary Origins of Earth's RNA Virome," *Science*, April 2022, 156–162.

7. See the World Health Organization at www.who.int.
8. See the United Nations at www.unep.org.
9. Victor M. Corman et al., "Link of a Ubiquitous Human Coronavirus to Dromedary Camels," *Proceedings of the National Academy of Sciences*, August 15, 2016, 9864–9869, https://doi.org/10.1073/pnas.1604472113. And Stacey L. Knobler, Alison Mack, Adel Mahmoud, and Stanley M. Lemon, "The Story of Influenza" (Washington, DC: National Academies Press, 2019), https://www.ncbi.nlm.nih.gov/books/NBK22148/.
10. A. A. Naqvi et al., "Insights into SARS-CoV-2 Genome, Structure, Evolution, Pathogenesis and Therapies: Structural Genomics Approach," *Biochimica et Biophysica Acta (Molecular Basis of Disease*), October 1, 2010, 165878, https://doi.org/10.1016/j.bbadis.2020.165878.
11. CSIRO Australia, "Bats May Hold Clues to Long Life and Disease Resistance," *ScienceDaily*, December 21, 2012, https://www.sciencedaily.com/releases/2012/12/121221114114.htm.
12. James Gorman, "How Do Bats Live with So Many Viruses?," *New York Times*, January 28, 2020, https://www.nytimes.com/2020/01/28/science/bats-coronavirus-Wuhan.html.
13. Giorgia G. Auteri and L. Lacey Knowles, "Decimated Little Brown Bats Show Potential for Adaptive Change," *Scientific Reports*, February 2020, 3023.
14. Javier Koh et al., "ABCB1 Protects Bat Cells from DNA Damage Induced by Genotoxic Compounds," *Nature Communications*, June 27, 2019, https://doi.org/10.1038/s41467-019-10495-4.
15. A. Banerjee et al., "Novel Insights into Immune Systems of Bats," *Frontiers in Immunology*, 2020, 26. Also see Aaron T. Irving et al., "Lessons from the Host Defenses of Bats, a Unique Viral Reservoir," *Nature*, January 2021, 363–370.
16. "Chiropteran Flight," University of California Museum of Paleontology, https://ucmp.berkeley.edu/vertebrates/flight/bats.html, n.d.
17. Ibid.
18. Rachael Rettner, "Why Bats Carrying Deadly Diseases Don't Get Sick," *LiveScience*, April 16, 2014, https://www.livescience.com/44870-bats-viruses-flight.html.
19. James Gorman, "How Do Bats Live with So Many Viruses?," *New York*

Times, January 28, 2020, https://www.nytimes.com/2020/01/28/science/bats-coronavirus-Wuhan.html.

20. Ibid.
21. G. Zhang et al., "Comparative Analysis of Bat Genomes Provides Insight into the Evolution of Flight and Immunity," *Science*, January 2013, 456–460.
22. Jennifer C. Felger, "Role of Inflammation in Depression and Treatment Implications," in *Handbook of Experimental Pharmacology: Antidepressants*, October 28, 2018, ed. Martin Michel (Berlin: Springer-Verlag), 255–286, https://doi.org/10.1007/164_2018_166.
23. Patrick Schultheiss et al., "The Abundance, Biomass, and Distribution of Ants on Earth," *Proceedings of the National Academy of Sciences*, September 19, 2022, https://doi.org/10.1073/pnas.2201550119.
24. David Attenborough, *Life on Earth: The Greatest Story Ever Told* (London: William Collins, 2018). Note that this quote was originally published in the 1979 first edition and based on the BBC television series.
25. Erik T. Frank, Marten Wehrhahn, and K. Eduard Linsenmair, "Wound Treatment and Selective Help in a Termite-Hunting Ant," *Proceedings of the Royal Society B: Biological Sciences*, February 2018, 2017–2457.
26. Alessandra Potenza, "These Termite-Hunting Ants Lick the Severed Legs of Their Friends to Treat Them," *Verge*, February 14, 2018, https://www.theverge.com/2018/2/13/17007916/termite-hunting-ants-megaponera-analis-wound-treatment-rescue-behavior.
27. To see some of this in action, see ibid.
28. Ibid.
29. M. Shibata et al., "Real-Space and Real-Time Dynamics of CRISPR-Cas9 Visualized by High-Speed Atomic Force Microscopy," *Nature Communications*, 2017.
30. Giedrius Gasiunas et al., "Cas9-crRNA Ribonucleoprotein Complex Mediates Specific DNA Cleavage for Adaptive Immunity in Bacteria," *Proceedings of the National Academy of Sciences USA*, September 2012, E2579-E2586. Also see Martin Jinek et al., "A Programmable Dual-RNA-Guided DNA Endonuclease in Adaptive Bacterial Immunity," *Science*, August 2012, 816–821.
31. Jinek et al., "A Programmable Dual-RNA-Guided DNA Endonuclease in Adaptive Bacterial Immunity."
32. Brad Plumer et al., "CRISPR, One of the Biggest Science Stories of the

Decade, Explained," *Vox*, July 23, 2018, https://www.vox.com/2018/7/23/17594864/crispr-cas9-gene-editing.

33. Ibid.
34. Matteo Antoine Negroni, Susanne Foitzik, and Barbara Feldmeyer, "Long-Lived Temnothorax Ant Queens Switch from Investment in Immunity to Antioxidant Production with Age," *Scientific Reports*, May 2019, 7270.
35. "What Can Ants, Bees, and Other Social Insects Teach Us about Aging?," *Science*, March 25, 2021, https://www.science.org/content/article/what-can-ants-bees-and-other-social-insects-teach-us-about-aging.
36. Janko Gospocic et al., "Kr-h1 Maintains Distinct Caste-Specific Neuro-Transcriptomes in Response to Socially Regulated Hormones," *Cell*, November 2021, 5807–5823.
37. Clarence Collison, "A Closer Look: Social Immunity," *Bee Culture*, May 25, 2015, https://www.beeculture.com/a-closer-look-social-immunity/.
38. Nathalie Stroeymeyt et al., "Social Network Plasticity Decreases Disease Transmission in a Eusocial Insect," *Science*, November 22, 2018, 941–945.
39. ScienMag Staff, "When Working Ants Take a Sick Day, the Whole Colony Benefits," *ScienMag*, November 22, 2018, https://scienmag.com/when-working-ants-take-a-sick-day-the-whole-colony-benefits/.
40. Mark C. Harrison et al., "Hemimetabolous Genomes Reveal Molecular Basis of Termite Eusociality," *Nature and Ecology Evolution*, March 2018, 557–566. Also see Daegan Inward, George Beccaloni, and Paul Eggleton, "Death of an Order: A Comprehensive Molecular Phylogenetic Study Confirms That Termites Are Eusocial Cockroaches," *Biology Letters*, June 2007, 331–335.
41. Daniel Elsner, Karen Meusemann, and Judith Korb, "Longevity and Transposon Defense: The Case of Termite Reproductives," *Proceedings of the National Academy of Sciences USA*, May 2018, 5504–5509.
42. Yella Hewings-Martin, "Jumping Genes Made Us Human, But Can They Cause Disease?," www.medicalnewstoday.com, August 17, 2017.
43. Joel Goh, Jeffrey Pfeffer, and Stefanos Zenios, "Exposure to Harmful Workplace Practices Could Account for Inequality in Life Spans across Different Demographic Groups," *Health Affairs*, October 2015, 1761–1768.

CHAPTER 8: Rhinos, Reproduction, and Running

1. Donald R. Prothero, *Rhinoceros Giants: The Paleobiology of Indricotheres* (Bloomington: Indiana University Press, 2013).

2. Kendra Meyer, "Andrews, Roy Chapman: Biographical or Historical Note," *American Museum of Natural History*, January 19, 2022, https://data.library.amnh.org/archives-authorities/id/amnhp_1000042.
3. For issues about fertility, see Shanna Swan, *Countdown: How Our Modern World Is Threatening Sperm Counts, Altering Male and Female Reproductive Development, and Imperiling the Future of the Human Race* (New York: Simon & Schuster, 2020).
4. Paolo Capogrosso et al., "One Patient Out of Four with Newly Diagnosed Erectile Dysfunction Is a Young Man—Worrisome Picture from the Every-day Clinical Practice," *Journal of Sexual Medicine*, July 2013, 1833–1841.
5. Parker M. Pennington et al., "Ovulation Induction in Anovulatory Southern White Rhinoceros (*Ceratotherium simum simum*) without Altrenogest," *Conservation Physiology*, June 2019. Also see Cyrillus Ververs et al., "Reproductive Performance Parameters in a Large Population of Game-Ranched White Rhinoceroses (*Ceratotherium simum simum*)," *PLoS One*, December 2017, e0187751.
6. Herman Pontzer et al., "Daily Energy Expenditure through the Human Life Course," *Science*, August 2021, 808–812.
7. "Endocrine Disruptors," National Institute of Environmental Health Sciences, 2018, https://www.niehs.nih.gov/health/topics/agents/endocrine/index.cfm.
8. EPA Press Office, "EPA Announces New Drinking Water Health Advisories for PFAS Chemicals, $1 Billion in Bipartisan Infrastructure Law Funding to Strengthen Health Protections," June 15, 2022, https://www.epa.gov/newsreleases/epa-announces-new-drinking-water-health-advisories-pfas-chemicals-1-billion-bipartisan.
9. D. J. Barker et al., "Weight in Infancy and Death from Ischaemic Heart Disease," *Lancet*, September 1989, 577–580.
10. A. Forsdahl, "Are Poor Living Conditions in Childhood and Adolescence an Important Risk Factor for Arteriosclerotic Heart Disease?," *British Journal of Preventive and Social Medicine*, June 1977, 91–95.
11. Cyrus Cooper, "David Barker Obituary," *Guardian*, September 11, 2013, https://www.theguardian.com/society/2013/sep/11/david-barker.
12. To access a library of data and published research on the developmental origins of disease, go to the International Society for Developmental Origins of Health and Disease at https://dohadsoc.org/. Also see J. J. Heindel and L. N. Vandenberg, "Developmental Origins of Health and Disease:

A Paradigm for Understanding Disease Cause and Prevention," *Current Opinion in Pediatrics*, April 2015, 248–253.

13. Victor Gabriel Clatici et al., "Diseases of Civilization—Cancer, Diabetes, Obesity and Acne—the Implication of Milk, IGF-1 and mTORC1," *Maedica*, December 2018, 273–281.
14. Heather B. Patisaul and Wendy Jefferson, "The Pros and Cons of Phytoestrogens," *Frontiers in Neuroendocrinology*, October 2010, 400–419, https://doi.org/10.1016/j.yfrne.2010.03.003.
15. Ibid.
16. Marieke Veurink, Marlies Koster, and Lolkje T. W. de Jong-van den Berg, "The History of DES, Lessons to Be Learned," *Pharmacy World and Science*, June 2005, 139–143, https://doi.org/10.1007/s11096-005-3663-z.
17. Laura S. Bleker et al., "Cohort Profile: The Dutch Famine Birth Cohort (DFBC): A Prospective Birth Cohort Study in the Netherlands," *BMJ Open*, March 2021, e042078.
18. Carl Zimmer, "The Famine Ended 70 Years Ago, But Dutch Genes Still Bear Scars," *New York Times*, January 31, 2018, https://www.nytimes.com/2018/01/31/science/dutch-famine-genes.html.
19. P. Ekamper et al., "Independent and Additive Association of Prenatal Famine Exposure and Intermediary Life Conditions with Adult Mortality between Age 18–63 Years," *Social Science and Medicine*, October 2014, 232–239.
20. Zimmer, "The Famine Ended 70 Years Ago."
21. Elmar W. Tobi et al., "DNA Methylation as a Mediator of the Association between Prenatal Adversity and Risk Factors for Metabolic Disease in Adulthood," *Science Advances*, January 2018, eaao4364.
22. "White Rhinoceros," *National Geographic*, November 11, 2010, https://www.nationalgeographic.com/animals/mammals/facts/white-rhinoceros.
23. Christopher Tubbs, Barbara Durrant, and Matthew Milnes, "Reconsidering the Use of Soy and Alfalfa in Southern White Rhinoceros Diets," *Pachyderm*, July 2016–June 2017, https://www.rhinoresourcecenter.com/pdf_files/151/1517208334.pdf.
24. See the Center for Food Safety at www.centerforfoodsafety.org.
25. Patisaul and Jefferson, "The Pros and Cons of Phytoestrogens."
26. Kristina S. Petersen, "The Dilemma with the Soy Protein Health Claim," *Journal of the American Heart Association*, June 27, 2019, https://doi org/10.1161/jaha.119.013202.

27. Patisaul and Jefferson, "The Pros and Cons of Phytoestrogens."
28. Wendy N. Jefferson, Heather B. Patisaul, and Carmen J. Williams, "Reproductive Consequences of Developmental Phytoestrogen Exposure," *Reproduction*, March 2012, 247–260, https://doi.org/10.1530/rep-11-0369.
29. Candace L. Williams et al., "Gut Microbiota and Phytoestrogen-Associated Infertility in Southern White Rhinoceros," *mBio,* April 2019, e00311–319.
30. Ibid.
31. Wendy N. Jefferson, "Adult Ovarian Function Can Be Affected by High Levels of Soy," *Journal of Nutrition*, December 2010, https://doi.org/10.3945/jn.110.123802.
32. Margaret A. Adgent et al., "A Longitudinal Study of Estrogen-Responsive Tissues and Hormone Concentrations in Infants Fed Soy Formula," *Journal of Clinical Endocrinology and Metabolism*, May 2018, 1899–1909.
33. "Babies Fed Soy-Based Formula Have Changes in Reproductive System Tissues," *Children's Hospital of Philadelphia News*, March 12, 2018, https://www.chop.edu/news/babies-fed-soy-based-formula-have-changes-reproductive-system-tissues.
34. Nina R. O'Connor, "Infant Formula," *American Family Physician,* April 2009, 565–570.
35. K. S. D. Kothapalli et al., "Positive Selection on a Regulatory Insertion–Deletion Polymorphism in FADS2 Influences Apparent Endogenous Synthesis of Arachidonic Acid," *Molecular Biology and Evolution,* July 2016, 1726–1739.
36. Srinivasan Beddhu et al., "Light-Intensity Physical Activities and Mortality in the United States General Population and CKD Subpopulation," *Clinical Journal of the American Society of Nephrology*, July 2015, 1145–1153. Also see Shigeru Sato et al., "Effect of Daily 3-s Maximum Voluntary Isometric, Concentric, or Eccentric Contraction on Elbow Flexor Strength," *Scandinavian Journal of Medicine and Science in Sports*, May 2022, 833–843.
37. Peter Schnohr et al., "Various Leisure-Time Physical Activities Associated with Widely Divergent Life Expectancies: The Copenhagen City Heart Study," *Mayo Clinic Proceedings*, December 2018, 1775–1785. Also see Pekka Oja et al., "Associations of Specific Types of Sports and Exercise with All-Cause and Cardiovascular-Disease Mortality: A Cohort Study of 80,306 British Adults," *British Journal of Sports Medicine*, May 2017, 812–817.

38. J. Graham et al., "Estimates of the Heritability of Human Longevity Are Substantially Inflated due to Assortative Mating," *Genetics,* October 3, 2018, 1109–1124, https://doi.org/10.1534/genetics.118.301613.
39. Ibid.

CHAPTER 9: Smart Suckers and Demented Dolphins

1. Lewis Thomas, *The Lives of a Cell: Notes of a Biology Watcher* (New York: Viking, 1974).
2. Carl Zimmer, "Yes, the Octopus Is Smart as Heck. But Why?," *New York Times*, November 30, 2018, https://www.nytimes.com/2018/11/30/science/animal-intelligence-octopus-cephalopods.html.
3. Tamar Gutnick et al., "Octopus Vulgaris Uses Visual Information to Determine the Location of Its Arm," *Current Biology*, March 2011, 460–462.
4. Lisa Hendry, "Octopuses Keep Surprising Us – Here Are Eight Examples How," Natural History Museum, https://www.nhm.ac.uk/discover/octopuses-keep-surprising-us-here-are-eight-examples-how.html, n.d.
5. Martin I. Sereno et al., "The Human Cerebellum Has Almost 80% of the Surface Area of the Neocortex," *Proceedings of the National Academy of Sciences USA*, August 2020, 19538–19543.
6. Peter Godfrey-Smith, *MetaZoa: Animal Life and the Birth of the Mind* (London: Williams Collins, 2020). Also see his previous work: *Other Minds: The Octopus, the Sea, and the Deep Origins of Consciousness* (New York: Farrar, Straus and Giroux, 2016). Also see Elle Hunt, "Alien Intelligence: The Extraordinary Minds of Octopuses and Other Cephalopods," *Guardian*, March 29, 2017, https://www.theguardian.com/environment/2017/mar/28/alien-intelligence-the-extraordinary-minds-of-octopuses-and-other-cephalopods.
7. Peter Godfrey-Smith, "The Mind of an Octopus," *Scientific American,* August 12, 2015, https://doi.org/10.1038/scientificamericanmind0117-62.
8. Roland C. Anderson et al., "Octopuses (*Enteroctopus dofleini*) Recognize Individual Humans," *Journal of Applied Animal Welfare Science*, 2010, 261–272. Also see Sy Montgomery, *The Soul of an Octopus: A Surprising Exploration into the Wonder of Consciousness* (New York: Atria, 2015).
9. P. B. Dews, "Some Observations on an Operant in the Octopus," *Journal of the Experimental Analysis of Behavior*, January 1959, 57–63. Also see his obituary: J. L. Katz and J. Bergman, "Obituary: Peter B. Dews (1922–2012)," *Psychopharmacology*, 2013, 193–194.

10. Jennifer Levine, "Why Octopuses Are Awesome," *Cell Mentor,* February 10, 2016, https://crosstalk.cell.com/blog/why-octopuses-are-awesome.
11. For a history of Lloyd Morgan's ideas, see R. J. Richards, "Lloyd Morgan's Theory of Instinct: From Darwinism to Neo-Darwinism," *Journal of the History of Behavioral Sciences*, January 1977, 12–32.
12. Piero Amodio et al., "Grow Smart and Die Young: Why Did Cephalopods Evolve Intelligence?," *Trends in Ecology and Evolution*, January 2019, 45–56.
13. Katherine Harmon Courage, "How the Freaky Octopus Can Help Us Understand the Human Brain," *Wired*, October 1, 2013, https://www.wired.com/2013/10/how-the-freaky-octopus-can-help-us-understand-the-human-brain/.
14. Zimmer, "Yes, the Octopus Is Smart as Heck."
15. Z. Yan Wang et al., "Steroid Hormones of the Octopus Self-Destruct System," *Current Biology*, May 12, 2022, 2572-2579.e4, https://doi.org/10.1016/j.cub.2022.04.043.
16. "Changes in Cholesterol Production Lead to Tragic Octopus Death Spiral," Press release, University of Chicago, May 12, 2022, https://www.eurekalert.org/news-releases/952033.
17. Wang et al., "Steroid Hormones of the Octopus Self-Destruct System."
18. "Changes in Cholesterol Production Lead to Tragic Octopus Death Spiral."
19. S. Piraino et al., "Reversing the Life Cycle: Medusae Transforming into Polyps and Cell Transdifferentiation in *Turritopsis nutricula* (Cnidaria, Hydrozoa)," *Biological Bulletin*, June 1996, 302–312.
20. "The Jellyfish That Never Dies," *BBC Earth,* https://www.bbcearth.com/news/the-jellyfish-that-never-dies, n.d.
21. Ibid.
22. Maria Pascual-Torner et al., "Comparative Genomics of Mortal and Immortal Cnidarians Unveils Novel Keys behind Rejuvenation," *Proceedings of the National Academy of Sciences*, September 2022, e2118763119.
23. Margaret Osborne, " 'Immortal Jellyfish' Could Spur Discoveries about Human Aging," *Smithsonian Magazine*, September 6, 2022, www.smithsonianmag.com/smart-news/immortal-jellyfish-could-spur-discoveries-about-human-aging-180980702/.
24. "Dolphin Brains Show Signs of Alzheimer's Disease," University of Oxford, October 22, 2017, https://www.ox.ac.uk/news/2017-10-23-dolphin-brains-show-signs-alzheimer%E2%80%99s-disease.

25. Danièlle Gunn-Moore et al., "Alzheimer's Disease in Humans and Other Animals: A Consequence of Postreproductive Life Span and Longevity Rather Than Aging," *Alzheimer's and Dementia*, February 2018, 195–204.
26. Owen Dyer, "Is Alzheimer's Really Just Type III Diabetes?," *National Review of Medicine*, December 2005, https://www.nationalreviewofmedicine.com/issue/2005/12_15/2_advances_medicine01_21.html. Also see S. M. de la Monte and J. R. Wands, "Alzheimer's Disease Is Type 3 Diabetes: Evidence Reviewed," *Journal of Diabetes Science and Technology*, November 2008, 1101–1113.
27. Saeid Safiri et al., "Prevalence, Deaths and Disability-Adjusted-Life-Years (DALYs) due to Type 2 Diabetes and Its Attributable Risk Factors in 204 Countries and Territories, 1990–2019: Results from the Global Burden of Disease Study 2019," *Frontiers in Endocrinology*, February 2022, https://doi.org/10.3389/fendo.2022.838027.
28. Stephanie Venn-Watson et al., "Blood-Based Indicators of Insulin Resistance and Metabolic Syndrome in Bottlenose Dolphins (*Tursiops truncatus*)," *Frontiers in Endocrinology*, October 2013, 136.
29. Victoria Gill, "Dolphins Have Diabetes Off Switch," *BBC News*, February 19, 2010, http://news.bbc.co.uk/2/hi/science/nature/8523412.stm.
30. Sarah Yarborough et al., "Evaluation of Cognitive Function in the Dog Aging Project: Associations with Baseline Canine Characteristics," *Scientific Reports*, August 2022, 13316.

CHAPTER 10: The Hitchhikers

1. Mary Bagley, "Cambrian Period: Facts & Information," *LiveScience*, May 27, 2016, https://www.livescience.com/28098-cambrian-period.html.
2. Ibid.
3. Emma Hammarlund, "Cancer Tumours Could Help Unravel the Mystery of the Cambrian Explosion," *Conversation*, January 23, 2018, https://phys.org/news/2018-01-cancer-tumours-unravel-mystery-cambrian.html.
4. Jochen J. Brocks et al., "The Rise of Algae in Cryogenian Oceans and the Emergence of Animals," *Nature*, August 16, 2017, 578–581, https://doi.org/10.1038/nature23457.
5. Hammarlund, "Cancer Tumours Could Help Unravel the Mystery."
6. Ibid.
7. Ibid.
8. Emma U. Hammarlund, Kristoffer von Stedingk, and Sven Påhlman,

"Refined Control of Cell Stemness Allowed Animal Evolution in the Oxic Realm," *Nature Ecology and Evolution*, February 2018, 220–228. To access Emma Hammarlund's work and published research, go to https://portal.research.lu.se/en/persons/emma-hammarlund.

9. Jordana Cepelewicz, "Oxygen and Stem Cells May Have Reshaped Early Complex Animals," *Quanta Magazine*, March 7, 2018, https://www.quantamagazine.org/oxygen-and-stem-cells-reshaped-animals-during-the-cambrian-explosion-20180307.
10. "Cancer Stem Cells—an Overview," *ScienceDirect*, https://www.sciencedirect.com/topics/neuroscience/cancer-stem-cell, n.d.
11. Hammarlund, "Cancer Tumours Could Help Unravel the Mystery."
12. Ibid.
13. Ibid.
14. "Japan Team Proves iPS-Based Cornea Transplant Safe in World-1st Trial," *Kyodo News*, April 4, 2022, https://english.kyodonews.net/news/2022/04/c8af6b7913b2-japan-team-proves-ips-based-cornea-transplant-safe-in-world-1st-trial.html.
15. Edward J. Steele et al., "Cause of Cambrian Explosion: Terrestrial or Cosmic?," *Progress in Biophysics and Molecular Biology*, August 2018, 3–23, https://doi.org/10.1016/j.pbiomolbio.2018.03.004.
16. Hammarlund, "Cancer Tumours Could Help Unravel the Mystery."
17. Steele, "Cause of Cambrian Explosion."
18. Laurette Piani et al., "Earth's Water May Have Been Inherited from Material Similar to Enstatite Chondrite Meteorites," *Science*, August 2020, 1110–1113.
19. Douglas Preston, "The Day the Dinosaurs Died," *New Yorker*, April 8, 2019, https://www.newyorker.com/magazine/2019/04/08/the-day-the-dinosaurs-died.
20. R. J. Worth, Steinn Sigurdsson, and Christopher H. House, "Seeding Life on the Moons of the Outer Planets via Lithopanspermia," *Astrobiology*, December 2013, 1155–1165.
21. Preston, "The Day the Dinosaurs Died."
22. A. Abbott, "Scientists Bust Myth That Our Bodies Have More Bacteria Than Human Cells," *Nature News*, January 2016. For more about the microbiome, follow the work of Rob Knight at UC San Diego: http://knightlab.ucsd.edu/.
23. "Stress and the Sensitive Gut—Harvard Health," *Harvard Health*

Publishing, August 21, 2019, https://www.health.harvard.edu/newsletter_article/stress-and-the-sensitive-gut.

24. Mark Kowarsky et al., "Numerous Uncharacterized and Highly Divergent Microbes Which Colonize Humans Are Revealed by Circulating Cell-Free DNA," *Proceedings of the National Academy of Sciences*, September 2017, 9623–9628.
25. Kenneth J. Locey and Jay T. Lennon, "Scaling Laws Predict Global Microbial Diversity," *Proceedings of the National Academy of Sciences*, May 24, 2016, 5970–5975, https://doi.org/10.1073/pnas.1521291113.
26. Brian R. C. Kennedy et al., "The Unknown and the Unexplored: Insights into the Pacific Deep-Sea following NOAA CAPSTONE Expeditions," *Frontiers in Marine Science*, August 2019, 480.
27. T. Cavalier-Smith, "Origin of Mitochondria by Intracellular Enslavement of a Photosynthetic Purple Bacterium," *Proceedings of the Royal Society B: Biological Sciences*, April 11, 2006, 1943–1952.
28. Tim Newman, "Mitochondria: Form, Function, and Disease," *Medical News Today*, February 8, 2018, https://www.medicalnewstoday.com/articles/320875.
29. Ibid.
30. Mitch Leslie, "Cholera Is Altering the Human Genome," *Science*, July 3, 2013, https://www.science.org/content/article/cholera-altering-human-genome.
31. Emilio Depetris-Chauvin and David N. Weil, "Malaria and Early African Development: Evidence from the Sickle Cell Trait," *Economic Journal*, May 2018, 1207–1234, https://doi.org/10.1111/ecoj.12433.
32. Leslie, "Cholera Is Altering the Human Genome."
33. Ibid.
34. Elinor K. Karlsson et al., "Natural Selection in a Bangladeshi Population from the Cholera-Endemic Ganges River Delta," *Science Translational Medicine*, July 2013, 192ra86. Also see Leslie, "Cholera Is Altering the Human Genome."

CHAPTER 11: Positivity, Personality, and Pain

1. Zaria Gorvett, "Why Pain Feels Good,"*BBC Future*, October 1, 2015, https://www.bbc.com/future/article/20151001-why-pain-feels-good.
2. Sarah E. Mills, Karen P. Nicolson, and Blair H. Smith, "Chronic Pain: A Review of Its Epidemiology and Associated Factors in Population-Based Studies," *British Journal of Anesthesia*, August 2019, e273–e283.

3. Patrick Skerrett, "Another Fight for Covid Long-Haulers: Having Their Pain Acknowledged," *STAT*, December 2, 2021, https://www.statnews.com/2021/12/02/long-covid-pain-not-acknowledged/.
4. See the National Institutes of Health's table, "Estimates of Funding for Various Research, Condition, and Disease Categories," at https://report.nih.gov/funding/categorical-spending#/, March 31, 2023.
5. Robert Jason Yong, Peter M. Mullins, and Neil Bhattacharyya, "The Prevalence of Chronic Pain among Adults in the United States," *Pain: The Journal of the International Association for the Study of Pain*, February 2022, https://doi.org/10.1097/j.pain.0000000000002291.
6. Yezhe Lin et al., "Chronic Pain Precedes Disrupted Eating Behavior in Low-Back Pain Patients," *PLoS One*, February 2022, e0263527.
7. Barbara L. Finlay and Supriya Syal, "The Pain of Altruism," *Trends in Cognitive Science,* December 2014, 615–617.
8. Yilu Wang et al., "Altruistic Behaviors Relieve Physical Pain," *Proceedings of the National Academy of Sciences USA*, January 2020, 950–958.
9. Eva Kahana et al., "Altruism, Helping, and Volunteering: Pathways to Well-Being in Late Life," *Journal of Aging and Health*, February 2013, 159–187.
10. Yilu Wang et al., "Altruistic Behaviors Relieve Physical Pain," *Proceedings of the National Academy of Sciences,* December 30, 2019, 950–958, https://doi.org/10.1073/pnas.1911861117.
11. Ibid.
12. See Bear.org.
13. Janet Bultitide, "Does the Brain Really Feel No Pain?," *Conversation*, September 5, 2018, https://theconversation.com/does-the-brain-really-feel-no-pain-102528.
14. Ibid.
15. Ibid.
16. Yudhijit Bhatacharjee, "Scientists Are Unraveling the Mysteries of Pain," *National Geographic,* December 17, 2019, https://www.nationalgeographic.com/magazine/article/scientists-are-unraveling-the-mysteries-of-pain-feature.
17. Access Irene Tracey's work and published papers at the University of Oxford: https://www.ndcn.ox.ac.uk/team/irene-tracey.
18. Bhatacharjee, "Scientists Are Unraveling the Mysteries of Pain."
19. Dale Purves et al., *Neuroglial Cells* (Sunderland, MA: Sinauer Associates, 2001), https://www.ncbi.nlm.nih.gov/books/NBK10869/.

20. Christof Koch, "Does Brain Size Matter?," *Scientific American*, January 1, 2016, 22–25, https://doi.org/10.1038/scientificamericanmind0116-22.
21. Ferris Jabr, "How Humans Evolved Supersize Brains," *Quanta Magazine*, November 10, 2015, https://www.quantamagazine.org/how-humans-evolved-supersize-brains-20151110/.
22. Christopher R. Donnelly et al., "Central Nervous System Targets: Glial Cell Mechanisms in Chronic Pain," *Neurotherapeutics*, July 2020, 846–860. Also see Parisa Gazerani, "Satellite Glial Cells in Pain Research: A Targeted Viewpoint of Potential and Future Directions," *Frontiers in Pain Research*, March 2021, 646068.
23. Yu Mu et al., "Glia Accumulate Evidence That Actions Are Futile and Suppress Unsuccessful Behavior," *Cell*, July 20, 2019, https://doi.org/10.1016/j.cell.2019.05.050.
24. Ibid.
25. Robert Puff, "Your Set Point for Happiness," *Psychology Today*, September 8, 2017, https://www.psychologytoday.com/us/blog/meditation-for-modern-life/201709/your-set-point-for-happiness.
26. F. Berthier and F. Boulay, "Lower Myocardial Infarction Mortality in French Men the Day France Won the 1998 World Cup of Football," *Heart*, May 2003, 555–556. Also see "Sports Victories Soothe Men's Hearts," *WebMD*, April 16, 2003, retrieved from https://www.webmd.com/heart-disease/news/20030416/sports-victories-soothe-mens-hearts? (This article is no longer available on the internet, unfortunately. Archived version: https://web.archive.org/web/20151019112537/http://www.webmd.com/heart-disease/news/20030416/sports-victories-soothe-mens-hearts).
27. "Fewer Heart Attack Deaths Reported during World Cup Win," *WebMD*, April 16, 2003, retrieved from https://www.webmd.com/heart-disease/news/20030416/sports-victories-soothe-mens-hearts? (This article is no longer available on the internet, unfortunately. Archived version: https://web.archive.org/web/20151019112537/http://www.webmd.com/heart-disease/news/20030416/sports-victories-soothe-mens-hearts).
28. T. Maruta et al., "Optimists vs. Pessimists: Survival Rate among Medical Patients over a 30-Year Period," *Mayo Clinic Proceedings*, February 2000, 140–143.
29. "Fewer Heart Attack Deaths Reported."

30. "Optimism and Your Health," *Harvard Health*, May 1, 2008, https://www.health.harvard.edu/heart-health/optimism-and-your-health, and for an overview on the subject of optimism and pain, see Burel R. Goodin and Hailey W. Bulls, "Optimism and the Experience of Pain: Benefits of Seeing the Glass as Half Full," *Current Pain and Headache Reports*, March 22, 2013, 329, https://doi.org/10.1007/s11916-013-0329-8.
31. Goodin and Bulls, "Optimism and the Experience of Pain: Benefits of Seeing the Glass as Half Full."
32. For an overview on the subject of optimism and pain, see ibid.
33. Melissa A. Wright et al., "Pain Acceptance, Hope, and Optimism: Relationships to Pain and Adjustment in Patients with Chronic Musculoskeletal Pain," *Journal of Pain*, August 2011, https://doi.org/10.1016/j.jpain.2011.06.002.
34. Mark Bekoff, "Pigs Are Intelligent, Emotional, and Cognitively Complex," *Psychology Today*, June 16, 2015, https://www.psychologytoday.com/us/blog/animal-emotions/201506/pigs-are-intelligent-emotional-and-cognitively-complex.
35. Lucy Asher et al., "Mood and Personality Interact to Determine Cognitive Biases in Pigs," *Biology Letters*, November 2016, 20160402.
36. University of Lincoln, "A Pig's Life: How Mood and Personality Affect the Decisions of Domestic Pigs," *ScienceDaily*, November 16, 2016, https://www.sciencedaily.com/releases/2016/11/161116101936.htm.
37. Jaclyn R. Aliperti et al., "Bridging Animal Personality with Space Use and Resource Use in a Free-Ranging Population of an Asocial Ground Squirrel," *Animal Behavior*, October 2021, 291–306.
38. Kat Kerlin, "Personality Matters, Even for Squirrels," UC Davis, September 10, 2021, https://www.ucdavis.edu/curiosity/news/personality-matters-even-squirrels-0.
39. Mario Incayawar, *Overlapping Pain and Psychiatric Syndromes: Global Perspectives* (London: Oxford University Press, 2020). Also see Tomiko Yoneda et al., "Personality Traits, Cognitive States, and Mortality in Older Adulthood," *Journal of Personality and Social Psychology*, April 2022.
40. Richard Stephens and Olly Robertson, "Swearing as a Response to Pain: Assessing Hypoalgesic Effects of Novel 'Swear' Words," *Frontiers in Psychology*, April 2020, 723.
41. Ibid.

42. Francesco Ventura et al., "Environmental Variability Directly Affects the Prevalence of Divorce in Monogamous Albatrosses," *Proceedings of the Royal Society B: Biological Sciences*, November 2021, 20212112.
43. Tess McClure, "Climate Crisis Pushes Albatross 'Divorce' Rates Higher—Study," *Guardian*, November 24, 2021, https://www.theguardian.com/environment/2021/nov/24/climate-crisis-pushes-albatross-divorce-rates-higher-study.
44. Bill Chappell, "Wisdom the Albatross, Now 70, Hatches Yet Another Chick," NPR, March 5, 2021, https://www.npr.org/2021/03/05/973992408/wisdom-the-albatross-now-70-hatches-yet-another-chick.

CHAPTER 12: Bonding, Sex, and the Law of Love

1. Follow Paul Zak's work and research at https://pauljzak.com/.
2. Paul J. Zak, *The Moral Molecule: The Source of Love and Prosperity* (New York: Dutton, 2012).
3. Tori DeAngelis, "The Two Faces of Oxytocin," *American Psychological Association*, February 2008, https://www.apa.org/monitor/feb08/oxytocin.
4. H. H. Dale, "The Action of Extracts of the Pituitary Body," *Biochemical Journal*, January 1909, 427–447, https://doi.org/10.1042/bj0040427.
5. Adam L. Penenberg, "Social Networking Affects Brains like Falling in Love." *Fast Company*, July 1, 2010, https://www.fastcompany.com/1659062/social-networking-affects-brains-falling-love.
6. Hasse Walum and Larry J. Young, "The Neural Mechanisms and Circuitry of the Pair Bond," *Nature Reviews Neuroscience*, October 9, 2018, 643–654, https://doi.org/10.1038/s41583-018-0072-6.
7. Christian Elabd et al., "Oxytocin Is an Age-specific Circulating Hormone That Is Necessary for Muscle Maintenance and Regeneration," *Nature Communications*, June 2014, 4082.
8. Abigail Tucker, "What Can Rodents Tell Us about Why Humans Love?," *Smithsonian Magazine*, February 2014, https://www.smithsonianmag.com/science-nature/what-can-rodents-tell-us-about-why-humans-love-180949441/?all=.
9. Follow Larry Young's work and research at https://www.larryjyoung.com/. Highlights of his studies are in the following papers: Robert C. Froemke and Larry J. Young, "Oxytocin, Neural Plasticity, and Social Behavior," *Annual Review of Neuroscience*, July 2021, 359–381, and Hasse Walum and Larry J. Young, "The Neural Mechanisms and

Circuitry of the Pair Bond," *Nature Reviews Neuroscience*, November 2018, 643–654.

10. Tucker, "What Can Rodents Tell Us about Why Humans Love?"
11. Ibid.
12. Ibid.
13. Tobias T. Pohl, Larry J. Young, and Oliver J. Bosch, "Lost Connections: Oxytocin and the Neural, Physiological, and Behavioral Consequences of Disrupted Relationships," *International Journal of Psychophysiology*, February 2019, 54–63. Also see Mariam Okhovat et al., "Sexual Fidelity Trade-Offs Promote Regulatory Variation in the Prairie Vole Brain," *Science*, December 2015, 1371–1374. Also see Tucker, "What Can Rodents Tell Us about Why Humans Love?"
14. Tucker, "What Can Rodents Tell Us about Why Humans Love?"
15. Ed Yong, "A Study of Unfaithful Voles Links Genes to Brains to Behaviour," *Science*, December 10, 2015, https://www.nationalgeographic.com/science/article/a-study-of-unfaithful-voles-links-genes-to-brains-to-behaviour.
16. Tucker, "What Can Rodents Tell Us about Why Humans Love?"
17. Ibid.
18. Larry Young and Brian Alexander, *The Chemistry Between Us: Love, Sex, and the Science of Attraction* (New York: Current, 2012).
19. Tucker, "What Can Rodents Tell Us about Why Humans Love?"
20. J. P. Burkett, "Oxytocin-Dependent Consolation Behavior in Rodents," *Science*, January 2016, 375.
21. Follow Tom Insel's work and research at https://www.thomasinselmd.com.
22. Jessica C. Burkhart et al., "Oxytocin Promotes Social Proximity and Decreases Vigilance in Groups of African Lions," *iScience*, March 2022, 104049.
23. Beth Azar, "Oxytocin's Other Side," *Monitor on Psychology*, March 2011, 40.
24. Nicholas M. Grebe et al., "Oxytocin and Vulnerable Romantic Relationships," *Hormones and Behavior*, April 2017, 64–74.
25. Vanessa Van Edwards, "How to Bond with Anyone with Dr. Paul Zak," *Science of People*, https://www.scienceofpeople.com/how-to-bond-with-anyone/, n.d.
26. Paul J. Zak et al., "Oxytocin Release Increases with Age and Is Associated

with Life Satisfaction and Prosocial Behaviors," *Frontiers in Behavioral Neuroscience*, April 2022, 846234.

27. Matthew A. Killingsworth, "Experienced Well-Being Rises with Income, Even above $75,000 per Year," *Proceedings of the National Academy of Sciences USA*, January 2021, e2016976118.
28. Claire Yang et al., "Social Relationships and Physiological Determinants of Longevity across the Human Life Span," *Proceedings of the National Academy of Sciences*, January 4, 2016, 578–583, https://doi.org/10.1073/pnas.1511085112.
29. Follow Robert Waldinger's work and research at http://www.robertwaldinger.com/. You can also follow Harvard's Adult Development study at https://www.adultdevelopmentstudy.org/.
30. Robert Waldinger, "What Makes a Good Life? Lessons from the Longest Study on Happiness," TED Talk, December 23, 2015, https://www.ted.com/talks/robert_waldinger_what_makes_a_good_life_lessons_from_the_longest_study_on_happiness.
31. Ibid.
32. Ibid.
33. Natascia Brondino et al., "Something to Talk About: Gossip Increases Oxytocin Levels in a Near Real-Life Situation," *Psychoneuroendocrinology*, March 2017, 218–224.
34. Van Edwards, "How to Bond with Anyone with Dr. Paul Zak."
35. Ibid.
36. Ibid.
37. "Experiences Menu-Sensei Lāna'i," n.d., Sensei, https://sensei.com/retreats/lanai/experiences-menu/.
38. Margaret M. Hansen, Reo Jones, and Kirsten Tocchini, "Shinrin-Yoku (Forest Bathing) and Nature Therapy: A State-of-the-Art Review," *International Journal of Environmental Research and Public Health*, July 2017, 851.
39. Roger S. Ulrich, "View through a Window May Influence Recovery from Surgery," *Science*, May 1984, https://www.researchgate.net/publication/17043718_View_Through_a_Window_May_Influence_Recovery_from_Surgery.
40. Jeffrey Lambert et al., "Taking a One-Week Break from Social Media Improves Well-Being, Depression, and Anxiety: A Randomized Controlled Trial," *Cyberpsychology, Behavior, and Social Networking*, May 2022, 287–293.
41. Marcia P. Jimenez et al., "Associations between Nature Exposure and

Health: A Review of the Evidence," *International Journal of Environmental Research*, May 2021.

ACKNOWLEDGMENTS

1. Jocelyn Dong, "Close of Hyatt Rickey's Sends Groups to New Locations," *Palo Alto Weekly*, June 8, 2005, www.paloaltoonline.com/weekly/morgue/2005/2005_06_08.rickeys08ja.shtml.

Image Credits

xx Collection of Lawrence J. Ellison. Photo by author.

xxii London Stereoscopic and Photographic Company (active 1855–1922). First published in *Borderland Magazine*, April 1896. Public domain.

xxii Wikimedia Commons. Author unknown. Public domain.

xxvi Charles Darwin's 1837 sketch is in the public domain and reproduced in various places for download, including this paper: Hugh M. B. Harris and Colin Hill, "A Place for Viruses on the Tree of Life," *Frontiers in Microbiology* 11 (January 2021): 604048.

4 Glenn Boghosian. Used with permission.

7 This image of a pancake batfish was taken by Sandra Raredon of the Smithsonian Institute in her role as an employee. As a work of the US federal government, the image is in the public domain.

13 This image, created by the author, is adapted from data published in the following paper: Kevin D. Hall et al., "Ultra-Processed Diets Cause Excess Calorie Intake and Weight Gain: An Inpatient Randomized Controlled Trial of Ad Libitum Food Intake," *Cell Metabolism* 30, no. 1 (July 2019): 67–77.

20 Photo by author.

35 Photo credit: Lenka Ulrichova. Used with permission.

46 Charles Darwin, 1890 (public domain). Division of Rare and Manuscript Collections, Cornell University Library.

52 Source of image: Richard M. Levenson et al., "Pigeons (*Columba livia*) as Trainable Observers of Pathology and Radiology Breast Cancer Images," *PLoS One* 10, no. 11 (November 2015): e0141357. Works published by PLOS are licensed under the Creative Commons Attribution (CC-BY) license.

55 Photo by author.

74 Photo by author, taken on Maasai Mara National Reserve, Kenya.

77 Leonardo da Vinci's *Vitruvian Man* (c. 1490) is a work of art in the public domain. The original drawing is housed at the Gallerie dell'Accademia in Venice, Italy. Downloadable at Wikimedia Commons.

77 Logo art provided by author. Ellison Institute, LLC.

100 Photo by author.

108 Image created by author. Adapted from: Tollis, Boddy, and Maley, "Peto's Paradox: How Has Evolution Solved the Problem of Cancer Prevention?," *BMC Biology* 15, no. 1 (July 2017): 60.

112 Cover of *Science* magazine 262, no. 5142 (December 24, 1993). Illustration by K. Sutliff and C. Faber Smith. Reprinted with permission from AAAS.

124 Photo credit of chimpanzee by Rishi Ragunathan on Unsplash. Published on December 18, 2018.

150 Photo credit of bat taken by Paramanu Sarkar. Wikimedia Commons. Licensed under the Creative Commons Attribution-Share Alike 4.0 International license. Created July 25, 2020. File at: https://commons.wikimedia.org/wiki/File:Bat_02.jpg#/media/File:Bat_02.jpg.

150 Photo credit of fire ants taken by Stephen Ausmus for the U.S. Department of Agriculture. Public domain.

155 Illustration of a bat head by Ernst Haeckel. Detail of the sixty-seventh plate from Ernst Haeckel's *Kunstformen der Natur* (1904). Public domain.

163 Photo credit of Matabele ants by Erik T. Frank. Reprinted with permission.

166 Cover of *Science* magazine 350, no. 6267 (December 18, 2015). Reprinted with permission from AAAS and Davide Bonaazi (illustrator).

178 Photo credit of white rhino by Keith Markilie on Unsplash. Published on May 12, 2019.

180 Illustration by Tim Bertelink. Wikimedia Commons. Licensed under the Creative Commons Attribution-Share Alike 4.0 International license. Created May 25, 2016. File at: https://commons.wikimedia.org/wiki/File:Indricotherium.png.

183 Cover of *Time* magazine featuring Roy Chapman Andrews (October 29, 1923). Used with permission. Https://content.time.com/time/magazine/0,9263,7601231029,00.html.

185 San Diego Zoo Wildlife Alliance. Reprinted with permission.

189 Image by author, adapted from public domain files on Wikimedia Commons. Chemical structure of equol: By Edgar181, uploaded February 11,

2008. Chemical structure of estradiol: By NEUROtiker, uploaded June 29, 2007. Image based on Figure 1 in: K. D. Setchell and A. Cassidy, "Dietary Isoflavones: Biological Effects and Relevance to Human Health," *Journal of Nutrition* 129, no. 3 (1999): 758S–767S.

210 Photo credit of octopus by Aquarium of Québec on Unsplash. Published March 24, 2021.

227 Cover of *Time* magazine (February 23, 2004). Used with permission.

234 Photo credit of Comet 67P/Churyumov-Gerasimenko taken on January 31, 2015. Image Credit: The European Space Agency (ESA)/Rosetta /NAVCAM—CC BY-SA IGO 3.0. (This work is licensed under the Creative Commons Attribution-ShareAlike 3.0 IGO license.) For more, go to www.esa.int.

238 Timeline of Earth chart created by author.

239 Horseshoe crab photo. Wikimedia Commons. This work is licensed under the Creative Commons Attribution-ShareAlike 2.0 Generic (CC BY-SA 2.0). Created May 24, 2016. This image was originally posted to Flickr by Plant Image Library at https://flickr.com/photos/138014579@N08/26923436154. File also at: https://upload.wikimedia.org/wikipedia/commons/e/ea/Limulus_polyphemus_%28Atlantic_Horseshoe_Crab%29_adult_underside_%2826923436154%29.jpg.

254 Gray squirrel yawning by Getty Images (iStock Photo). Credit: Dgwildlife (https://www.dgwildlife.com/). Stock photo ID:473012660. Upload date: May 9, 2015. Standard license.

265 Brain size chart created by author. Adapted from: F. Jabr, "How Humans Evolved Supersized Brains," *Quanta Magazine*, November 10, 2015.

274 Photo of pig. Wikimedia Commons. This work is licensed under the Creative Commons Attribution-Share Alike 4.0 International license. Created April 27, 2020. File at: https://commons.wikimedia.org/wiki/File:Historia-de-los-cerdos.jpg#/media/File:Historia-de-los-cerdos.jpg.

277 Photo credit of short-tailed albatross taken by James Lloyd Place. Wikimedia Commons. Licensed under the Creative Commons Attribution 2.5 Generic (CC BY 2.5). Created August 25, 2007.

282 Photo credit by Nick Fewings on Unsplash. Published on January 26, 2018.

294 Photo courtesy of Tom Insel.

312 Cover of *Time* magazine featuring Andy Grove (December 29, 1997). Used with permission.

Index

Note: Page numbers followed by "n" indicate footnotes. *Italicized* page numbers indicate photographs and other illustrations.

About the Author

DAVID B. AGUS is one of the world's leading doctors and pioneering biomedical researchers. He is the founding director and co-CEO of the Ellison Institute of Technology, a professor of medicine and engineering at the University of Southern California, and a visiting professor at the University of Oxford. A medical oncologist, Dr. Agus leads a multidisciplinary team of researchers dedicated to the development and use of technologies to guide doctors in making health care decisions tailored to individual needs. An international leader in global health and approaches for personalized health care, Dr. Agus serves in leadership roles at the World Economic Forum and is co-chair of the Global Health Security Consortium. He is also a CBS News contributor. Dr. Agus's three books, *The End of Illness*, *A Short Guide to a Long Life*, and *The Lucky Years: How to Thrive in the Brave New World of Health*, are all *New York Times* and international bestsellers. He is a 2017 recipient of the Ellis Island Medal of Honor. He lives in California with his wife, two children, and their dog, Georgie.